Bioadhesive Drug Delivery Systems

Editors

Vincent Lenaerts, Ph.D.
Professor
Faculty of Pharmacy
University of Montreal
Montreal, Quebec, Canada

Robert Gurny, Ph.D.
Professor
School of Pharmacy
University of Geneva
Geneva, Switzerland

CRC Press, Inc.
Boca Raton, Florida

Library of Congress Cataloging-in Publication Data

Bioadhesive drug delivery systems / editors, Vincent Lenaerts, Robert
  Gurny
       p. cm.
    Includes bibliographies and index.
    ISBN 0-8493-5367-X
    1. Bioadhesive drug delivery systems. I. Lenaerts, Vincent.
II. Gurny, Robert.
[DNLM: 1. Dosage Forms. 2. Drug Administration Routes. QV 785
B6114]
RS201.B54B56 1990
615.5′8—dc20
DNLM/DLC
for Library of Congress   89-7256
                                                                        CIP

This book represents information obtained from authentic and highly regarded sources. Reprinted material is quoted with permission, and sources are indicated. A wide variety of references are listed. Every reasonable effort has been made to give reliable data and information, but the author and the publisher cannot assume responsibility for the validity of all materials or for the consequences of their use.

Direct all inquiries to CRC Press, Inc., 2000 Corporate Blvd., N.W., Boca Raton, Florida, 33431.

International Standard Book Number 0-8493-5367-X

Library of Congress Card Number 89-7256
Printed in the United States

PREFACE

Over the last decade, controlled drug delivery and site-specific drug delivery have made rapid advances. Bioadhesive systems now play a major role in this field, due to their interesting potentialities. Besides acting as platforms for sustained release dosage forms, bioadhesive polymers can themselves exert some control over the rate and amount of drug release, and thus contribute to the therapeutic efficacy of such systems. In the last few years, many researchers have benefited from these properties in their efforts to find answers to biopharmaceutical problems.

Although the polymer and biomedical literature contains some publications on bioadhesive systems, and several symposia around the world have given attention to this new area, there have thus far been few efforts to present the whole subject methodologically in a textbook. It was therefore with great pleasure and enthusiasm that we accepted the invitation of CRC Press to edit a book on bioadhesive drug delivery systems.

The 12 chapters of this book are contributions from researchers around the world who have been working for years in this field. It was impossible, however, to cover all aspects of bioadhesion. Adhesives used in the area of transdermal systems have intentionally not been included, since they have been discussed extensively elsewhere. The chapters offer a very good introduction to uninitiated scientists, and an in-depth analysis of some basic concepts.

Chapter 1 presents the basics on the physiology and pathology of mucus and discusses their implications for drug delivery. In Chapter 2 the scaling concepts and molecular theories of adhesion of synthetic polymers to the glycoproteinic network are discussed. Chapter 3 includes test methods now available for evaluation of bioadhesion and parameters which are important for testing and designing new bioadhesives. In Chapter 4, we start with pharmaceutical applications and give an extensive overview of the possibilities of bioadhesives/ mucoadhesives in oral drug delivery. Chapter 5 discusses the potential of nanoparticles as gastroadhesive drug delivery systems. Mucoadhesive buccal patches for peptide delivery are presented in Chapter 6. Chapter 7 is devoted to tablet-like bioadhesive dosage forms for buccal/gingival administration of prostaglandins and many other substances, whereas Chapter 8 deals with the use of semisolid dosage forms at the same site of application. Nasal administration of drugs combined with bioadhesive systems, discussed in Chapter 9, has attracted considerable research interest in recent years as a route of choice for numerous bioactive materials, especially polypeptides. Chapters 10 and 11 give an excellent introduction to ocular bioadhesive systems. Finally, Chapter 12 is devoted to the vaginal and intrauterine route of administration.

The chapters of this multi-authored book should not be read as isolated contributions. The editors tried to introduce cross-listing of chapters and there is a subject index at the end of the book to facilitate its use.

The colleagues who have agreed to contribute to this book are warmly thanked for their contributions and for accepting the deadlines. Special thanks are also due to the editorial staff of CRC Press, and especially Marsha Baker, for their assistance during the past two years.

Robert Gurny
Vincent Lenaerts

EDITORS

Vincent Lenaerts, Ph.D., is professor of pharmaceutical technology at the University of Montreal, Canada. He graduated in 1979 from the University of Louvain, Belgium, with a B.Sc. in pharmacy, and obtained his Ph.D in pharmaceutical sciences from the same institution in 1984. In that same year he joined the company UPSA in Rueil-Malmaison, France, as a manager of the pharmaceutical technology division. He assumed his present position in 1986.

Dr. Lenaerts is a member of the Controlled Release Society, the Arbeitsgemeinschaft für Pharmazeutische Verfahrenstechnik, and a co-founder and former secretary of the Groupement Thématique de Recherche sur les Vecteurs.

He has been the recipient of a Proficiency Fellowship from the Institut pour l'Aide à la Recherche Scientifique dans l'Industrie et l'Agriculture and of grants from the Medical Research Council of Canada, the North Atlantic Treaty Organization, and the Cancer Research Society.

Dr. Lenaerts has authored over 50 papers and communications. His major research interests relate to the medical and pharmaceutical applications of controlled release drug delivery systems.

Dr. Robert Gurny, Ph.D., is a professor in the Department of Biopharmaceutics and Physical Pharmacy at the University of Geneva, Switzerland, where he earned both his B.S. in pharmacy and his Ph.D. in physical pharmacy. He later earned a degree in statistics and computer science and from 1973 to 1977 was a co-worker for the Swiss Pharmacopoeia. Subsequently he was a research associate in the Department of Industrial and Physical Pharmacy at Purdue, West Lafayette, Indiana.

Dr. Gurny's major research interests include pharmaceutical processing and the use of polymers in the design of new controlled drug-release systems, in which he has authored some 50 publications and 7 book chapters. He consults in pharmaceutical technology for several pharmaceutical companies and is an editorial advisor for several European and American journals. Dr. Gurny is also a member of several important pharmaceutical and chemical associations.

CONTRIBUTORS

Reinhold Anders, Dr. rer. nat.
Galenic Department
Hoechst AG
Frankfurt, West Germany

Patrick Couvreur, Ph.D.
Professor
Department of Pharmacy
University of Paris XI
Chatenay-Malabry, France

N. P. Gregory
Department of Pharmacy
Brighton Polytechnic
Brighton, Sussex, England

Luc Grislain, Ph.D.
Manager
Department of Metabolism
Bio-Pharmacie Servier
Orleans, France

Pardeep K. Gupta
School of Pharmacy
University of Wisconsin
Madison, Wisconsin

Robert Gurny, Ph.D.
Professor
School of Pharmacy
University of Geneva
Geneva, Switzerland

Ryoji Konishi
Vice President
Teikoku Seiyaku Co., Ltd.
Kagawa, Japan

Jörg Kreuter, Ph.D.
Professor
Institute of Pharmacological Technology
J. W. Goethe University
Frankfurt, West Germany

Vincent Lenaerts, Ph.D.
Professor
Faculty of Pharmacy
University of Montreal
Montreal, Quebec, Canada

Sau-Hung S. Leung, Ph.D.
Columbia Research Labs
Madison, Wisconsin

Yoshiharu Machida, Ph.D.
Associate Professor
Department of Pharmaceutics
Hoshi University
Tokyo, Japan

Ph. Maincent
Professor
Galenic Pharmacy
Faculty of Pharmaceutical Sciences
Nancy, France

Christopher Marriott, D.Sc.
Professor
Department of Pharmacy
Brighton Polytechnic
Brighton, Sussex, England

Hans P. Merkle, Dr.sc.nat.
Professor
Department of Pharmacy
Swiss Federal Institute of Technology
  Zurich (ETH)
Zurich, Switzerland

David L. Middleton, M.S.
The UpJohn Company
Kalamazoo, Michigan

Antonios G. Mikos, Ph.D.Ch.E.
School of Chemical Engineering
Purdue University
West Lafayette, Indiana

Tsuneji Nagai, Ph.D.
Professor
Department of Pharmaceutics
Hoshi University
Tokyo, Japan

Haesun Park, Ph.D.
Research Associate
School of Pharmacy
Purdue University
West Lafayette, Indiana

Kinam Park, Ph.D.
Assistant Professor
School of Pharmacy
Purdue University
West Lafayette, Indiana

Nikolaos A. Peppas, D.Eng.
Professor
School of Chemical Engineering
Purdue University
West Lafayette, Indiana

Joseph R. Robinson, Ph.D.
Professor
School of Pharmacy
University of Wisconsin
Madison, Wisconsin

Aloys Wermerskirchen, Dr. rer. nat.
Pharmaceutical Institute
University of Bonn
Bonn, West Germany

TABLE OF CONTENTS

Chapter 1

MUCUS PHYSIOLOGY AND PATHOLOGY

Christopher Marriott and N. P. Gregory

TABLE OF CONTENTS

I. INTRODUCTION

The route from the mouth to the anus, including the diverticulum that forms the respiratory tract, is lined with mucus, and this represents the potential site of attachment of any bioadhesive delivery system. The other two sites to which such systems might be applied, the eye and the female reproductive tract, are similarly coated with mucus gel. Consequently, the interface to which a bioadhesive drug delivery system must adhere will consist of an epithelial surface coated with a layer of mucus. The nature and thickness of this layer of mucus may alter significantly during disease, which might in turn lead to a change in the behavior of a delivery system. Therefore, it is appropriate to consider the secretion, nature, and physical properties of mucus together with the changes that occur in disease.

Mucus is found in a wide range of Phyla performing a protective and lubricative function; in mammals, it is normally found in the gastrointestinal tract (GIT), the urinogenital tract, and the airways, as well as the nose, ear, and eye. One would expect the physical and chemical properties of the gel to differ from species to species and from site to site if only because the environment into which it is secreted varies. In the GIT, for example, the gel is mixed with microorganisms, secreted and leached protein, and is bathed in a solution of continually changing ionic strength and pH. To date, there is a considerable body of literature which suggests that there is at least an underlying uniformity of structure of mucus from different sources based on a large molecular weight glycoprotein. To understand mucus, both in the normal and the pathological state, it is necessary to understand the structure of the glycoprotein molecule. However, this has proved to be one of the major challenges of structural molecular biology.

Without a detailed knowledge of the structure, it is very difficult to discuss with confidence mechanisms of mucus secretion and how mucus performs its protective and lubricative function. Until we are able to do this, we will not effectively understand the pathology of mucus in diseases in which abnormalities in mucus secretion and function are a primary manifestation. More in context with this volume, an understanding of mucus is important if we are to attempt to exploit mucus as a substrate for bioadhesive formulations.

II. MUCUS NOMENCLATURE

Unfortunately, the terminology used to describe the different components of the mucus glycoprotein molecule is confusing. Mucus has been studied by scientists in many different disciplines and what may be appropriate in histology, for example, may not be so in biochemistry. To avoid this, a nomenclature has been developed[1] and is being adopted by those working in the field. A summary of the scheme is given below:

- Mucus — the general term for the heterogeneous secretion found on epithelial surfaces
- Mucin — histological term to describe the stainable components of mucus
- Mucus glycoprotein — the principal biochemical component of mucus (a large molecular weight molecule, which is highly glycosylated)
- Subunits — glycopeptides with a molecular weight of 500 kDa that are covalently bonded together to form the mucus glycoprotein macromolecule
- Apomucin — the peptide component of the subunits after the carbohydrate has been chemically removed (This is an *in vitro* preparation, but the term may be used to describe the posttranslational product prior to glycosylation now that researchers are beginning to unravel this aspect of the biosynthesis of glycoprotein.)

Although the scheme cannot be considered to be totally comprehensive, it will be used for the purposes of this chapter; where anomalies occur, they will be commented upon.

III. THE STRUCTURE OF MUCUS GLYCOPROTEIN

Mucus glycoprotein is the principal molecular component of mucus. Studies on the rheology of the purified molecule indicate that it is this component which confers upon mucus the gelling properties that are so important if the secretion is to function.[2] How the molecule is constructed remains a subject of debate. There is general agreement that the principal unit is a relatively high molecular weight glycopeptide, often called a subunit, which is known to be covalently bound to other subunits through disulfide bonds, and probably interacts intermolecularly with other subunits through ionic bonds and entanglements.

The subunit of mucus glycoprotein has been isolated from mucus secretions of various species and sites. These include rat small intestine,[3,4] pig stomach,[5] intestine,[6] colon,[7] human airway,[8] stomach,[9] and cervix.[10] Estimates of M_r ranging from 380 to 720 kDa have been reported depending upon the source of the subunit. From the results of these studies, it has been possible to propose models of the subunit and, to date, two such models have been described.

The "bottle brush" model views the subunit as a peptide with a region of dense glycosylation. The glycosylated region is set to one end of the peptide, like the hairs on a bottle brush, leaving a region of nonglycosylated peptide (the brush handle) at the other end. The "rolling pin" model is similar in that it represents the subunit as a glycosylated peptide, but with the glycosylated region at the center, thus leaving both ends as nonglycosylated peptide.[11] The immediate attraction of this model is that it allows for disulfide bonding at each unglycosylated terminal, unlike the bottle brush model that only allows bonding at one end. The rolling pin model can, therefore, best explain how the subunits may "polymerize". However, polmerization of the "bottle brush" structure could be achieved through a linking peptide.

The subunit, whether it is a bottle brush or a rolling pin, is a highly glycosylated peptide. This extensive glycosylation in fact accounts directly for the majority of the sugar on the whole mucus glycoprotein molecule, except perhaps for a small amount of glycosylation that has recently been reported in the peptide links between subunits.[12] The peptide component of the subunit can, therefore, be conveniently divided into the glycosylated and the nonglycosylated regions. However, despite using subunits from various sources, attempts to elucidate the primary structure continue to be frustrated by the difficulty in totally deglycosylating the peptide without disturbing its primary structure.

Recently this has been achieved with submaxillary mucus glycoprotein, being almost completely deglycosylated (>90%) of the N-acetyl-hexosamines. Using the naked peptide, the apomucin, Bhavanandan and Hegarty[13] were able to raise antibodies and identify translation products in a cell free system. The translation product was a 60 kDa protein, although it is not known whether further processing of this protein occurs. The glycoprotein used in this study, however, is one of the simplest structurally, and at present it is impossible to know whether the primary structure of the apoprotein is common to all subunits, or if there are variations from site to site or species to species. To date, a number of amino acid analyses have been performed on the subunit and the whole mucus glycoprotein, and although the data do not permit prediction of the primary structure, they do indicate the degree of variation. Most notable is the high molar ratio of the amino acids threonine and serine, to which the carbohydrate moieties are linked. From a study based on amino acid analysis, it has already been proposed that human intestinal mucus glycoproteins contain two distinct core peptides.[14]

Studies on the glycopeptide have shown that although only five monosaccharides are found, namely galactose (Gal), fucose (Fuc), N-acetyl-galactosamine (GalNac), N-acetyl-glucosamine (GlcNac), and N-acetyl-neuraminic acid (AcNeu, sialic acid), these monosaccharides are assembled in a variety of ways. The average chain length for oligosaccharides attached to the subunit core peptide is 8 with a range from 2 to 14: the chains may be either

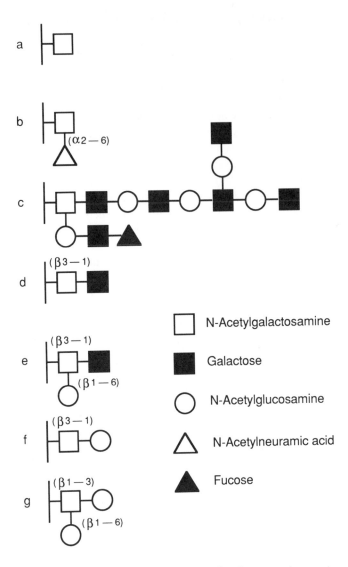

FIGURE 1.   Generalized carbohydrate structures found on mucus glycoprotein.

linear or branched. Despite the complexity of the oligosaccharide structures available, from the studies carried out so far, a number of guidelines to their construction can be formulated. It is inappropriate to call these "rules" at this point, because mucus glycoprotein has been known to reveal another aspect of its structure just when it is thought to be understood.

Briefly, the guidelines are

1.   The initial monosaccharide is always covalently bound to either a threonine or serine residue by an α-*O*-glycosidic bond (Figure 1a). This is different to the majority of serum glycoproteins and proteglycans, which are normally *N*-glycosidically linked, though this is not exclusive as IgA and glycophorin A also use the α-*O*-glycosidic bond.

2.   The beta anomeric linkage is found between all intrachain monosaccharides. If the anomer occurs, except at the sugar-protein bond, then chain elongation ceases. Fuc and AcNeu are linked to the previous monosaccharides, and these are always sites of chain termination, though a chain need not terminate in either of these monosaccharides (Figure 1b).

3. Where branching does occur, it is always 1-3β and 1-6β from either Gal or GalNac. Gal branching occurs inside the chain, whereas GalNac branching occurs at the preliminary monosaccharide (Figure 1c). Branching other than the linkage does occur (in the α form), but this is only at terminating residues (Figure 1b.)

4. The intrachain sections, or core structures, can be classified into four major groups containing GalNac, Gal, and GlcNac (Figures 1d, e, f, and g).

Any of the sugars can bear sulfate residues, which together with the AcNeu confer a negative charge on the molecule. The biosynthetic pathways of oligosaccharide construction have been reviewed by a number of authors,[15-18] and although a detailed description is outside the scope of this chapter, it is worth examining the system briefly because one of the results could be of great relevance to possible bioadhesive systems.

A. MUCUS BIOSYNTHESIS

Mucus glycoproteins are synthesized in specialized cells that are embedded in the mucosa of the surface onto which they are to be secreted. The biosynthesis of the two components, the peptide and the oligosaccharide, uses processes that are common to protein synthesis and O-glycosidically linked oligosaccharides, respectively. The synthesis of the protein follows the familiar DNA-makes-RNA-makes-protein scheme, but the gene or genes are yet to be isolated. Some work, as already mentioned, has reported success in the isolation of the RNA. It is unknown at the present time how the core peptides of the whole molecule are constructed, so it is not only convenient to consider the biosynthesis of just one core peptide, but also necessary.

The biosynthesis of the carbohydrate component is more thoroughly understood because of the similarities with other glycoproteins and glycolipids, particularly those that constitute the blood group antigens, and it is the desire to understand these antigens that appears to have increased the interest in the glycosylation of the O-linked oligosaccharides.

The initiation of mucus and other O-glycosidically linked glycoproteins, can be contrasted with the majority of proteins that use the N-glycosidic linkage. In this group, initiation occurs by the addition of the first monosaccharide reticulum.[19,20] The majority of the oligosaccharide structure is independently assembled onto a dolicholpyrophosphate backbone[21] from where it is grafted to the initiated glycoprotein.

The initiation of the O-linked glycoproteins, however, occurs on the smooth endoplasmic reticulum after the nascent peptide has left the ribosome,[22] and does not utilize a lipid intermediate to construct the oligosaccharide.[23] Once the initiation has been completed, the elongation of the oligosaccharides appears to be determined by the specificities and availability of enzymes, and by the availability of the monosaccharide substrate.

The initiation of the glycosylation occurs in the same way for each of the many oligosaccharide chains, namely the action of UDP — GalNac:Polypeptide N-acetylgalactosamyltransferase (GalNac:GalNacTrans) on the core peptide following the scheme:

$$UPD\text{-}GalNac + Ser(Thr)\text{-}peptide — GalNac\text{-}\alpha O\text{-}Ser(Thr)Peptide + UDP$$

Attempts to determine if any peptide primary structure is required for glycosylation initiation have used ovine submaxillary gland mucus[24] glycoprotein, which has been progressively shortened by digestion with pronase, and synthetic peptides. From these studies, a generality has emerged which suggests that no primary structure per se is required. Apart from Ser and Thr, the other amino acid necessary for initiation is proline. This is assumed to disrupt any secondary structure that may otherwise form and thus allow access to the peptide by GalNac:GalNacTrans. The minimum peptide length required for the successful incorporation of GalNac is difficult to determine. The use of synthetic peptides has revealed an octapeptide,

Val–Thr–Pro–Arg–Thr–Pro–Pro–Pro,[25] to be active as a GalNac acceptor using GalNac:GalNacTrans purified from porcine submaxillary glands.

The assembly of the carbohydrate chains onto the initiated peptide is achieved by the action of a set of enzymes collectively known as glycosyltransferases. It is thought that there is a unique glycosyltransferase for each type of monosaccharide added to the growing chain by a particular bond.[26] The monosaccharide substrates for the transferases are the nucleotide sugars, USP–GalNac, UDP–Gal, GDP-Fuc, and CMP–NeuAc, a common modification in carbohydrate biosynthesis that is required to overcome the inherent unreactivity of monosaccharides. The nucleotide moiety, except in the case of CMP–NeuAc which is synthesized in the nucleus,[27] is also required to transport the nucleotide-sugar across the endoplasmic reticulum membrane. This process is thought to be a one-for-one exchange for the free nucleoside (e.g., UMP) and not an active transport process.[28]

The growing oligosaccharide chains have been divided into three portions:[28] the core, composed of the initial two or three monosaccharides; the backbone containing the repeating units of Gal–GlcNac, and the terminal region, which includes the final two or three monosaccharides on the chain. Four types of core structure, two types of backbone structure, and a number of terminal structures have been described. The control mechanisms that dictate the way in which oligosaccharide chains are constructed are diverse. At the genetic level, there is control on the availability of the glycosyltransferases, and at the substrate level, a variety of feedback mechanisms occurs. Changes in the monosaccharide composition can be swift in response to diseased states, as also can be the degree of sulfation. These responses are discussed later.

Once the mucus glycoprotein is complete, budding-off from the Golgi apparatus membrane occurs to form a vacuole enclosing the molecule from which it will be secreted. It is unknown how the glycoprotein is processed other than the glycosylation before it is enclosed in the vacuole. Once in the vacuole, it is thought that the molecule is dehydrated to allow tighter packing. This may involve calcium ions being used to form a complex with the glycoprotein. Studies on the secretion of mucus glycoprotein are very limited because of the lack of suitable experimental material. However, studies have been carried out on the secretion of mucus glycoprotein from the terrestial slug *(Ariolimax columbianus)*, which indicates that there is a massive efflux of Ca^{2+} immediately prior to the release of the glycoprotein.[30]

B. ANTIGENICITY

In addition to the biochemical and physical investigations on mucus glycoproteins, probing of the molecule with antibodies has also proved to be very productive. Two types of immunological activity can be identified, which are defined as unspecific activity and specific activity.

Unspecific activity refers to the antigenic determinants that mucus glycoproteins share with other glycoproteins, glycolipids, and simple excreted oligosaccharides. The most studied of these, though not the most abundant, are the carbohydrate structures that constitute the ABO(H) blood groups. Specific activity refers to the antigenic determinants that have been discovered using antibodies to the mucus glycoprotein, particularly monoclonal antibodies. The antigenic determinants in this group are located on the carbohydrate and the peptide region of the glycoprotein. Such a classification will have anomalies, but it illustrates the two tiers at which antigenic determinants occur.

1. Unspecific Activity

The antigenic determinants in this division are the blood group antigens, so-called because they were originally found on the surface of erythrocytes. Although these antigens have now been described on the surfaces of many cell types as well as in secreted glycoproteins, their function has yet to be identified.

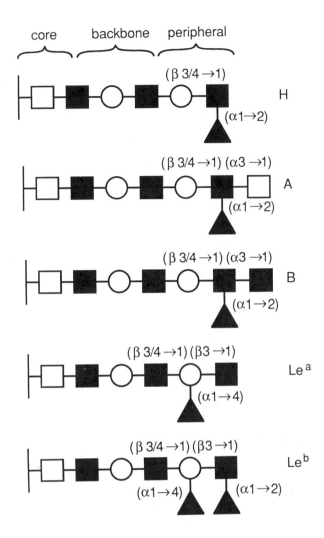

FIGURE 2. Major blood group ideotypes found on mucus glycoprotein (key is the same as Figure 1).

A recent hypothesis[31,32] suggests that they are binding for endogenous ligands, which may regulate nearby receptors of, for example, epithelial growth factor. A further speculation of this hypothesis, and one which is pertinent to mucus glycoproteins, is that the antigens act as receptors for infective agents. It is unlikely that the antigens on the mucus glycoprotein will play a part in any endogenous ligand binding, except in association with immunoglobulins that are secreted onto the epithelial surface and are important in the ability of mucus to remove infective agents.[33] The use of the ideotypes as "hooks" to catch infective agents is, however, feasible and evidence to suggest that *Streptococcus sanguis*[34] and *Pseudomonas aeruginosa*[35] adherence, to buccal cells and tracheal cells, respectively, can be inhibited by salivary gland and tracheal mucus glycoprotein lends weight to this hypothesis. However, no structural analysis of the receptor structures for these microorganisms has been performed, except that sialic acid is thought to be an important constituent.[35]

All the determinants in this group are expressed on the carbohydrate portion of the mucus glycoprotein molecule. In many instances, for example, with the ABO(H) system, the appearance of a determinant can remove a preceding determinant (Figure 2). The sequential nature of these antigens is important because degradation of the mucus glycoprotein *in vivo* will change the antigenicity of the glycoprotein. No studies have been performed on the *in vivo* disappearance of the antigens so it is impossible to say whether or not the erosion is random. It is conceivable that selective degradation by the bodies' own secretions or by the enzymes of the microflora associated with the site of secretion may cause a nonrandom and, consequently, predictable degradation.

Of greater importance is the control of secreted mucus glycoprotein blood group antigens by the allomorphic secretor gene, *Sese*. These genes[36] are expressed in 70% of the population as *Sese* or *Sese*,[35] the so-called secretors; the remaining 30%, homozygous *sese*, are nonsecretors. The secretor/nonsecretor classification refers only to the carbohydrate structures that are expressed as the component antigens of the ABO(H) system and to their appearance on secreted glycoproteins. The action of this gene does not influence the expression of the ABO(H) structures on the cell surfaces. Although nonsecretors do not produce significant amounts of the ABO(H) antigens, some can be detected, and they do secrete other blood group antigens. The secretogene appears not to code for a specific glycosyl transferase; rather it controls, in an as yet undefined way, the function of the α $(1 - >2)$ fucosyl transferase that creates the H determinant.[37] This process illustrates dramatically the sequential nature of these determinants, showing clearly that if the H determinant is not synthesized, then the succeeding A and B determinants also cannot be expressed. Conversely, the removal of GalNac (for A) or Gal (for B) will reveal the H determinant.

2. Specific Activity

The determinants that collectively make up the specific activity are found on both the oligosaccharide and peptide portions of the mucus glycoprotein molecule. It is too early to say whether the information obtained by studying the distribution of the specific determinants will have more than a research interest. Monoclonal antibodies have been raised against the whole glycoprotein to test whether or not the same site of secretion is able to deliver onto the epithelia more than one type of glycoprotein molecule. A recent report[38] of such a strategy using antibodies raised against human colonic mucus glycoprotein suggests that there are differences in the molecules at this site. This confirms and expands an earlier report of two distinct colonic glycoproteins.[39] Other workers, however, have described immunological similarities between sites of production and between certain species.[40,41] Caution must, therefore, be exercised when considering immunological data because the continual turnover of mucus glycoprotein may lead to misinterpretation of the antigenic significance. Considerably more research needs to be done on the specific antigens before any permanent and exploitable trends in their distribution can be defined.

C. MACROMOLECULAR STRUCTURE

The discussion so far on the mucus glycoprotein molecule has been centered on the basic glycoprotein subunit. However, estimates of the total molecular weight vary between 2×10^6 and 14×10^6 Da. The unusually [42-47] large molecular weights recorded for the glycoprotein are a result of polymerization of the basic 5×10^5 Da subunit (Figure 3).

Two schools of thought emerge when describing how the subunits are polymerized, which can be grouped into those who believe it is achieved with the aid of a link-peptide, and those who think that any link-peptide is an artifact of the preparative procedure.

The first model to be proposed for the structure of the glycoprotein considers four subunits covalently bound to a central 70,000 Da link-peptide by disulfide bonds: the so-called windmill structure.[48] However, the size and conformation of the pig stomach molecule, from which the data for this model were taken, cannot be supported by data from electron microscopy studies.[49] As a structural feature, the link-peptide has been investigated in a variety of different mucus glycoproteins. From these studies, it can be suggested that although the peptide is a discrete structural entity, there are chemical differences between peptides

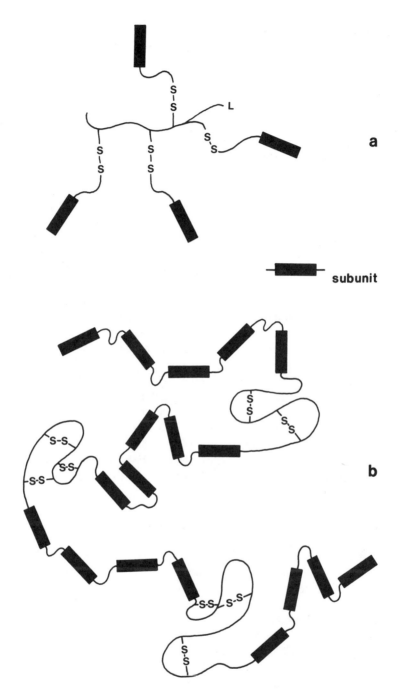

FIGURE 3. Proposed macromolecular structures for mucus glycoprotein; (a) the nonlinear model that may involve a link peptide (L) from which subunits branch off, and (b) the linear model containing four groups of multiple subunit assembly.

isolated from different sources. The link-peptide of pig and human stomach glycoprotein[50] is reported to have a molecular weight of 70 kDa and to be unglycosylated. Pig small intestinal glycoprotein link-peptide molecular weight has been estimated at 90 kDa,[6] and human intestinal mucus glycoprotein at 118 kDa.[51] Human mucus peptide obtained from sputum has a molecular weight of 70 kDa, the same as that for human stomach. However, this peptide did exhibit some degree of glycosylation.[8] Arguably, the link-peptide could be an artifact of the preparative procedure. This has been tested using three commonly reported procedures: gel exclusion chromatography, CsCl density gradient ultracentrifugation, and CsCl ultracentrifugation with guadinium chloride.[12] In each procedure, the link-peptide was identified using immunological techniques. A second possibility is that glycoprotein from different sites has a different link-peptide, a possibility that may also include some mucus glycoproteins that do not have the link-protein at all. The presence and function of the link-peptide has been questioned, and an alternative interpretation proposed.

The "non-link-peptide" model of mucus glycoprotein considers the molecule as a linear polymer of subunits in which there is a conformational order. On a length of core peptide, four regions of glycosylation occur,[10] and these regions are equivalent to four subunits. The four subunit assembly is covalently bound by disulfide bridges to another assembly of four subunits, and it is suggested there are four such assemblies in each mucus glycoprotein molecule. The appearance of the link-peptide is attributed to the way that the disulfide bonds between assemblies are reduced and how the nonglycosylated regions are digested by proteases. Intramolecular disulfide bonds are thought to be part of the nonglycosylated peptide region.

Digestion by protease, it is suggested, first liberates the nonglycosylated region, and subsequent reduction of disulfide bonds could liberate what appears on electrophoresis gels and upon ultracentrifugation as a discrete protein component. Recently it has been reported[52] that there are structural differences between intracellular mucus glycoprotein and secreted glycoprotein. Interestingly, the previously reported 118 kDa link-protein of the secreted preparation appears to be the product of reduction of a much larger 200 kDa protein, found intracellularly. Thus one could speculate that the link-proteins are indeed intramolecular features.

Whatever the macromolecular architecture, it is certain that mucus glycoproteins are of high molecular weight and are capable of producing viscoelastic gels at low concentrations. The gel thus contains a high concentration of water ($>95\%$), which is held in contact with the membrane from which it was secreted. This water makes a significant contribution to the homeostatic function of mucus secretions.

IV. MUCUS SECRETION

Although the mucus secreted may not appear to differ according to the site of secretion, the cells in which it is produced do in fact vary. It is, therefore, convenient to discuss the individual regions separately.

A. RESPIRATORY TRACT

The mucus that overlies the respiratory epithelium is produced by surface cells and submucosal glands. In the normal human lung, mucus is only secreted down to the terminal bronchioles, which are about 1 mm in diameter. Submucosal glands are only found in the cartilage containing airways (trachea and bronchi) although some species (e.g., birds) do not have glands at all.

1. Epithelial Cells

Eight epithelial and one migratory cell have been found in the human surface epithelium. Of these, four are secretory, namely goblet cells, Clara cells, serous cells, and the "special type" cells. Ciliated cells are also found and are important in that they are involved in mucus clearance.[53]

a. Serous Cells

This cell has only been identified in the human lung at the fetal stage. Little is known of its fate postnatally although it is likely that it transforms into a mucus secreting cell.[54] However, in some animals, particularly specific pathogen-free (SPF) rats, the serous cell is the most common cell found in the upper airway. It has been suggested that these cells may produce the serous fluid that bathes the cilia.

b. Goblet Cells

The chalice-like shape from which these cells derive their name is produced by the distension due to the packing with dense secretory granules. Those cells that contain granules, but are not distended, should not strictly be referred to as goblet cells and are probably better referred to as mucous cells. In the human airway, these cells all produce acid glycoprotein and this may be either sialoglycoprotein or a mixture of sialo- and sulphoglycoprotein.[55]

The cytoplasm of the goblet cell is electron-dense and, as with the serous cell, the nucleus is irregular. The rough endoplasmic reticulum is located mainly in the base of the cell. The secretory granules are electron-lucent and sometimes have an electron-dense core. Because each granule often has an incomplete membrane, fusion between them regularly occurs.

Goblet cells maintain a slow, "baseline" secretory rate that involves the intermittent release of single secretory granules, which are constantly replaced. Greater mucus secretion is achieved by compound exocytosis that temporarily depletes intracellular granules.

c. Clara Cells

These cells also have an irregular nucleus, but the cytoplasm is not electron-dense and is similar to the ciliated cells. The secretory granule is electron-dense and irregular in outline. There is, however, an abundance of endoplasmic reticulum, which is smooth and without ribosomes. The apex of the cell projects into the lumen, and it produces a secretion that is different from those of goblet or serous cells. In man, these cells appear to be confined to the terminal bronchioles, although they have been found as high as the hilum in the rat and the trachea and nose of the mouse.

Histochemical studies have shown that the secretory granules stain with periodic acid-Schiff (PAS), which indicates a neutral glycoprotein, but that this could be digested by pepsin. Some studies have suggested that the Clara cells may produce lung surfactant (dipalmitoyl lecithin), but it is known that the alveolar type II pneumocyte is the prime source of this material. The proposal was focused on the fact that Clara cells take up leucine, galactose, and acetate, and they have ultrastructural similarities with testicular interstitial cells, which produce steroids based on cholesterol.[55]

d. Ciliated Cells

Ciliated cells are found throughout the respiratory tract with the exception of the anterior nose and the alveoli.[56] They are usually found in fields together with goblet cells and gland ducts; each ciliated field is separated by regions where ciliated cells are absent. Although the total number has been estimated to be 3×10^{12} cells, it is not clear whether their incidence increases or decreases with progression down the respiratory tract.[54]

Ciliated cells are characterized by their long cellular projections containing fibrils surrounded by cytoplasm and enclosed by the membrane of the cell. Numerous microvilli are also present. The cilia are densely packed at about $8/\mu m^2$ or 200 per cell, and the length varies at different airway levels being longer in the trachea (5 to 7 μm) than in the small bronchi (3 to 4 μm).[57] They are normally 0.25 μm in diameter and a crown of short projections has been demonstrated on the ciliary tips. The cilia beat at about 10 to 20 Hz, and it has been reported that in the peripheral airways cilia beat faster.

2. Tracheobronchial Submucosal Glands

The tracheobronchial submucosal glands are found in all airways with cartilage in the wall.[53] They normally lie between the epithelium and the plates of cartilage and have a density of about one gland per square millimeter of epithelium. It is usually stated that in the normal human lung, 40 times more mucus is secreted by the glands than the goblet cells.

There are four distinct regions that have been identified within the gland.[55] These are the ciliated duct, the collecting duct, the mucous tubule, and the serous tubule. The ciliated duct is continuous with the lumen of the airway, typically nonbranching and lined with ciliated mucus-secreting epithelium, which contains fewer goblet cells than the surface epithelium. This ciliated duct leads into the collecting duct where the ciliated epithelium is replaced by tall, nonciliated cells. These cells, which are highly eosinophilic and packed with mitochondria increase from 30 to 70 μm along this duct, which is about 1mm in length and runs obliquely to the surface epithelium. The lumen is 100 μm in diameter at the widest point, and it narrows towards its distal end.

The cells possess high metabolic activity, and it has been proposed that they regulate water and ionic flux in the gland secretion. It may be of significance in this respect that blood capillaries are more numerous around the collecting duct than the secretory tubules, which arise abruptly, the junction coinciding with the point of branching. The epithelium that arises first is normally lined with mucous cells. Each branch is approximately 500 μm long, and a typical gland might contain 13 major branches. The mucous tubules are packed with secretion. The serous tubules are located at the ends of the mucous tubules and may occur individually or in groups. Each tubule is 50 to 180 μm in length, and the lumen is small. The anatomical arrangement of the secretory tubules is such that their secretion must flow over the mucous epithelium presumably enhancing mucus hydration and removal. The ratio of mucous to serous tubules is 1:1, and their joint secretion passes into the collecting duct.

Mucus gland cells, like goblet cells, contain large amounts of alcian blue-positive material (acidic glycoproteins) whereas serous cells contain a chiefly alcian blue-negative (neutral glycoproteins). In contrast, epithelial secretions contain more sialic acid relative to galactose and *N*-acetylglucosamine; submucosal secretion is more highly sulfated.

Myoepithelial cells are found beneath the mucous, serous, and the collecting duct cells. These contain fibrils and are considered to be contractile. It is likely that gland discharge is facilitated by contraction of such cells.

Both cholinergic and adrenergic innervation of the submucosal glands has been demonstrated.[58] Each type of cell within the gland receives both types of innervation although the differential responsiveness of the cells to a variety of neurohumoral substances has been observed. Mucous cell secretion is stimulated more potently by β-adrenergic and cholinergic agonists than by α-adrenergic agonists. In contrast, serous cells are stimulated most potently by α-adrenergic and cholinergic agonists. Considering both serous and mucous cells, the ratio of cholinergic to adrenergic innervation is 9:1, but serous cells receive a considerably greater number of both axon types: there is no evidence of selective innervation. Antibodies raised to serous cell contents do not react with mucous cells and vice versa. It is possible that one of the manifestations of disease is a change in the relative sensitivity of individual cell types to a particular agonist.

3. Mucociliary Clearance

In the lung, nose, ear, and cervix, ciliated cells are present in the surface epithelium. In these regions, they function together with the overlying layer of secreted mucus as a means of removing, for example, discrete particles and microorganisms. Such agents become entrapped in the mucus due to either its inherent "stickiness", or receptor mediated effects, or by interaction with immunoglobulins. In the human airway, secretory IgA is the most common immunoglobulin, and it has been suggested that it orientates in the surface of the mucus layer with the hydrophilic region embedded in the mucus and the hydrophobic groups in the airway. This not only maximizes the chances of interacting with bacteria and viruses, but also makes the most economical use of the immunoglobulin.

The two layer concept of mucociliary clearance was proposed by Lucas and Douglas[59] who suggested that a mucus layer or blanket floated upon a layer of watery fluid, the sol layer. This latter layer is only 3 to 5 μm in depth, and the mucus layer is of the order of 2 to 4 μm. The cilia are 7 μm in length when fully extended, but can assume a folded configuration that approximately halves their length. It is this flexibility that is the key to the mucus clearance: each cilium undergoes a relatively fast effective stroke when it is extended so that its tip protrudes through the sol layer and pushes into the mucus, thus propelling it forwards or upwards. At the end of the effective stroke, the cilia take on the folded conformation when they withdraw from the mucus layer and thus make their recovery stroke immersed only in the sol layer. By such means, the mucus is only moved in one direction. The cilia are able to interact with the mucus due to the presence of a crown of "hooks" that exist around the tip of each cilium.[55]

The beating of the cilia is generally coordinated such that waves move along the epithelium and plaques of mucus are transported. A continuous blanket does not exist in the normal airway, and the rafts or plaques move from one area of ciliated epithelium to another in a nonlinear manner.[60] The overall outcome in the airway is for the mucus to be conducted cephalad until it reaches the oropharynx from which it gains access to the GIT by swallowing. The rate of mucus transport in man is genetically determined and lies within the range of 4 to 10 mm min^{-1} in the trachea of nonsmokers. The rate is lower in the periphery and and is reduced at night.[61]

In the nose, the cilia also carry mucus towards the oropharynx.[56] Ciliated cells are not found in the eye or the GIT.

B. GASTROINTESTINAL TRACT

For convenience, the GIT will be considered as three distinct areas, namely the stomach, the small intestine, and the colon. Since the majority of drug molecules are absorbed in the former two regions, these will be dealt with in the greatest detail.

1. The Stomach

The stomach wall is composed of four principal coats. From the outside these are

1. The serous coat composed of loose connective tissue and simple squamous epithelium together with blood and lymph vessels;
2. The muscular coat composed of three muscle layers: the outer longitudinal, middle circular, and inner oblique;
3. The submucous coat composed of loose connective tissue supporting the large blood vessels and lymphatics; and
4. The mucous coat consisting of the muscularis mucosa, a layer of outer longitudinal and inner circular smooth muscle, the lamina propria composed of loose connective tissue, some collagenous and reticular fibers with blood and lymph vessels, and an epithelial lining of columnar cells. The mucous coat is thrown into large, predominantly longitudinal folds known as nigre, which are mostly readily visible in the empty stomach, but which almost disappear upon distension with food. The epithelial lining has numerous invaginations that penetrate the lamina propria to form the gastric glands. These are of three main types: cardiac, parietal (or oxyntic), and pyloric, and each is specialized for a different secretory function. The parietal glands are found in the fundus and corpus while the other two types occur most frequently in those regions of the stomach from which they derive their names.

The main secretory cells of the stomach are contained in these gastric glands and may be divided into parietal (or oxyntic) cells that secrete acid, chief cells that secrete pepsinogen, an inactive precursor of pepsin, and mucous cells that secrete mucus and endocrine cells. Parietal cells occur exclusively in the parietal glands of the fundus and body of the stomach. They have an extensive intracellular network of interconnecting membranes in the form of vesicles, tubules, asterns, and canaliculi, which serve to increase manifestly the surface area over which acid secretion can occur.[62] Parietal cells can secrete acid at a maximum concentration of 160 mM against a concentration gradient of approximately 1,000,000:1. The secretory process has a large oxygen requirement and involves metabolism via the citric acid pathway. H^+ and HCO_3^- ions are generated intracellularly by carbonic anhydrase, and each diffuses out of the cell in opposite directions at the same rate, H^+ ions entering the lumen and HCO_3^- ions crossing the basolateral membrane in exchange for Cl^- ions. H^+ ions traverse the apical membrane of the parietal cell by means of an electronegative pump and by an electroneutral mechanism involving a K^+ dependent ATP-ase.[63] Chloride ions pass into the lumen in association with the H^+ ions down an electrochemical gradient and aslo by an electrogenic pump. Water, which represents the principal component of gastric juice, is thought to enter the lumen by passing down an osmotic gradient created by H^+ and Cl^+ ion secretion.

Acid secretion is stimulated by histamine, acetylcholine, and gastrin: the parietal cell has receptors for all three of these agonists. Stimulation of these receptors is thought to increase the rate of secretion by increasing intracellular calcium and cyclic AMP levels. Putative inhibitors of acid secretion include somatostatin, some prostaglandins, secretin, vasoactive intestinal peptide, gastric inhibitory peptide, glucagon, serotonin, and dopamine.[62] Physiologically, the prostaglandins and somatostatin are probably the most important.

Gastric pepsins are secreted principally from chief cells found in close association with parietal cells in the base of the oxyntic glands. These proteases are secreted as inactive pepsinogens with a molecular weight of 42 kDa, and these precursors undergo cleavage at a pH below 5 to produce the active enzymes (32 kDa).[64] On the basis of immunological evidence, two types of pepsinogens have been identified. They are synthesized via the cellular rough endoplasmic reticulum and Golgi bodies and stored as zymogen granules in vacuoles. The same stimulants of acid secretion cause pepsin release and on prolonged demand, the granular store is depleted, but a high proportion of maximum output can be maintained by *de novo* synthesis.

Mucus-secreting cells are ubiquitous throughout the stomach, forming the surface columnar epithelium as well as lining the neck region of the oxyntic glands and composing the principal cell type in the cardiac and pyloric glands. Secretion across the apical membrane occurs by a combination of exocytosis, apical expulsion, and cell exfoliation. Once released, the mucus gel anneals to form a continuous layer adhering to the surface epithelium.[65]

It has been proposed that this mucus layer is the site where H^+ ions are neutralized by HCO_3^-, and that consequently a pH gradient exists across the mucus layer.

A number of hormones are secreted by the gastric mucosa that include gastrin (from G cells), histamine (from mast-like cells), intrinsic factor (from parietal cells), and somatostatin (from D cells).

2. The Small Intestine

The small intestine is divided into three parts, the duodenum, the jejunum, and the ileum although there is a general similarity in the structure of each. The innermost layer of the intestine is known as the mucosa, which has a lining of epithelium specialized according to site and function. It is separated from the muscularis mucosa by the lamina propria mucosa, which contains cells of the lymphoreticular system.

Mucus secreting Brunner's glands are found only in the duodenum.[66] The intestinal surface epithelium is thrown into folds and covered with finger-like villi, 0.5 to 1.5 mm in length. Approximately 10 to 40 villi are found per square millimeter, and their surface is composed of columnar cells, the luminal surface of which are composed of microvilli. The mucus-containing goblet cells lie between the columnar cells. Crypts of Lieberkühn are found at the base of the villi; there are three crypts to every villi, which are simple tubes 0.3 to 0.5 mm deep. They contain the precursor cell populations known as enteroblasts, which provide the replacement mucosal cells. The cells continually move closer to the villus tip, maturing into their ultimate form as they emerge from the crypt. Once they reach the tip of the villus they are sloughed off, and the entire epithelium is replaced every 3 to 6 days.[67] This shedding has been associated with the leakiness of the gut with respect to plasma proteins. The cells are shed at a rate of 50 to 100 million/d, and it has been calculated that up to 50 g of endogenous protein migrates into the gut lumen every day. The villi of the human intestinal mucosa are finger-like as they are in the mouse, but rat villi are tongue-shaped. Duodenal villi are shorter and broader and all villi can be modified by diet or environment.[66]

Goblet cells are most numerous in the crypts and form the second most numerous cell type of the villi in the jejunum.[66] In contrast, the colon has an almost flat mucosal surface. Goblet cells represent 25% of the surface epithelial cells in the duodenum rising in number with progression down the gut so that in the colon 60% of the surface cells are goblet cells. Only acetylcholine and cholinomimetic agents have been shown to act as goblet cell secretogogues in normal intestinal tissue. However, this only applies as the cell matures in the crypt, and once it has migrated to the villus or mucosal surface, this sensitivity is lost. It is suggested that this is due to the loss of acetylcholine receptors on migration.

The distribution of subepithelial cholinergic nerve endings is not known, but they are separated from migrating epithelial cells by the basal lamina, so classical neuroeffector functions do not form directly on epithelial cell basal membranes. Although this would involve variable diffusion distances for neurotransmitters, these nerves appear to be capable of accelerating mucus secretion from crypt goblet cells; this response may be very rapid.

The lymphoid tissue of the mucosa becomes especially prominent in the ileum forming the aggregated lymphoid masses termed Peyer's patches, which are overlain by M cells. The striated border of the epithelium bears a glycocalyx, which is a glycoprotein coat that stains with PAS reagent. A coat of fine filaments extending about 0.1 m from the microvilli tips is also present (sometimes referred to as the "fuzzy coat"). The material forming the cell coat is continually produced by the Golgi apparatus; the role of the glycocalyx is unclear, but many digestive enzymes are found in its vicinity. The glycocalyx is less compact in the small intestine than in the small bowel.

The goblet cell is similar to that of the airway except that its shape is determined by the forces created by the surrounding enterocytes. They are unicellular and are produced from stem cell precursors in the crypts. Mucus granules detach from the elaborate Golgi apparatus at the rate of one every 2 to 4 min. The granules are stored for discharge in the merocrine mode, one or two at a time. In addition to the normal baseline secretion, explosive discharge occurs in response to irritants. The microvilli that are present on goblet cells become less distinct as the cell swells. A protective and lubricative coating of mucus covers the intestinal epithelium, and it is thought that this may not only represent a barrier to antigens and toxins but also drug molecules.

3. The Colon

The large intestine is not covered with villi, but contains deep tubular pits that increase in depth towards the rectum. The epithelium is composed of one layer of tall prismatic cells. Goblet cells are more numerous than in the small intestine both on the surface and in the pits, and some goblet cells possess microvilli. The glycocalyx is less compact than in the small intestine consisting of loosely arranged radial filaments extending perpendicularly to the surface membrane.

4. Control of Secretion

Mild irritation may result in the release of mucus such that even passing saline through the rat colon causes depletion of goblet cell reserves. Thus mechanical stimulation of the gut may account for a substantial proportion of the basal secretion from surface goblet cells. However, it does appear that intestinal goblet cell secretion is chiefly under cholinergic control, but only while they are within the crypts. Adrenergic agents do not promote mucus secretion although they may have an effect on synthesis of the mucus glycoprotein.[68]

C. MUCUS SECRETION IN THE EYE

Mucus is produced by the goblet cells in the conjunctiva. It has been shown[69] that goblet cells are most abundant in the inner canthral region and the lower fornix with a greater density on the palpebral conjunctiva. The mucus is secreted onto the surface of the conjunctiva and is wiped over the surface of the cornea by the upper lid. Both acid and neutral mucin granules have been demonstrated within the cells. The lacrimal gland also contains mucous and serous cells, and a glycocalyx is also believed to be present.

Mucus from the lacrimal glands has been shown to differ in amino acid and carbohydrate content from typical epithelial glycoproteins. Their molecular weight has been shown to be of the order of 10^5 Da. Conjunctival mucus has been shown to be made up of a mixture of different molecular sizes, the highest being of 10^6 Da.

D. MUCUS SECRETION BY THE CERVIX

The human female cervix, in conjunction with the mucus that it secretes, serves a number of functions. These may be summarized as:[70]

1. The provision of receptive environment to sperm penetration around the time of ovulation while inhibiting penetration at other stages of the cycle
2. The provision of a sperm reservoir
3. The provision of an energy source for spermatozoa
4. The protection of spermatozoa from the hostile environment of the vagina and from being phagocytosed
5. The filtration of defective and immotile spermatozoa
6. The provision of a site for the capacitation of spermatozoa

The cervix forms the connection between the uterus and the vagina. The supravaginal cervix lies above the level of the vaginal vault while the portis extrema is the lower portion exposed to the vagina and lined with vaginal epithelium. The endocervical canal, although variable is, on average, 2.5 cm in length, flattened from front to back and fusiform in shape. It is encroached upon by cervical folds and in cross-section represents a complex branching structure. The external os changes with the stages of the menstrual cycle, and this is accompanied by changes in the tissue vascularity, the dimensions of the cervical canal, and the volume and consistency of the mucus. These all increase in the proliferative phase of the cycle, reaching a peak at ovulation to create the optimum conditions for sperm transport. The external os reaches a diameter of 3 mm at this time and decreases to a minimum of 1mm during the luteal phase.

The cervical mucosa is an involved system of clefts, grooves, and crypts. The endocervical crypts lie within the villus of the cervical epithelium. They are composed of columnar cells of two types, mucous cells and ciliated cells, which waft mucus and other secretions towards the vagina. There are few ciliated cells on the ectocervix, but they are particularly abundant at the uterocervical junction.

Three cytologically distinct mucous cell populations have been identified. Two of these are rich in secretory granules (vacuolated and nonvacuolated cells) that may occupy 80% of the cytoplasm. A vacuolated cell that has few granules has also been observed, and this may represent a depleted secretory cell. Three types of granule have been identified in mucous cells, one of which only contains neutral glycoproteins. Furthermore, the central core of one of the latter type of granules contains only the neutral type of glycoprotein.[71] It is felt that these differences represent different stages of maturation although the co-secretion of lysozyme may indicate different functionality of cells.

Release of mucus by endocervical mucous cells is believed to be under hormonal control.[70] A secretory cycle has been proposed for mucus cells that implies the occurrence of storage and secretory phases. This proposal is based on increase in mucus volume, which occurs as a result of increasing estrogen levels at midcycle. However, the release of mucus granules occurs continuously under the influence of both progesterone and estrogen, but increases slightly during acute estrogen administration.[72] There is little evidence to suggest that the amount of mucin stored in the cells alters during the menstrual cycle.[73] The release of mucin normally occurs exocytotically although apocrine release may occur during excessive stimulation.

The amount of mucus glycoprotein present in the secretion has been shown to be constant throughout the cycle with a slight increase occurring during midcycle.[74-76] The viscoelastic properties of the cervical mucus start to decrease about 6 d before ovulation and reach a minimum at that time. This can be detected by an increase in both Spinnbarkeit (thread formation) and ferning (when a sample of cervical mucus is allowed to dry in air). This mucus is receptive to spermatozoa, which are able to pass quickly in large numbers. One in 2000 spermatozoa are found in the cervical mucus 15 min after ejaculation, and a continuous stream of spermatozoa arrive at the fallopian tubes over the following 30 min. Although the spermatozoa must be motile, their progress is mainly controlled by the properties of the cervical mucus. At phases of the cycle other than the ovulatory stage, spermatozoa reaching the cervix are promptly immobilized.[77] The functional changes in mucus viscoelasticity and penetrability by spermatozoa are due to the changing water content. This has been reported to be 95 to 98% at ovulation, falling to 85 to 90% at other stages of the cycle.[76,77]

The hostility of the thickened cervical mucus to sperm penetration has been exploited as a means of contraception, and the low-dose oral contraceptive depends largely on this action for its effectiveness. Sequential oral contraceptives do not affect the mucus and, like estrogens, may even increase sperm penetration. Only high doses of progestogens increase the passage of spermatozoa across the cervix.[78]

Cervical mucus contains a wide range of substances in addition to mucus glycoproteins including plasma proteins, other proteins (e.g., lactoferrin), enzymes, amino acids, cholesterol, lipids, and a range of inorganic ions, the concentration of which are known to fluctuate during the cycle.[77,78]

V. MUCUS IN PATHOLOGICAL STATES

A. DISEASES OF THE AIRWAYS

Diseases have been recognized that are due either to an excess or a paucity of mucus. Such diseases include, for example, dry eye, glue ear (secretory otitis media), chronic obstructive airways disease, and asthma. Extremes of seriousness are represented by the common cold and the most common inherited disease in Caucasian populations, cystic fibrosis, where all mucus-secreting epithelia are affected. In general, conditions where mucus hypersecretion occurs are more common than those associated with its absence.

The commonest hypersecretory disease is that concerned with the respiratory tract and is usually referred to as chronic obstructive airways disease. Studies in experimental animals exposed to cigarette smoke or sulfur dioxide have indicated that the initial stages of the disease involve an increase in the number of sugar side chains on the glycoprotein molecule that bear acidic groupings from 50 to approximately 80%. Both sialic acid and sulfate groups increase, and the number of the former that are resistant to removal by sialidase treatment also increases. Neither the chemical basis for this change in resistance nor the physiological significance of the change in acidity is understood.

If the exposure to the irritant continues, then mucus cell hyperplasia occurs. The number of goblet cells in the epithelium increase (usually at the expense of ciliated cells), and the submucosal glands enlarge. The resultant increase in mucus output rapidly overloads the mucociliary transport system since the inflammation results in the concomitant secretion of immunoglobulins, plasma proteins, and DNA, all of which have been shown to contribute significantly to the viscoelasticity of the mucus.[79,80] A reduction in mucus clearance occurs, and at this point, cough takes over as the primary clearance mechanism. The material that is expectorated is usually referred to as sputum, which is composed of the total lung secretion together with saliva.

Complete blockage of parts of the airway can result, and this has obvious implications for the use of pharmaceutical aerosols. With cystic fibrosis patients, who probably exhibit the most extensive form of chronic obstructive airways disease, regular physiotherapy is the only way that the airways can be kept clear of mucus. The sputum from this disease is particularly rubbery and sticky, and it has been the subject of some debate as to whether this is due to an abnormal glycoprotein. Recent studies have shown that while the sputum shows abnormally high rheological parameters compared with other infected sputum, the glycoprotein purified from such sputum is essentially normal in terms of its rheological and biochemical characteristics.[81] However, it has also been shown that this purified glycoprotein interacts in an unusual manner with DNA and that the combination is responsible for the elevated elasticity. Furthermore, the DNA that is bound to the glycoprotein when it is secreted in sputum is in fact host derived and does not originate from bacterial cells.[81]

The classification of sputum is extremely difficult because of its variability, much of which can be attributed to the effects of infection. The mean dry weight increases to the order of 6 to 8%, and the pH increases. The sialic acid content increases in chronic bronchitis, asthma, bronchiestasis, and cystic fibrosis. Purulent sputum also exhibits increased levels of sulfate. Since fucose levels do not alter appreciably during disease, sialic acid fucose ratios have also been shown to increase. This may well be due to the occurrence of infection and reflects serum transudation rather than a change in mucus glycoprotein type. The amount of both IgA and IgG is elevated in chronic pulmonary disease, and this has been shown to correlate with the degree of infection.

B. DISEASES OF THE GASTROINTESTINAL TRACT

There is little doubt that mucus glycoprotein, a secretion primarily concerned with protecting the mucosal epithelia, will change in diseases of GIT. However, the extent to which the changes represent a response to trauma, as opposed to an alteration in mucosal physiology caused by the trauma, is unclear.

In the first instance, however, mucus glycoproteins prevent damage caused to the mucosa by bacteria, viruses, noxious agents, and digestive juices by a passive and active process. Passively the mucus gel acts as a continuous barrier that is replaced either at a steady basal rate, or as a sudden surge in response to stimuli, such as the binding of antibody complexes to the goblet cell membrane. It has been suggested that the control mechanisms for these two types of mucus glycoprotein secretion are separate.[82] The active protection afforded by mucus glycoprotein involves the interaction of molecule with the agents causing damage. In almost every case the structural feature of the mucus glycoprotein involved is the carbohydrate component.

The carbohydrate structure of secreted mucus glycoprotein is to a great extent the same as that of the glycoproteins and glycolipids embedded in the epithelial cell membranes. Thus mucus glycoproteins act as "dummy receptors" for carbohydrate binding ligands. Such ligands are widespread in nature and are used particularly by microorganisms and parasites to establish themselves on the gut wall. Other ligands, ingested lectins in food, for example, can innocently provoke responses as they bind to the cell membrane. The similar or identical structure of mucus glycoprotein carbohydrates will effectively intercept these ligands. Once bound to the mucus glycoprotein, the ligands and the associated infective agent can be efficiently removed from the mucosa by sloughing off of the mucus and subsequent excretion. This combination of active and passive protection of the mucosa is likely to be a major problem when designing bioadhesive devices that use mucus glycoprotein as a substrate, or which attempt to use receptors on the cell membrane that mucus glycoproteins mimic.

Apart from the replication of receptor structures on mucus glycoproteins, other features of the carbohydrate composition confer on the macromolecule a resistance to proteolytic digestion. The degree of protection correlates with the amount of sulfated monosaccharides in the glycoprotein and has led to the suggestion that sulfated mucus glycoproteins are antiulcerogenic because they prevent autodigestion of the mucosa.[74]

The physical and chemical properties of mucus glycoproteins are known to change markedly in disease. The change is a result of two factors acting either independently or in combination, and the result may often compromise the ability of mucus glycoprotein to perform its protective function. The physical properties, quantified by the secretions' viscoelasticity, are affected by the addition of molecules not normally present in mucus glycoprotein to any great extent. DNA from cell debris[75] and albumin[76] that leaches into the GIT in inflammation is known to thicken the mucus gel by interaction with the glycoprotein. Changes in the molecular composition of mucus glycoproteins have been studied in order to understand the role of the glycoproteins in specific diseases. This is not an easy task, and it is apparent that no generalizations can be made. The integrity of the gastrointestinal mucosa is usually regarded as being determined by the balance between protective functions and damaging agents. In all examples of GIT disease, the way in which this balance is disturbed is unknown. Because mucus glycoproteins are an integral part of the protective function, it is likely that factors that affect its structure will also affect this balance. In peptic ulcers, for example, it is reported that the mucus glycoprotein contains more acidic glycoproteins,[77] and it is also reported that they are more degraded.[78]

Adenocarcinomas have also been shown to produce more acidic (sialic acid containing) glycoproteins as well as mimicking some of the antigenic determinants associated with the cell surface glycoproteins of the tumor.[88] In cystic fibrosis, the sialic acid content of the glycoproteins remains the same as in control groups, but exhibits an increase in sulfated glycoproteins.[89] Goblet cells continue to produce mucus glycoproteins in Crohn's disease but they are absent in ulcerative colitis.[90] Fundamentally, it is unknown whether such changes in mucus secretion and structure are the cause of the disease or a manifestation of it. This lack of understanding, however, should not prevent us from attempting to utilize the protection afforded the mucus glycoprotein either by stimulating its production or possibly introducing synthetic polymers with similar characteristics. The former approach is indeed common, being the mode of action of a number of antiulcer drugs, with investigations into more potent glycoprotein synthesis stimulants such as prostaglandins currently under development.

C. DISEASES OF THE EYE

A shortage of mucus in the eye leads to breakup of the tear film and dry spot formation although it is likely that concomitant changes in the epithelial surface are also involved. Excess of mucus is a symptom of a number of diseases including keratoconjunctivitis sicca

(KCS), neuroparalytic keratitis, and vernal catarrh. Inflammation with the associated increase in the passage of plasma proteins may be equally important since this will result in increased mucus viscoelasticity. Less is known of the changes that occur in the type of mucin that is secreted in diseases of the eye. However, a tendency for the degree of sulfation to increase has been observed.[69]

D. DISEASES OF THE CERVIX

It is beyond the scope of this book to deal with the wide range of diseases that can occur in the lower female reproductive tract. Bacterial and fungal infections obviously represent the majority of conditions, and local treatment with anti-infective agents in the form of creams, ointments, and pessaries is usually effective.

Mucus-related conditions are usually concerned with conception and are due either to insufficient mucus being secreted or it not being able to support the passage of sperm. This is usually referred to as cervical factor infertility although cervical mucus hostility is only one aspect of this diffuse condition. If the mucus is thick, it is probably due to low water content, and it can be treated by removal of the cervical plug followed by artificial insemination. In some cases, the mucus may be of suitable quality for just 1 d of the cycle, and fertilization can only result if spermatozoa arrive at the cervix at the optimum time. A complete absence of mucus can result in infertility, and mucus transplantation has been offered.[91] In the case of cystic fibrotics, who often present with thick cervical mucus, treatment with a locally applied mucolytic agent, *N*-acetylcysteine, has been attempted.[77]

Some cervical mucus is lethal to the sperm of the partner, and this is usually due to immunologic factors. Sometimes antisperm antibodies can be demonstrated in the serum. Cytotoxic antibodies may be present in the cervical mucus, and then many immobilized sperm are seen in what appears to be normal mucus.

Intrauterine contraceptive devices are usually fitted with locating threads that lead out to the cervix so that they traverse the cervical mucus plug. The presence of such threads has been implicated in the occurrence of pelvic inflammatory disease where bacteria are thought to use the thread as a means of access to the uterus since the cervical mucus plug normally prevents such access. It has recently been demonstrated that the polymeric threads are capable of supporting bacterial growth and encouraging their upward transmission. The microrugosity of the thread is thought to be a significant factor in this respect.[92] The administration of orally active mucolytic (or perhaps more correctly termed mucoregulatory) agents, which are normally used to treat chronic obstructive airways disease, has been shown to reduce cervical mucus viscoelasticity and permit bacterial access to the uterus.[93] It is, therefore, feasible that a side effect of such treatment of airways disease could be pregnancy.

VI. CONCLUSIONS

The epithelia to which bioadhesive delivery systems are to be attached are covered with a layer of mucus that is continually produced and constantly changing. Major differences occur in disease states, and it is certain that variation occurs from individual to individual. There are also many differences that exist between species, and if experimental systems are to be tested in animals, it is important that an appropriate model be used. It is desirable that at least two species are used, and it must be remembered that there are few good animal models of the disease states.

REFERENCES

1. **Reid, L. M. and Clamp J. R.**, The biochemical and histochemical nomenclature of mucus, *Br. Med. Bull.*, 34 (1), 5, 1978.
2. **Allen, A., Bell A., Mantle, M., and Pearson, J. P.**, in *Mucus in Health and Disease*, Chantler, E. N., Elder, J. B., and Elstein, M., Eds., Plenum Press, New York, 1982, 115.
3. **Fahim, R. E. F., Forstner, G. G., and Forstner, J. F.**, Hetrogeneity of rat goblet cell mucin before and after reduction, *Biochem. J.*, 209, 117, 1983.
4. **Smits, H. L., Van Kerkof, P. J. M., and Kramer, M. F.**, Isolation and partial characterization of rat duodenal gland mucus glycoprotein, *Biochem. J.*, 203, 779, 1982.
5. **Scawen, M. and Allen, A.**, The action of proteolytic enzymes on glycoprotein from pig gastric mucus, *Biochem. J.*, 163, 363, 1977.
6. **Mantle, M., Mantle, D., and Allen A.**, Polymeric structure of pig small-intestinal mucus glycoprotein, *Biochem. J.*, 195, 277, 1981.
7. **Marshall, T. and Allen, A.**, The isolation and characterization of the high molecular weight glycoprotein from pig colonic mucus, *Biochem. J.*, 173, 569, 1978.
8. **Tabachnik, N. F., Blackburn, P., and Cerami, A.**, Biochemical and rheological characterization of sputum mucins from patients with cystic fibrosis, *J. Biol. Chem.*, 256, 7161, 1981.
9. **Pearson, J. P., Allen, A., and Venables, C. W.**, Gastric mucus: isolation and polymeric structure of the undergraded glycoprotein: its breakdown by pepsin, *Gastroenterology*, 78, 709, 1980.
10. **Carlstedt, I., Lindgren, H., and Sheehan, J. K.**, The macromolecular structure of human cervical mucus glycoproteins, *Biochem. J.*, 213, 427, 1983.
11. **Silberberg, A. and Meyer F.**, in *Mucus in Health and Disease*, Chantler, E. N., Elder, J. B., and Elstein, M., Eds., Plenum Press, New York, 1982, 53.
12. **Fahim, R. E. F, Specian, R. D., Forstner, G. G., and Forstner, J. F.**, Characterization and localization of the putative link component in rat small-intestinal mucin, *Biochem. J.*, 243, 631, 1987.
13. **Bhavanandan, V. P. and Hegarty, J. D.**, Identification of the mucin core protein by cell-free translation of messenger RNA from bovine submaxillary glands, *J. Biol. Chem.*, 262 (12), 5913, 1987.
14. **Wesley, A., Mantle, M., Man, D., Qureshi, R., Forstner, G., and Forstner, J.**, Neutral and acidic species of human intestinal mucin, *J. Biol. Chem.*, 260, 7955, 1985.
15. **Schachter, H. and Williams, D.**, in *Mucus in Health and Disease*, Chantler, E. N., Elder, J. B., and Elstein, M., Eds., Plenum Press, New York, 1982, 3.
16. **Phelps, C. F.**, Biosynthesis of mucus glycoprotein, *Br. Med. J.*, 34, 43, 1978.
17. **Carlstedt, I., Sheehan, J. K., Corfield, A. P., and Gallagher, J. T.**, Mucus a gel of a problem, in *Essays in Biochemistry*, Campbell, P. N. and Marshall, R. D., Eds., Academic Press, New York, 1985, 20.
18. **Hughes R. C.**, in *Glycoproteins*, Chapman & Hall, London, 1983, chap. 3.
19. **Kiely, M. L., McKnight, G. S., and Schimke, R. T.**, Studies on the attachment of carbohydrate to ovalbumin nascent chains in hen oviduct, *J. Biol. Chem.*, 251, 5490, 1976.
20. **Bergman, L. W. and Kuehal, W. M.**, Addition of glucosamine and mannose to nascent immunoglobulin heavy chains, *Biochemistry*, 16, 4490, 1977.
21. **Struck, D. K. and Lennarz, W. J.**, The function of saccharide lipids in synthesis of glycoproteins, in *The Biochemistry of Glycoproteins and Proteoglycans*, Lennarz, W. J., Ed., Plenum Press, London, 1980, 2.
22. **Kim, Y. S., Perdomo, J., and Nordberg, J.**, Glycoprotein biosynthesis in small intestinal mucosa. I. A study of glycosyl transferases in microsomal subfractions, *J. Biol. Chem.*, 246, 5466, 1971.
23. **Hanover, J. A., Lennarz, W. J., and Young, J. D.**, Synthesis of N and O linked glycopeptides in oviduct membrane preparations, *J. Biol. Chem.*, 255, 6713, 1980.
24. **Hill, H. D., Jr., Schwyzer, M., Steinman, H. M., and Hill, R. L.**, Ovine submaxillary mucin. Primary structure and peptide substrates of UDP-N-acetylgalactosamine: mucin transferases, *J. Biol. Chem.*, 252, 3799, 1977.
25. **Young, J. D., Tsuchiya, D., Sandlin, D. E., and Holroyde, M. J.**, Enzymic O-glycosylation of synthetic peptides from sequences in basic myelin protein, *Biochemistry*, 18, 4444, 1979.
26. **Brockhausen, I., Matta, K. L., Orr, J., Schachter, H., Koenderman, A. H. L., and Van den Eijnden, D. H.**, Mucin synthesis, *Eur. J. Biochem.*, 157, 463, 1986.
27. **Kean, E. L.**, Nuclear cytidine S^1-monophosphosialic acid synthetase, *J. Biol. Chem.*, 245, 2301, 1970.
28. **Hirschberg, C. B. and Snider, M. D.**, Topography of glycosylation in the rough endoplasmic reticulum and Golgi apparatus, in *Annu. Rev. Biochem.*, 63, 1987, 56.
29. **Feizi, T., Gool, H. C., Childs, R. A., Picard, J. K., Uemura, K., Loomes, L. M., Thorpe, S. J., and Hounsell, E. F.**, Mucin type glycoproteins, *Biochem. Soc. Trans.*, 12, 591, 1984.
30. **Verdugo, P., Deyrup-Olsem, I., Aitken, M., Villalon, M., and Johnson, D.**, Molecular mechanisms of mucin secretion. I. The role of intragranular charge shielding, *J. Dent. Res.*, 66 (2), 506, 1987.

31. **Feizi, T. and Childs, R.,** Carbohydrate structures of glycoproteins and glycolipids as differentation antigens, tumour associated antigens and components of receptor systems, *Trends Biochem. Sci.*, 10, 24, 1985.

32. **Feizi, T. and Childs, R.,** Carbohydrates as antigenic determinants of glycoproteins, *Biochem. J.*, 245, 1, 1987.

33. **Lee, G. B. and Ogilvie, B. M.,** The intestinal mucus layer in *Trichinella spiralis* infected rats, in *Recent Advances in Mucosal Immunity*, Strober, W., Hanson, L. A., and Sell, K. W., Eds., Raven Press, New York, 1982, 319.

34. **Williams, R. C. and Gibbons, R. J.,** Inhibition of streptococcal attachment to receptors on human buccal epithelial cells by antigenically similar salivary glycoprotes, *Infect. Immun.*, 11, 711, 1975.

35. **Ramphal, R. and Pyle, M.,** Evidence for mucins and sialic acid as receptors for *Pseudomonas aeruginosa* in the lower respiratory tract, *Infect. Immun.*, 41, 339, 1983.

36. **Watkins, W. M.,** Biochemistry and genetics of the ABO, Lewis, and P blood group systems, in *Advances in Human Genetics*, Vol. 10, Harris, H. and Hirshhorn, K., Eds., Plenum Press, New York, 1980, 1.

37. **Schachter, H. and Roseman S.,** Mammalian glycosyl transferases: their role in the synthesis and function of complex carbohydrates and glycolipids, in *The Biochemistry of Glycoproteins and Proteoglycans*, Lennarz, W. J., Ed., Plenum Press, London, 1980, 2.

38. **Podoisky, D. K., Fournier, D. A., and Lynch, K. E.,** Development of anti human colonic mucin monoclonal antibodies, *J. Clin. Invest.*, 77(4), 1251, 1986.

39. **Gold, D. V., Schochat, D., and Miller, F.,** Protease digestion of colonic mucin, *J. Biol. Chem.*, 256, 6354, 1981.

40. **Qureshi, R., Forstner, G., and Forstner, J.,** Radioimmunoassay of human intestinal goblet cell mucin, *J. Clin. Invest.*, 64, 1149, 1979.

41. **Mukkur, T., Watson, D., Saini, K., and Lascelles, A.,** Purification and characterization of goblet cell mucin of high M_r from small intestine of sheep, *Biochem. J.*, 229, 419, 1985.

42. **Woodward, H., Horsey, B., Bhavanandan, V. P., and Davidson, E. A.,** Isolation, purification and properties of respiratory mucins glycoproteins, *Biochemistry*, 21, 694, 1982.

43. **Creeth, J., Bhaskar, K. R., Horton, J. R., Das, I., Lopez-Vidriero, M., and Reid, L.,** Separation and characterisation of bronchial glycoproteins by density gradient methods, *Biochem. J.*, 167, 557, 1977.

44. **Mantle, M. and Allen, A.,** Isolation and characterization of native glycoprotein from pig small intestinal mucus, *Biochem. J.*, 195, 267, 1987.

45. **Carlstedt, I. and Sheehan, J. K.,** Macromolecular properties and polymeric structure of mucus glycoproteins, *Ciba Found. Symp.* 109, Pitman, London, 1984, 157.

46. **Meyer, F. A. and Paradossi, G.,** The mechanism of thermal degradation of a high molecular weight glycoprotein complex from bovine cervical mucus, *Biochem. J.*, 209, 565, 1983.

47. **Harding, S. E., Rowe, A. J., and Creeth, J. M.,** Further evidence for a flexible and highly expanded spheroidal model for mucus glycoproteins in solution, *Biochem. J.*, 209, 893, 1983.

48. **Allen, A.,** Mucus — a protective secretion of complexity, *Trends Biochem. Sci.*, 169, 9, 1983.

49. **Sheehan, J. K., Oates, K., and Carlstedt, I.,** Electron microscopy of cervical, gastric and bronchial mucus glycoprotein, *Biochem. J.*, 239, 147, 1986.

50. **Pearson, J. P., Allen A., and Parry, S.,** A 70,000 molecular weight protein isolated from purified pig gastric mucus glycoprotein by reduction of disulphide bridges and its implications in polymeric structure, *Biochem. J.*, 197, 155, 1981.

51. **Mantle, M., Forstner, G., and Forstner F.,** Biochemical characterization of the component parts of intestinal mucin from patients with cystic fibrosis, *Biochem. J.*, 224, 345, 1984.

52. **Fahim, R. E. F., Forstner, G. G., and Forstner, J. F.,** Structural and compositional differences between intracellular and secreted mucin of rat small intestine, *Biochem. J.*, 248, 389, 1987.

53. **Jeffery, P. K. and Reid, L. M.,** New features of rat airway epithelium a quantitative and electron-microscopic study, *J. Anat.*, 120, 295, 1975.

54. **Lopez-Vidriero, M. T.,** Lung secretions, in *Aerosols and the Lung*, Clarke S. W. and Pavia, D., Eds., Butterworths, London, 1984, chap. 2.

55. **Jeffery, P. K. and Reid, L. M.,** The respiratory mucous membrane, in *Respiratory Defense Mechanisms* (Part 1), Brain, J. D., Proctor, D. F., and Reid, L. M., Eds., Marcel Dekker, New York, 1977, chap. 7.

56. **Sleigh, M. A.,** The nature and action of respiratory tract cilia, in *Respiratory Defense Mechanisms* (Part 1), Brain, J. D., Proctor, D. F., and Reid, L. M., Eds., Marcel Dekker, New York, 1977, chap. 8.

57. **Serafini, S. M. and Michaelson, E. D.,** Length and distribution of cilia in human and canine airways, *Bull. Eur. Physiopathol. Respir.*, 13, 551, 1977.

58. **Basbaum, C. B.,** Regulation of secretion from serous and mucous cells in the trachea, in *Mucus and Mucosa*, Ciba Found. Symp. 109, Pitman, London, 1984, 4.

59. **Lucas, A. M. and Douglas, L. C.,** Principles underlying ciliary activity in the respiratory tract, *Arch. Ototaryngol.*, 20, 518, 1934.

60. **Iravani, J. and van As, A.,** Mucus transport in the tracheobronchial tree of normal and bronchitic rats, *J. Pathol.*, 106, 81, 1972.

61. **Konietzko, N.,** Mucus transport and inflammation, *Eur. J. Respir. Dis.,* 69 (S147), 72, 1986.
62. **Rees, W. D. W. and Turnberg, L. A.,** Biochemical aspects of gastric secretion, *Clin. Gastroenterol.,* 10, 521, 1981.
63. **Forte, J. G., Machen, T. E., and Obrink, K. J.,** Mechanisms of gastric H$^+$ and Cl$^-$ transport, *Annu. Rev. Physiol.,* 42, 111, 1980.
64. **Samloff, I. M.,** Pepsinogens, pepsins and pepsin inhibitors, *Gastroenterology,* 60, 586, 1971.
65. **Allen, A.,** The structure and function of gastrointestinal mucus, in *Basic Mechanisms of Gastrointestinal Mucosal Cell Injury and Protection,* Harmon, J. W., Ed., William & Wilkins, London, 1981, 351.
66. **Carr, K. E. and Toner, P. G.,** Morphology of the intestinal mucosa, in *Pharmacology of Intestinal Permeation,* Csaky, T. Z., Ed., Springer-Verlag, Berlin, 1984, chap. 1.
67. **Davenport, H. W.,** *Physiology of the Digestive Tract,* 4th ed., Year Book Medical Publishers, Chicago, 1977, chap. 11.
68. **Neutra, M. R., Phillips, T. L., and Phillips, T. E.,** Regulation of intestinal goblet cells *in situ,* in mucosal explants and in the isolated epithelium, in *Mucus and Mucosa,* Ciba Found. Symp. 109, Pitman, London, 1984, 20.
69. **Wright, P. and Mackie, I. A.,** Mucus in the healthy and diseased eye, *Trans. Ophthalmol. Soc. U.K.,* 91, 1, 1977.
70. **Elstein, M.,** Functions and physical properties of mucus in the female genital tract, *Br. Med. Bull.,* 34, 83, 1978.
71. **Nicosia, S. V.,** Physiology of cervical mucus production, *Semin. Reprod. Endocrinol.,* 4, 313, 1986.
72. **Nicosia, S. V.,** An *in vivo* and *in vitro* structural-functional analysis of cervical mucus secretion, *Reproduction,* 5, 261, 1981.
73. **Topkins, P.,** The histological appearance of the endocervix during the menstrual cycle, *Am. J. Obstet. Gynecol.,* 58, 654, 1949.
74. **Wolf, D. P., Blasco, L., Khan, M. A., and Litt, M.,** Human cervical mucus. II. Changes in viscoelasticity during the ovulatory menstrual cycle, *Fertil. Steril.,* 28, 47, 1977.
75. **Wolf, D. P., Sokoloski, J., Khan, M. A., and Litt, M.,** Human cervical mucus. III. Isolation and characterisation of rheologically active mucin, *Fertil. Steril.,* 28, 53, 1977.
76. **Wolf, D. P., Blasco, L., Khan M. A., and Litt, M.,** Human cervical mucus. IV. Viscoelasticity and sperm penetrability during the ovulatory menstrual cycle, *Fertil. Steril.,* 30, 163, 1978.
77. **Blasco, L.,** Clinical approach to the evaluation of sperm-cervical mucus interactions, *Fertil. Steril.,* 28, 1133, 1977.
78. **Hafez, E. S. E.,** The cervix and sperm transport, in *Human Reproduction, Conception and Contraception,* 2nd ed., Hafez, E. S. E., Ed., Harper & Row, Hagerstown, 1980, chap. 9.
79. **Marriott, C.,** Mucus: its structure function and evaluation, in *Drug Delivery to the Respiratory Tract,* Ganderton, D. and Jones, T., Eds., Ellis Horwood, Chichester, 1987, chap. 7.
80. **Marriott, C., Beeson, M. F., and Brown, D. T.,** Biopolymer induced changes in mucus viscoelasticity, *Adv. Exp. Med. Biol.,* 144, 89, 1982.
81. **Lethem, M. I., Smedley, Y., James, S. L., Burke, J., and Marriott, C.,** The contribution of non-mucin components to the increased viscoelasticity of cystic fibrosis sputum, *Pediatr. Pulmonol.,* Suppl.1, 121, 1987.
82. **Specian, R. D. and Neutra, M. R.,** Mucus granule transport and secretion: effects of colchicine and cytochalasin B, *J. Cell. Biol.,* 87, 278, 1980.
83. **Mikuni-Takagaki, Y. and Hotta, K.,** Characterization of peptide inhibitory activity associated with sulphated glycoproteins isolated from gastric mucosa, *Biochim. Biophys. Acta,* 584, 288, 1979.
84. **List, S. J., Findlay, B. P., Forstner G. G., and Forstner, J. F.,** Enhancement the viscosity of mucin by serum albumin, *Biochem. J.,* 175, 565, 1978.
85. **Lethem, M. I., Marriott, C., and James, S. L.,** Abnormal interactions of cystic fibrosis mucus glycoproteins with DNA, *Eur. J. Respir. Dis.,* 71 (Suppl. 153), 276, 1987.
86. **Guslandi, M. and Ballarin, E.,** Assessment of the mucus-bicarbonate barrier in the stomach of patients with chronic gastric disorders, *Clin. Chim. Acta,* 144, 133, 1984.
87. **Younan, F., Pearson, J. Allen, A., and Venables, C.,** Changes in the structures of mucous gel on the mucosal surface of the stomach in association with peptic ulcer disease, *Gastroenterology,* 82, 827, 1982.
88. **Forstner, G. and Wesley, A. W.,** Clinical aspects of gastrointestinal mucus, in *Mucus in Health and Disease,* Chantler, E. N., Elder, J. B., and Elstein, M., Eds., Plenum Press, London, 1982, 199.
89. **Wesley, A. W., Qureshi, A. R., Forstner, G. G., and Forstner, J. F.,** Differences in mucous glycoproteins of small intestine from subjects with and without cystic fibrosis, in *Mucus in Health and Disease,* Chantler, E. N., Elder, J. B., and Elstein, M., Eds., Plenum Press, New York, 1982, 145.
90. **Bouchier, I. A. D.,** Inflammatory bowel disease, in *Gastroenterology,* Balliere Tindall, London, 14, 164.
91. **Check, J. H. and Rakoff, A. E.,** Treatment of cervical factor by donor mucus insemination, *Fertil. Steril.,* 28, 113, 1977.

92. **Wilkins, K. M., Hanlon, G. W., Martin, G. P., and Marriott, C.,** The influence of surface free energy and microrugosity on the adhesion of bacteria to polymer microfilaments, *J. Pharm. Pharmacol.*, 27, 65P, 1985.
93. **Malhi, J. S., Gard, P. R., Hanlon G. W., and Marriott, C.,** The effects of bromhexine hydrochloride and S-carboxymethyl-L-cysteine on guinea-pig uterine microflora, *J. Pharm. Pharmacol.*, 38, 1025, 1987.

Chapter 2

SCALING CONCEPTS AND MOLECULAR THEORIES OF ADHESION OF SYNTHETIC POLYMERS TO GLYCOPROTEINIC NETWORKS

Antonios G. Mikos and Nikolaos A. Peppas

TABLE OF CONTENTS

I. INTRODUCTION

Bioadhesion is the phenomenon of interfacial force interactions between two biological bodies.[1] Bioadhesion occurs between biological objects such as in cell fusion and platelet aggregation, or biological objects and artificial substrates as in cell adhesion to culture dishes and platelet adhesion to biomaterials, or artificial materials and biological substrates as in adhesion of hydrogels to soft tissues and adhesion of sealants to tooth surfaces.[2]

Bioadhesive systems have been used for many years in dentistry and orthopedics[3-6] as well as in ophthalmology[7] and for surgical applications.[8,9] However, recently there has been also a significant interest in the use of bioadhesives in other areas, such as soft tissue-based artificial replacements[10] and controlled release systems for local release of bioactive agents.[11] Such applications include systems for release of drugs in the buccal or nasal cavity,[12,13] for intestinal or rectal administration,[14,15] and even for urinary bladder applications.[16] Many of these applications are discussed in other chapters of this book.

Controlled release polymeric systems for drug delivery are often designed in order to target drugs in specific areas of the body. Bioadhesive controlled release systems may be the solution to this problem, since strong interactions between chemical groups of the polymer and the mucous lining of tissue may keep a device in contact with tissue for a period of time. The turnover of mucus determines its maximum transit time as shown by Leung et al. in Chapter 4.

In this chapter, the fundamentals of phenomena that relate to the adhesion of synthetic polymers, hydrocolloids, or mixtures thereof with a biological surface, and particularly a soft tissue, are examined. The mechanistic and structural aspects of bioadhesion and *novel molecular* theories are presented.

II. MECHANISMS OF BIOADHESION

A. THE BIOADHESIVE INTERFACE

Adhesive bonds between a polymer and a soft tissue require contributions from the surface of the potentially bioadhesive polymer, the first layer of the natural tissue, and the interfacial layer between adhesive and tissue (Figure 1). Recently, we have presented detailed reviews of the fundamental aspects of bioadhesion[1,17] with special emphasis on the mechanisms involved during the development of these bonds. Thus here we will present only a brief review of this subject, and we will concentrate predominantly on new theories.

As discussed by Marriott and Gregory in Chapter 1 of this book, mucus is a highly viscous product, which coats the lining of hollow organs in contact with external media.[18,19] The main components of the mucous layer are glycoproteins or mucins, inorganic salts, proteins, lipids, and mucopolysaccharides, and its composition varies depending on its source. The mucin composition also depends on the pathological conditions. It was found that mucins secreted by abnormal tissues are histochemically different from the corresponding mucins produced by the normal tissues of these tumors.[20] This is important for targeting of controlled release systems to cancerous tissues.

From a mechanistic point of view, the *glycoprotein fraction* is responsible for its gel-like characteristics. Mucous glycoproteins consist of a protein core with carbohydrate side chains covalently attached. Submaxillary gland glycoproteins consist of approximately 20% protein and 80% sugar,[21] with an average molecular weight of 2×10^6. About 25% of the polypeptide backbone is bare, whereas the remaining is densely glycosylated,[22] and the conformation of these regions is quite different.

Branched oligosaccharides are attached to the peptide backbone predominantly by *O*-glycosidic linkages via the serine and threonine amino acid components.[20] The number of sugar residues at each side chain varies from 2 to 20 with an average value of 8.[23,24] Each

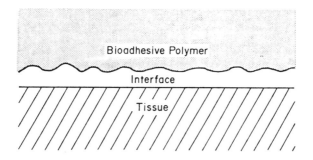

FIGURE 1. Basic geometry of a bioadhesive controlled release system in contact with a soft tissue. (From Peppas, N. A. and Buri, P. A., *J. Controlled Release,* 2, 257, 1985. With permission.)

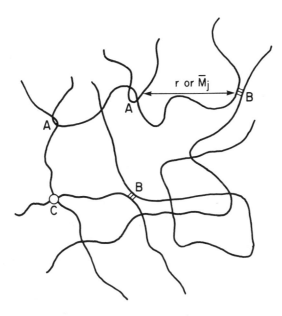

FIGURE 2. Representation of the cross-linked structure of the intestinal mucus network. Possible junctions include entanglements (A), molecular associations (B), and permanent cross-links (C). An average end-to-end distance between two junctions, r, corresponds to a molecular weight, $\bar{M}_j$. (From Peppas, N. A. and Buri, P. A., *J. Controlled Release,* 2, 257, 1985. With permission.)

carbohydrate chain terminates either in a sialic acid group, having a value of pK_a equal[25] to 2.6, or in a L-fucose group. Therefore, the mucin molecule behaves essentially as an anionic polyelectrolyte for pH larger than 2.6. The mucous gel is held together by either primary (disulfide bonds) or secondary bonds (electrostatic and hydrophobic interactions).

Figure 2 presents a simplified view of the glycoproteinic macromolecular structure of mucus.[26] Park et al.[15] have offered other possible simplified structures of the mucus network.

B. CHEMICAL AND PHYSICAL INTERACTIONS

Adhesion of polymers to tissues may be achieved by (1) primary ionic or covalent chemical bonds, (2) secondary chemical bonds, or (3) physical or mechanical bonds.[27-31]

Primary chemical bonds are the result of chemical reaction of functional groups of the adhesive material with the substrate.[32] They are hardly desirable for most soft tissue uses where a semipermanent adhesive bond strength is needed lasting from a few minutes to a few hours. These bonds will not be further discussed.

Secondary chemical bonds contribute to bioadhesive bonds through van der Waals dispersive interactions or hydrogen bonding. The van der Waals forces can be classified as: (1) Debye forces due to permanent dipole-induced dipole interactions, (2) Keesom forces due to permanent dipole-permanent dipole interactions, and (3) London forces due to induced dipole-induced dipole interactions. Hydrogen bonds are also important in bioadhesion as in other form of adhesion. Hydrophilic functional groups forming hydrogen bonds are hydroxylic groups (–OH), carboxyl groups (–COOH), sulfate groups (–SO$_4$H), amino groups (–NH$_2$), and others.[8,33]

Physical or mechanical bonds are obtained by inclusion of the adhesive material in the crevices of the tissue. Thus the surface roughness of the substrate becomes an important factor in bioadhesion.[32] Only highly fluid materials or suspensions that can be incorporated within these anomalies of the tissue can be considered successful adhesive systems. Therefore, the viscosity of liquid bioadhesive controlled release formulations is important in the development of satisfactory bioadhesive stability.[34]

III. THEORIES OF BIOADHESION

The theoretical framework for polymer-polymer adhesion can be easily extended to describe the bioadhesion of polymeric materials with biological surfaces. Pertinent theories include the electronic, the adsorption, the wetting, the diffusion, and the fracture theory.

A. ELECTRONIC THEORY

The electronic theory proposed by Derjaguin and Smilga[35] indicates that there is likely to be electron transfer on contact of the bioadhesive polymer and the glycoproteinic network, which have different electronic structures, which will in turn lead to the formation of a double layer of electrical charge at the bioadhesive interface. The electrostatic and molecular components of bioadhesion have been discussed recently by Derjaguin et al.[36]

B. ADSORPTION THEORY

According to the adsorption theory, bioadhesive systems adhere to tissue because of van der Waals, hydrogen bonding, and related forces.[37,38] The adsorption theory has been set forth over a period of many years by numerous investigators, and it is best analyzed in the works of Kinloch[32] and Huntsberger.[30]

C. WETTING THEORY

Intimate molecular contact is a prerequisite for development of strong adhesive bond, requiring examination of the wetting equilibrium and dynamic behavior of the bioadhesive-candidate material with the mucus.[10,39,40] Some important characteristics for liquid bioadhesive materials (the Sharpe-Schonhorn criteria) include (1) a zero or near zero contact angle, (2) a relatively low viscosity, and (3) an intimate contact that excludes air entrapment.

The specific work of adhesion, W_{bt}, between a bioadhesive controlled release system (subscript b) and the tissue (subscript t) is equal to the sum of the two surface tensions, γ_b and γ_t, less the interfacial tension, γ_{bt}, according to the Dupré equation.

$$W_{bt} = \gamma_b + \gamma_t - \gamma_{bt} \qquad (1)$$

Therefore, the interfacial energetics are responsible for the contact of the two surfaces and for the adhesive strength.[41]

It is, therefore, possible to express the adhesive behavior under static conditions in terms

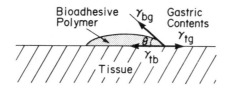

FIGURE 3. A liquid bioadhesive formulation spreading over a soft tissue section. (From Peppas, N. A. and Buri, P. A., *J. Controlled Release*, 2, 257, 1985. With permission.)

of the spreading coefficient, $S_{b/g}$, of a liquid or gel bioadhesive formulation with the tissue substrate in a physiological environment (subscript g), which is given by Equation 2 (Figure 3).

$$S_{b/g} = \gamma_{gt} - \gamma_{bt} - \gamma_{bg} \tag{2}$$

For a bioadhesive material to displace the physiological milieu and adhere spontaneously on the tissue, the spreading coefficient must be positive.

Characterization of the interfacial tension of tissue and gastric fluid, γ_{tg}, could be done *in vitro* or *in situ* using excised sections of tissue from animals and applying the classical Zisman analysis.[42,43] Good and Girifalco[44] offered a relationship that can be applied to bioadhesive systems to calculate the interfacial tension, γ_{bt}.

$$\gamma_{bt} = \gamma_b + \gamma_t - 2\Phi(\gamma_b\gamma_t)^{1/2} \tag{3}$$

The value of the parameter Φ is available in previous publications.[45,46]

It is well known that the interfacial tension γ may be expressed in terms of its dispersion (subscript d) and polar (subscript p) components:[47]

$$\gamma = \gamma^d + \gamma^p \tag{4}$$

Thus the interfacial tensions γ_{bt}, γ_{bg}, and γ_{gt} can be written as follows.[48,49]

$$\gamma_{bt} = [(\gamma_b^d)^{1/2} - (\gamma_t^d)^{1/2}]^2 + [(\gamma_b^p)^{1/2} - (\gamma_t^p)^{1/2}]^2 \tag{5}$$

$$\gamma_{bg} = [(\gamma_b^d)^{1/2} - (\gamma_g^d)^{1/2}]^2 + [(\gamma_b^p)^{1/2} - (\gamma_g^p)^{1/2}]^2 \tag{6}$$

$$\gamma_{gt} = [(\gamma_g^d)^{1/2} - (\gamma_t^d)^{1/2}]^2 + [(\gamma_g^p)^{1/2} - (\gamma_t^p)^{1/2}]^2 \tag{7}$$

The interfacial properties of two immiscible polymers were studied by Helfand and Tagami[50-52] using a mean field theory. They predicted that the interfacial tension scales to $\chi^{1/2}$, where χ is the polymer-polymer Flory interaction parameter.

$$\gamma_{bt} \sim \chi^{1/2} \tag{8}$$

Thus low values of the χ-factor, corresponding to structural similarities of the bioadhesive polymer and the mucous glycoproteins, result in high values of the work of adhesion. Helfand and Tagami have also concluded that in the absence of any solvent the interfacial properties are independent of the polymer molecular weight, the chain ends are more concentrated at the interface, and a solute molecule being adsorbed at the interface enhances the interpenetration of polymer chains. These conclusions are reexamined in Section IV of this chapter in view of our novel scaling law concepts.

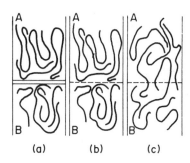

FIGURE 4.   Molecular model of chain interpenetration during bioadhesion of a polymer (A) with the mucus (B). (From Peppas, N. A. and Buri, P. A., *J. Controlled Release*, 2, 257, 1985. With permission.)

D. DIFFUSION THEORY

Interpenetration of the chains of polymer and mucus may lead to formation of a sufficiently deep layer of chains. This diffusion mechanism was first discussed by Voyutskii[53] for the intimate contact of two polymers (adhesion) or two pieces of the same polymer (autohesion). Recent work by Prager and Tirrell,[54] de Gennes,[55,56] and Mikos and Peppas[57] has advanced our understanding of this interpenetration process.

During chain interpenetration (Figure 4), the molecules of the polymer and the dangling chains of the glycoproteinic network are brought in intimate contact. Due to the concentration gradient, the bioadhesive polymer chains penetrate at rates that are dependent on the diffusion coefficient of a macromolecule through a cross-linked network and the chemical potential gradient. Typical values of the polymer diffusion coefficient through the glycoproteinic network of the mucus may be in the range of 10^{-10} to 10^{-16} cm²/s as discussed by Reinhart and Peppas,[58] Peppas and Lustig,[59] Gilmore et al.,[60] and Tirrell.[61] Effectively, one visualizes the transport of long polymer chains across the bioadhesive interface by regular diffusion or by reptation into a loosely cross-linked network of glycoproteins.[62,63]

In addition to topological characteristics, good solubility of the bioadhesive medium in the mucus[32] is required in order to achieve bioadhesion. Thus the difference of the solubility parameters of the bioadhesive medium and the glycoprotein should be as close to zero as possible. Thus the bioadhesive medium must be of similar chemical structure to the glycoproteins.

E. FRACTURE THEORY

The fracture theory of bioadhesion relates the difficulty of separation of two surfaces after adhesion to the adhesive bond strength. We have recently offered a new way of analyzing this phenomenon. In the work of Ponchel et al.,[64-66] we have used a mechanical (tensile) approach and a fracture model to express the fracture energy as a function of structural characteristics of the polymer and the glycoproteins. In our work,[57] we have developed a stochastic model to investigate the effect of chain entanglements on the polymer fracture properties. Theoretical predictions of the variation of the fracture energy and strength with the polymer molecular weight were in good agreement with experimental measurements.

The tensile fracture strength, σ_F, which is equivalent to the bioadhesive bond strength may be calculated by Equation 9, where E is the Young modulus of elasticity, G_F is the fracture energy, and L is the critical crack length upon separation of the two surfaces.

$$\sigma_F = \left(\frac{2EG_F}{\pi L}\right)^{1/2} \tag{9}$$

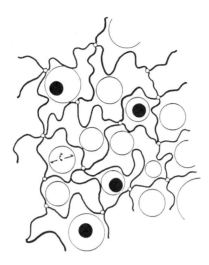

FIGURE 5.   The effective area for diffusion (open circle) of a solute
(dark circle) through a polymer gel is characterized by an average mesh
size, ξ.

Thus the stiffness of the material (i.e., elastic modulus) can be used as a measure of
bioadhesion.

Further analysis of these theories can be found in standard references by Peppas and
Buri,[1] Mikos and Peppas,[17] Duchêne et al.,[67] and Robinson and collaborators.[2] In the
remaining portion of this chapter, we will introduce novel models and theoretical predictions
of the bioadhesive process.

IV. SCALING CONCEPTS AND NEW DIFFUSION MODELS FOR BIOADHESION

A. SCALING CONCEPTS IN BIOADHESION

Scaling analysis is a relatively novel approach of representation of polymer phenomena,[68]
where the functional dependence of a set of parameters on a given quantity is given in the
form of one or more proportionalities without particular concern for the numerical coefficients. Only certain constants of proportionality may be material dependent. Among many
other applications, scaling concepts have been used to understand the relationships between
structure and diffusive transport through polymers.

Phenomena involving gels can be represented in scaling concepts by the general picture
of Figure 5. An average correlation length or mesh size characterizes the network and the
effective space available for diffusion, and it can be measured by neutron or quasi-elastic
light scattering. The *blob* models as proposed by de Gennes can be used to quantify the
degree of swelling of a polymer. Inside one blob or *sphere of influence*, the chain does not
interact with other chains.

The formation of a bioadhesive bond between a polymer and a mucin gel can be studied
using scaling concepts of polymer diffusion and relaxation. The mucin gel can be simulated
with a polymer gel, according to the models of de Gennes.[68]

The interpenetration of macromolecules at the interface results in the formation of *bridges*
between the two biomaterials. The interpenetration mechanism calls for the diffusion of few
free polymer chains trapped in the polymer network and also the relaxation of chain ends
of the polymeric network. Thus, for the bioadhesion of gels, the existence of gel defects in
their structure is necessary for the formation of an adhesive bond.

Adhesion or healing of two gels can be described in terms of the fracture energy at contact time t, $G_F(t)$, which scales to (is proportional to) the number of effective polymer chain crossings, $N_{eff}(t)$, per unit area; a polymer chain crossing is considered effective if the chain crosses the interface and is entangled about it.[57]

$$G_F(t) \sim N_{eff}(t) \tag{10}$$

The value of N_{eff} is calculated here as a function of the polymer structural characteristics. We have recently completed a detailed analysis of bioadhesion using scaling concepts.[69]

In our analysis, it is assumed that the two polymers in contact have exactly the same structural characteristics. If two different compatible polymers are in contact — which is the case in bioadhesion of biomaterials on mucin gels — the fracture energy will be the sum of the additive contributions due to the interpenetration of the macromolecular chains from both polymers.

A polymer chain of degree of polymerization N much larger than the degree of polymerization between entanglements, N_e, is now considered. The chain is confined in a tube that is formed by the topological constraints of neighboring polymer chains. The tube diameter is equal to the mesh size between entanglements, ξ, and the tube length, $L_t(N)$, is

$$L_t(N) = \left(\frac{N}{g_t}\right)\xi_t \tag{11}$$

where g_t is the number of monomers between entanglements.

The diffusion of a polymer chain results in the destruction of part of the original tube and the formation of a new tube of equal length, $L_t(n)$, being

$$L_t(n) = \left(\frac{n}{g_t}\right)\xi_t \tag{12}$$

that confines a chain segment of degree of polymerization n as shown in Figure 6. The length of the new tube at time t is

$$L_t(n) = (2D_t t)^{1/2} \tag{13}$$

where D_t is the tube diffusion coefficient expressed as[68]

$$D_t = D_b\left(\frac{g_b}{N}\right) \tag{14}$$

Here D_b is the blob diffusion coefficient and g_b is the number of monomers per blob. From Equations 13 and 14 we derive that

$$L_t(n) \cong g_b^{1/2}D_b^{1/2}N^{-1/2}t^{1/2} \tag{15}$$

Also, the volume of the new tube is

$$V_t(n) \cong L_t(n)\xi_t^2 \tag{16}$$

When two polymeric materials are brought in contact, the macromolecular chains start penetrating across the interface. The interpenetration thickness d is calculated as

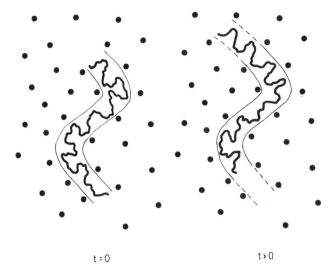

t = 0   t > 0

FIGURE 6.   A polymer chain diffuses along its tube, which is formed by the topological constraints (●) imposed by adjacent polymer chains. The motion of the chain results in the destruction of a portion of the original tube and the formation of a new one of equal length.

$$d \cong \xi_t \left(\frac{n}{g_t}\right)^{1/2} \cong g_b^{1/4}\xi_t^{1/2}D_b^{1/4}N^{-1/4}t^{1/4} \tag{17}$$

The total number of tubes, $N_{tot}(t)$, that cross a unit interface at time t is obtained as

$$N_{tot}(t) \cong \phi_e d \tag{18}$$

The parameter ϕ_e is the volume fraction of tube ends, which is related to the polymer volume fractions, v_2, and the degree of polymerization of the polymer chains, N, as follows:

$$\phi_e = \frac{v_2\phi_f}{N} \tag{19}$$

Here ϕ_f is the volume fraction of free chains trapped inside a polymer network on a dry basis. For uncross-linked polymers, the value of ϕ_f is one. The volume fraction, ϕ_t, of the tubes that cross the interface is expressed in terms of $N_{tot}(t)$ by

$$\phi_t \cong \frac{N_{tot}(t)V_t(n)}{d} \tag{20}$$

The surface tube crossing density scales to ϕ_t. Therefore, the number of tube crossings per unit interface — which is equal to N_{eff} — at time t is obtained as

$$N_{eff}(t) \cong \frac{\phi_t}{\xi_t^2} \tag{21}$$

The number of tube crossings, $v(t)$, of a tube that passes through the interface is calculated as the ratio of N_{eff} over N_{tot}.

$$\nu(t) = \frac{N_{eff}(t)}{N_{tot}(t)} \cong \left(\frac{n}{g_t}\right)^{1/2} \tag{22}$$

Combining the previous equations, the following scaling law is derived for the number of effective chain crossings:

$$N_{eff}(t) \cong \upsilon_2 \phi_f g_b^{1/2} D_b^{1/2} N^{-3/2} t^{1/2} \tag{23}$$

The time required for a polymer chain to diffuse along its tube, designated as τ_r, is called the terminal relaxation time and is defined in Equation 24.

$$\tau_r = \frac{L_t^2(N)}{2D_t} \tag{24}$$

Using Equations 11 and 14, Equation 24 is modified to yield:

$$\tau_r \cong g_b^{-1} g_t^{-2} D_b^{-1} N^3 \tag{25}$$

At a contact time, τ_r, the polymer chains have escaped from their original tubes and the number of tubes crossing the interface obtains its maximum equilibrium value.

$$N_{eff}(\tau_r) \cong \upsilon_2 \phi_f g_t^{-1} \xi_t \tag{26}$$

The parameter $N_{eff}(t)$ can be also written as a function of $N_{eff}(\tau_r)$ as follows:

$$\frac{N_{eff}(t)}{N_{eff}(\tau_r)} = \left(\frac{t}{\tau_r}\right)^{1/2} \qquad (t \leq \tau_r) \tag{27}$$

The value of the parameters D_b, g_b, g_t, and ξ for swollen gels depends on the solvent quality. To apply this analysis to bioadhesion, we treat first those cases of potentially bioadhesive polymers that are swollen in a poor solvent (Section B), and then we discuss the case of swollen bioadhesive gels by good solvents (Section C). For polymer gels in contact with biological fluids, the solvent is a very dilute aqueous electrolytic solution.

B. ADHESION (HEALING) OF TWO POORLY SWOLLEN HYDROGELS
In a poorly swollen hydrogel, the blob is the same as the monomer repeating unit. Therefore, the number of monomers per blob is one.

$$g_b = 1 \tag{28}$$

The blob diffusion coefficient scales to the absolute temperature,[68] T.

$$D_b \cong T \tag{29}$$

The number of monomers between entanglements is constant equal to N_e.

$$g_t = N_e \tag{30}$$

The mesh size between entanglements is related to the degree of polymerization between entanglements, N_e, and the polymer volume fraction, υ_2, as follows:

$$\xi_t = bN_e^{1/2}v_2^{-1/3} \tag{31}$$

Here b is the statistical chain length.

In the detailed analysis,[69] we have also developed expressions for the interpenetration length, the terminal relaxation time, and the equilibrium number of effective chain crossings from the values of the aforementioned parameters.

C. ADHESION (HEALING) OF TWO SWOLLEN HYDROGELS

The degree of swelling of a hydrogel determines the configuration of a linear polymer chain trapped in the polymer network. Partial disentanglement or even dissolution of the polymer chain may occur depending on the relative magnitude of the degree of polymerization between cross-links, N_c, compared to the values of the parameters N and N_e. For values of N_c larger than N_e, partial disentanglement is possible to occur. Furthermore, if N_c is larger than N, a linear polymer chain might be dissolved in the solvent forming one blob. In that case, linear polymer chains cannot bridge the two polymers in contact.

The polymer volume fractions corresponding to the onset of disentanglements and chain dissolution, designated as v_2^+ and v_2^*, respectively, can be calculated from the scaling theory of de Gennes,[68]

$$v_2^+ \cong (1 - 2\chi)^{-3/5}N_e^{-4/5} \tag{32}$$

$$v_2^* \cong (1 - 2\chi)^{-3/5}N^{-4/5} \tag{33}$$

Here χ is the polymer-solvent interaction parameter. Obviously, v_2^* is much smaller than v_2^+. Nevertheless, the occurence of partial disentanglement or even dissolution of the linear polymer chains depends on the value of the minimum polymer volume fraction, $v_{2,min}$, which corresponds to equilibrium swelling of the hydrogel.

$$v_{2,min} \cong (1 - 2\chi)^{-3/5}N_c^{-4/5} \tag{34}$$

In the following analysis, both cases of $v_2^+ \leq v_2 < 1$ and $v_2 \leq v_2 \leq v_2^+$ will be examined.

The number of monomers per blob and the blob mesh size obey the following scaling laws:[68]

$$g_b \cong v_2^{-5/4}(1 - 2\chi)^{-3/4} \tag{35}$$

$$v_b \cong bv_2^{-3/4}(1 - 2\chi)^{-1/4} \tag{36}$$

The number of monomers between entanglements depends on the value of the polymer volume fraction and is derived as

$$g_t = \begin{cases} N_e & (v_2^+ \leq v_2 < 1) \\ \\ g_b & (v_2^* \leq v_2 \leq v_2^+) \end{cases} \tag{37}$$

The mesh size between entanglements is also obtained as

$$\xi_t = \begin{cases} \xi_b \left(\dfrac{g_t}{g_b} \right)^{1/2} & (v_2^+ \leqslant v_2 < 1) \\\\ \xi_b & (v_2^* \leqslant v_2 \leqslant v_2^+) \end{cases} \tag{38}$$

The blob diffusion coefficient is a function of the blob mesh size[68]

$$D_b \cong \frac{T}{\eta_s \xi_b} \tag{39}$$

with η_s being the solvent viscosity.

Again, the various fracture properties can now be calculated as a function of the various structural parameters as described in our recent work.[69]

D. FRACTURE CRITERIA

The fracture energy, as previously discussed, scales to the number of polymer chain segments, which are entangled on either sides of the fracture plane. The proportionality constants involved in the power law of Equation 10 depend on the fracture mechanism. In brittle polymers, the polymer chain segments between entanglements are stretched upon deformation and eventually break.[57] Also, the degree of polymerization between entanglements does not change with deformation.

However, in rubbery polymers, as with swollen hydrogels, the polymer chains can relax and relieve the applied stress through partial disentanglement. Therefore, the fracture mechanism calls for the sliding of linear polymer chains, one next to each other, without chain rupture.

The necessary force, f_t, to pull out a chain from its tube with constant velocity, v, is proportional to this velocity.

$$f_t = \frac{v}{\mu_t} \tag{40}$$

The velocity v is equal to the applied deformation rate. The parameter μ_t is the tube mobility and can be expressed in terms of the tube diffusion coefficient by an Einstein relationship.[68]

$$\mu_t = \frac{D_t}{T} \tag{41}$$

Then Equation 40 is modified as follows:

$$f_t(N) = \frac{vTN}{g_b D_b} \tag{42}$$

The work, G_{t_p}, required to *pull out* a polymer chain of degree of polymerization n from its tube of length $L_t(n)$ — which is the same as the work required to remove a tube from the chain — is derived as

$$G_{t_p}(t) = f_t(n) L_t(n) \tag{43}$$

From the definition of the force, $f_t(n)$, and the tube length, $L_t(n)$, we also obtain that

$$G_{t_p}(t) \cong v g_t \xi_t^{-1} T N^{-1} t \qquad (t \leqslant \tau_r) \tag{44}$$

Consequently, the fracture energy at contact time t, which corresponds to chain pullout at the fracture plane is calculated as

$$G_{F_p}(t) = N_{tot}(t)G_{t_p}(t) \cong \nu\upsilon_2\phi_f g_b^{1/4} g_t \xi_t^{-1/2} D_b^{1/4} TN^{-9/4} t^{5/4} \quad (t \leq \tau_r) \tag{45}$$

Thus the fracture energy at contact time t is related to the corresponding value at time τ_r through Equation 46.

$$\frac{G_{F_p}(t)}{G_{F_p}(\tau_r)} = \left(\frac{t}{\tau_r}\right)^{5/4} \quad (t \leq \tau_r) \tag{46}$$

The equilibrium fracture energy $G_{F_p}(\tau_r)$ is derived as

$$G_{F_p}(\tau_r) \cong \nu\upsilon_2\phi_f g_b^{-1} g_t^{-3/2} \xi_t^2 D_b^{-1} TN^{3/2} \tag{47}$$

From Equation 47, it is concluded that for high deformation rates and/or high molecular weight polymers the fracture energy goes to infinity. Nevertheless, this is not realistic, and it is expected that for such high values of the ν and/or N the polymer chains crossing the fracture plane break at fracture rather than slide next to each other. In that case, the fracture criterion becomes chain scission instead of chain pullout.

The energy, G_{t_r}, required to *rupture* a macromolecular bridge crossing the fracture plane is proportional to the number of monomers per bridge.[57]

$$G_{t_r} \cong g_t \tag{48}$$

Then the fracture energy at contact time t is given by

$$G_{F_r} = N_{eff}(t)G_{t_r} \cong \upsilon_2\phi_f g_b^{1/2} g_t D_b^{1/2} N^{-3/2} t^{1/2} \quad (t \leq \tau_r) \tag{49}$$

Alternatively, the value of $G_{F_r}(t)$ is expressed in terms of $G_{F_r}(\tau_r)$ as

$$\frac{G_{F_r}(t)}{G_{F_r}(\tau_r)} = \left(\frac{t}{\tau_r}\right)^{1/2} \quad (t \leq \tau_r) \tag{50}$$

The equilibrium value of the fracture energy at contact time equal to the terminal relaxation time is given by

$$G_{F_r}(\tau_r) \cong \upsilon_2\phi_f \xi_t \tag{51}$$

V. UTILITY OF NEW SCALING LAWS: EFFECT OF STRUCTURAL CHARACTERISTICS ON BIOADHESION AND DESIGN OF NOVEL BIOADHESIVE SYSTEMS

A. CONCENTRATION OF BIOADHESIVE MATERIAL

In most soft tissue applications of bioadhesion, the bioadhesive material is dispersed in a polymer matrix. The variation of the adhesive bond strength with the concentration of the polymeric material responsible for bioadhesion is very important in controlled drug release technology. Our theory predicts that the equilibrium fracture energy, $G_F(\tau_r)$, which is a

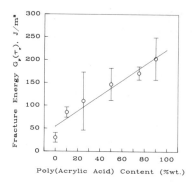

FIGURE 7.   Variation of the equilibrium fracture energy, $G_F(\tau_r)$, between drug-free poly(acrylic acid)-hydroxypropyl methylcellulose tablets and bovine sublingual mucus at 26°C with the dry poly(acrylic acid) content, for systems with water-preswollen surface.

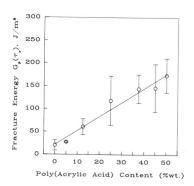

FIGURE 8.   Variation of the equilibrium fraction energy, $G_F(\tau_r)$, between metronidazole-containing poly(acrylic acid)-hydroxypropyl methylcellulose tablets and bovine sublingual mucus at 26°C with the dry poly(acrylic acid) content, for systems with water-preswollen surface. The amount of metronidazole was kept constant at 50 wt%.

measure of the adhesive bond strength, is proportional to the volume fraction, ϕ_f, of the bioactive adhesive compound on a dry basis. Recent experimental studies of Ponchel et al.[64,66] of bioadhesion of poly(acrylic acid) containing systems on bovine sublingual mucus indeed support this scaling law as shown in Figures 7 and 8.

B. EQUILIBRIUM POLYMER VOLUME FRACTION

Obviously the degree of swelling plays a very important role in bioadhesive phenomena. For poorly swollen hydrogels it is predicted that[69]

$$G_{F_r}(\tau_r) \sim \upsilon_2^{2/3} \tag{52}$$

For equilibrium swollen hydrogels, the value of the minimum polymer volume fraction determines the applicability of the pertinent scaling law.[69]

$$G_{F_r}(\tau_r) \sim \begin{cases} \upsilon_2^{7/8} & (\upsilon_2^+ \le \upsilon_2 < 1) \\ \\ \upsilon_2^{1/4} & (\upsilon_2^* \le \upsilon_2 \le \upsilon_2^+) \end{cases} \tag{53}$$

Despite the increased chain mobility for low values of the polymer volume fraction, the fracture energy decreases because the concentration of free chains responsible for bioadhesion also decreases. The following scaling law is derived for the tube diffusion coefficient.

$$D_t \sim \frac{g_b}{\xi_b} \sim \upsilon_2^{-1/2}(1 - 2\chi)^{-1/2} \qquad (54)$$

Consequently, highly cross-linked materials should be candidates for bioadhesion on gly-coproteinic networks. These conclusions agree with experimental findings of Chen and Cyr[70] that the adhesive properties of hydrocolloids for intraoral applications decrease drastically with excessive hydration.

C. HYDROGEL-WATER INTERACTION PARAMETER

The χ-factor is related to the thermodynamic interactions between the polymer and the solvent.[71] The lower the value of χ, the better the solvent. The threshold value of χ is one half, as larger values result in phase separation. For swollen hydrogels, it has been calculated[69] that the terminal relaxation time, which corresponds to the time necessary for the development of a maximum adhesive bond, decreases for values of χ close to one half.

$$\tau_r \sim \begin{cases} (1 - 2\chi)^{3/4} & (\upsilon_2^+ \leqslant \upsilon_2 < 1) \\ \\ (1 - 2\chi)^{3/2} & (\upsilon_2^* \leqslant \upsilon_2 \leqslant \upsilon_2^+) \end{cases} \qquad (55)$$

This is justified because the tube diffusion coefficient increases as the hydrogel-water quality decreases based on Equation 54. Thus hydrogels with χ-factors in the vicinity of one half will be biomaterials of choice for formation of fast adhesive bonds.

D. POLYMER MOLECULAR WEIGHT

The fracture energy is predicted from Equation 47 to scale to $N^{3/2}$ up to a critical chain length. Thereafter the fracture energy does not vary with the degree of polymerization as shown in Equation 51. This critical chain length, N_{cr}, is higher than N_e and can be estimated[69] by equating the values of G_{F_p} and G_{F_r}. Chen and Cyr[70] reported that the molecular weight of various hydrocolloids, such as potassium carrageenate, guar gum, and karaya, should exceed 100,000 and that their adhesive properties do not change for higher molecular weights. Smart et al.[72] also found that the molecular weight of sodium carboxymethyl cellulose, which is a potential bioadhesive material, does not affect bioadhesion for values higher than 78,600.

E. MOLECULAR WEIGHT BETWEEN ENTANGLEMENTS

The maximum value of the fracture energy, which corresponds to the scission of all effective chain segments crossing the fracture plane, has been found to scale to the mesh size between entanglements, ξ_t, according to Equation 51. This result is similar to that of the Lake and Thomas theory[73] for cross-linked polymers, i.e., the fracture energy scales to the mesh size between cross-links.

F. CONTACT TIME

The fracture energy at contact time t has been found to scale to either $t^{5/4}$ or $t^{1/2}$. For low deformation rates and degrees of polymerization, it is calculated that the fracture energy is proportional to $t^{5/4}$. For large deformation rates, which is required in good bioadhesives, the fracture energy is predicted to scale to the square root of the contact time. Jud et al.[74]

measured the fracture energy of brittle polymers as a function of time and reported that the work of fracture (or healing) indeed scales to $t^{1/2}$ in agreement with theoretical results of Prager and Tirrell[54] and de Gennes[55]. Finally, the results of the work of Ponchel et al.[64] with swollen hydrogels also agree with these scaling arguments.

VI. CONCLUSIONS

In this chapter, we have offered a thorough analysis of polymer-mucus bioadhesion in terms of recent molecular theories, some of which (Section IV) are presented for the first time. We conclude that various structural parameters of the polymer and the glycoproteinic network are important in the development of the bioadhesive bond. They include the equilibrium polymer volume fraction, v_2, the number of repeating units (monomers) between entanglements, N_e, the size of the chain, N, and the size of each link, b. In addition, the polymer solvent interaction parameter, χ, the concentration of the bioadhesive polymer, ϕ_f, the viscosity of the biological fluid, η_s, and the temperature, T, also play an important role. Finally, the adhesive force is developed according to the adhesion time, t.

ACKNOWLEDGMENTS

This work was supported by a National Science Foundation grant (No. CBT-86-17719) and by a David Ross Fellowship to A. G. M.

REFERENCES

1. **Peppas, N. A. and Buri, P. A.,** Surface, interfacial and molecular aspects of polymer bioadhesion on soft tissues, *J. Controller Release,* 2, 257, 1985.
2. **Park, K., Cooper, S. L., and Robinson, J. R.,** Bioadhesive hydrogels, in *Hydrogels in Medicine and Pharmacy,* Vol. 3, Peppas, N. A., Ed., CRC Press, Boca Raton, FL, 1987, 151.
3. **Manly, R. S., Ed.,** *Adhesion in Biological Systems,* Academic Press, New York, 1970.
4. **Mutimer, M., Riffkin, C., Hill, J., Glickman, M. E., and Cyr, G. N.,** Modern ointment base technology. II. Comparative evaluation of bases, *J. Am. Pharm. Assoc. Sci. Ed.,* 45, 212, 1956.
5. **Wright, P. S.,** Composition and properties of soft lining materials for acrylic dentures, *J. Dent.,* 9, 210, 1981.
6. **Ducheyne, P., van der Perre, G., and Aubert, A. E., Eds.,** *Biomaterials and Biomechanics 1983,* Elsevier, Amsterdam, 1984.
7. **Refojo, M. F., Dohlman, C. H., and Koliopoulos, J.,** Adhesives in ophthalmology, *Surv. Ophthalmol.,* 15, 217, 1971.
8. **Gross, L. and Hoffman, R.,** Medical and biological adhesives, in *Handbook of Adhesives,* 2nd ed., Skeist, I., Ed., Van Nostrand-Reinhold, New York, 1977, 818.
9. **Wang, P. Y.,** Surgical adhesives and coatings, in *Medical Engineering,* Ray, C. D., Ed., *Year Book Medical Publishers,* Chicago, 1974, 1123.
10. **Baier, R. E.,** Conditioning surfaces to suit the biomedical environment: recent progress, *J. Biomech. Eng.,* 104, 257, 1982.
11. **Banker, G. S.,** Pharmaceutical applications of controlled release, in *Medical Applications of Controlled Release,* Vol. 2, Langer, R. S. and Wise, D. L., Eds., CRC Press, Boca Raton, FL, 1984, 1.
12. **Gurny, R., Meyer, J. M., and Peppas, N. A.,** Bioadhesive intraoral release systems: design, testing and analysis, *Biomaterials,* 5, 336, 1984.
13. **Ishida, M., Nambu, N., and Nagai, T.,** Ointment-type oral mucosal dosage form of carbopol containing prednisolone for treatment of aphtha, *Chem. Pharm. Bull.,* 31, 1010, 1983.
14. **Banker, G. S.,** Bioadhesive and controlled retension systems for oral and rectal administration, in *Emploi des Polymères dans l'Elaboration de Nouvelles Formes Mèdicamenteuses,* Buri, P., Doelker, E., and Pasquier, P., Eds., University of Geneva, Geneva, 1980, 129.

15. **Park, K., Ch'ng, H. S., and Robinson, J. R.,** Alternative approaches to oral controlled drug delivery: bioadhesives and in situ systems, in *Recent Advances in Drug Delivery Systems,* Anderson, J. M. and Kim, S. W., Eds., Plenum Press, New York, 1984, 163.

16. **Peppas, N. A., Teillaud, E., and Nelson, L.,** Controlled release microparticle systems for urinary tract applications, *Proc. Int. Symp. Controlled Release Bioact. Mater.,* 11, 63, 1984.

17. **Mikos, A. G. and Peppas, N. A.,** Systems for controlled release of drugs. V. Bioadhesive systems, *S. T. P. Pharma,* 2, 705, 1986.

18. **Jeffery, P. K. and Reid, L. M.,** The respiratory mucus membrane, in *Respiratory Defense Mechanisms,* Vol. 5, Brain, J. D., Proctor, D. F., and Reid, L. M., Eds., Marcel Dekker, New York, 1977, 193.

19. **Phalen, R. B.,** *Inhalation Studies: Foundations and Techniques,* CRC Press, Boca Raton, FL, 1984.

20. **Horowitz, M. I.,** Gastrointestinal glycoproteins, in *The Glycoconjugates,* Vol. 1, Horowitz, M. I. and Pigman, W., Eds., Academic Press, New York, 1977, 189.

21. **Bloomfield, V. A.,** Hydrodynamic properties of mucous glycoproteins, *Biopolymers,* 22, 2141, 1983.

22. **Scawen, M. and Allen, A.,** The action of proteolytic enzymes on the glycoprotein from pig gastric mucus, *Biochem. J.,* 163, 363, 1977.

23. **Boat, T. F. and Cheng, P. W.,** Biochemistry of airway mucus secretions, *Fed. Proc.,* 39, 3067, 1980.

24. **Roussel, P., Lamblin, G., Degand, P., Walker-Nasir, E., and Jeanloz, R. W.,** Heterogeneity of the carbohydrate chains of sulfated bronchial glycoproteins isolated from a patient suffering from cystic fibrosis, *J. Biol. Chem.,* 250, 2114, 1975.

25. **Johnson, P. M. and Rainsford, K. D.,** The physical properties of mucus: preliminary observations on the sedimentation behaviour of porcine gastric mucus, *Biochim. Biophys. Acta,* 286, 72, 1972.

26. **Peppas, N. A., Hansen, P. J., and Buri, P. A.,** A theory of molecular diffusion in the intestinal mucus, *Int. J. Pharm.,* 20, 107, 1984.

27. **Feijen, J., Beugeling, T., Bantjes, A., and Smit-Sibinga, C. T.,** Biomaterials and interfacial phenomena, *Adv. Cardiovasc. Phys.,* 3, 100, 1979.

28. **Hench, L. L. and Ethridge, E. C.,** *Biomaterials: An Interfacial Approach,* Academic Press, New York, 1982.

29. **Huntsberger, J. R.,** Mechanism of adhesion, in *Treatise on Adhesion and Adhesives,* Vol. 1, Patrick, R. L., Ed., Marcel Dekker, New York, 1967, 120.

30. **Huntsberger, J. R.,** Mechanisms of adhesion, *J. Paint Technol.,* 39, 199, 1967.

31. **Huntsberger, J. R.,** Surface energy, wetting and adhesion, *J. Adhes.,* 12, 3, 1981.

32. **Kinloch, A. J.,** The science of adhesion. I. Surface and interfacial aspects, *J. Mater. Sci.,* 15, 2141, 1980.

33. **Pritchard, W. H.,** The role of hydrogen bonding in adhesion, *Aspects Adhes.,* 6, 11, 1971.

34. **Davis, S. S. and Khanderia, M. S.,** Rheological characterization of plastibases and the effect of formulation variables on the consistency of these vehicles, *Int. J. Pharm. Tech. Prod. Manuf.,* 1, 11, 1980.

35. **Derjaguin, B. V. and Smilga, V. P.,** *Adhesion: Fundamentals and Practise,* McLaren, London, 1969.

36. **Derjaguin, B. V., Toporov, Y. P., Mueler, V. M., and Aleinikova, I. N.,** On the relationship between the electrostatic and the molecular component of the adhesion of elastic particles to a solid surface, *J. Colloid Interface Sci.,* 58, 528, 1977.

37. **Good, R. J.,** Surface free energy of solids and liquids: thermodynamics, molecular forces and structure, *J. Colloid Interface Sci.,* 59, 398, 1977.

38. **Tabor, D.,** Surface forces and surface interactions, *J. Colloid Interface Sci.,* 58, 2, 1977.

39. **Frisch, E. E.,** The interface of implants with tissue, *Org. Coat. Appl. Polym. Sci. Proc.,* 48, 374, 1983.

40. **Wang, P. Y. and Bazos, M. J.,** Polymer surface interactions in the biological environment, in *Physico-chemical Aspects of Polymer Surfaces,* Mittal, K. L, Ed., Plenum Press, New York, 1983, 943.

41. **Kammer, H. W.,** Adhesion between polymers, *Acta Polym.,* 34, 112, 1983.

42. **Fox, H. W. and Zisman, W. A.,** The spreading of liquids on low energy surfaces. I. Polytetrafluoro-ethylene, *J. Colloid Sci.,* 5, 514, 1950.

43. **Sharfrin, E. G. and Zisman, W. A.,** Constitutive relations in the wetting of low-energy surfaces and the theory of the retraction method of prepared monolayers, *J. Phys. Chem.,* 64, 519, 1960.

44. **Good, R. J. and Girifalco, L. A.,** A theory for estimation of surface and interfacial energies. III. Estimation of surface energies of solids from contact angle data, *J. Phys. Chem.,* 64, 561, 1960.

45. **Good, R. J.,** Spreading pressure and contact angle, *J. Colloid Interface Sci.,* 52, 308, 1975.

46. **Wu, S.,** Surface and interfacial tensions of polymer melts. II. PMMA, PBM and polystyrene, *J. Phys. Chem.,* 74, 632, 1970.

47. **Schultz, J., Tsutsumi, K., and Donnet, J. B.,** Surface properties of high energy solids, *J. Colloid Interface Sci.,* 59, 277, 1977.

48. **Kaelbe, D. H. and Uy, K. C.,** Reinterpretation of organic liquid-PTFE surface interactions, *J. Adhes.,* 2, 50, 1970.

49. **Owens, D. K. and Wendt, R. C.,** Estimation of the surface free energy of polymers, *J. Appl. Polym. Sci.,* 13, 1740, 1969.

50. **Helfand, E. and Tagami, Y.**, Theory of the interface beween immiscible polymers, *Polymer Lett.*, 9, 741, 1971.
51. **Helfand, E. and Tagami, Y.**, Theory of the interface between immiscible polymers, *J. Chem. Phys.*, 56, 3592, 1972.
52. **Helfand, E. and Tagami, Y.**, Theory of the interface between immiscible polymers, *J. Chem. Phys.*, 57, 1812, 1972.
53. **Voyutskii, S. S.**, *Autohesion and Adhesion of High Polymers*, John Wiley & Sons, New York, 1963.
54. **Prager, S. and Tirrell, M.**, The healing process at polymer-polymer interfaces, *J. Chem. Phys.*, 75, 5194, 1981.
55. **de Gennes, P. G.**, Sur la soudure des polymères amorphes, *C. R. Acad. Sci. Paris Sér. B*, 291, 219, 1980.
56. **de Gennes, P. G.**, Couples de polyméres compatibles: propriétes spéciales en diffusion et en adhésion, *C. R. Acad. Sci. Paris Sér. II*, 292, 1505, 1981.
57. **Mikos, A. G. and Peppas, N. A.**, Polymer chain entanglements and brittle fracture, *J. Chem. Phys.*, 88, 1337, 1988.
58. **Reinhart, C. T. and Peppas, N. A.**, Solute diffusion in swollen membranes. II. Influence of crosslinking on diffusive properties, *J. Membr. Sci.*, 18, 227, 1984.
59. **Peppas, N. A. and Lustig, S. R.**, The role of crosslinks, entanglements and relaxations of the macromolecular carrier in the diffusional release of biologically active materials: conceptual and scaling relationships, *Ann. N.Y. Acad. Sci.*, 44, 26, 1985.
60. **Gilmore, P. T., Falabella, R., and Laurence, R. L.**, Polymer/polymer diffusion, *Macromolecules*, 13, 880, 1980.
61. **Tirrell, M.**, Polymer self-diffusion in entangled systems, *Rubber Chem. Technol.*, 57, 523, 1984.
62. **Lustig, S. R. and Peppas, N. A.**, Scaling concepts in controlled release, *Proc. Int. Symp. Control. Rel. Bioact. Mater.*, 11, 104, 1984.
63. **Morris, E. R. and Rees, D. A.**, Principles of biopolymer gelation: possible models for mucus gel structure, *Br. Med. Bull.*, 34, 49, 1978.
64. **Ponchel, G., Touchard, F., Duchêne, D., and Peppas, N. A.**, Bioadhesive analysis of controlled-release systems. I. Fracture and interpenetration analysis in poly(acrylic acid)-containing systems, *J. Controlled Release*, 5, 129, 1987.
65. **Peppas, N. A., Ponchel, G., and Duchêne, D.**, Bioadhesive analysis of controlled-release systems. II. Time-dependent bioadhesive stress in poly(acrylic acid)-containing systems, *J. Controlled Release*, 5, 143, 1987.
66. **Ponchel, G., Touchard, F., Wouessidjewe, D., Duchêne, D., and Peppas, N. A.**, Bioadhesive analysis of controlled-release systems. III. Bioadhesive and release behavior of metronidazole-containing poly(acrylic acid)-hydroxypropyl methylcellulose systems, *Int. J. Pharm.*, 38, 65, 1987.
67. **Duchêne, D., Touchard, F., and Peppas, N. A.**, Pharmaceutical and medical aspects of bioadhesive systems for drug administration. *Drug Dev. Ind. Pharm.*, 14, 283, 1988.
68. **de Gennes, P. G.**, *Scaling Concepts in Polymer Physics*, Cornell University Press, Ithaca, 1979.
69. **Mikos, A. G. and Peppas, N. A.**, Healing and fracture at the interface between two gels, *Europhys. Lett.*, 6, 403, 1988.
70. **Chen, J. L. and Cyr, G. N.**, Compositions producing adhesion through hydration, in *Adhesion in Biological Systems*, Manly, R. S., Ed., Academic Press, New York, 1970, 163.
71. **Flory, P. J.**, *Principles of Polymer Chemistry*, Cornell University Press, Ithaca, 1953.
72. **Smart, J. D., Kellaway, I. W., and Worthington, H. E. C.**, An in-vitro investigation of mucosa-adhesive materials for use in controlled drug delivery, *J. Pharm. Pharmacol.*, 36, 295, 1984.
73. **Lake, G. J. and Thomas, A. G.**, The strength of highly elastic materials, *Proc. R. Soc. London Ser. A*, 300, 108, 1967.
74. **Jud, K., Kausch, H. H., and Williams, J. G.**, Fracture mechanics studies of crack healing and welding of polymers, *J. Mater. Sci.*, 16, 204, 1981.

Chapter 3

TEST METHODS OF BIOADHESION

Kinam Park and Haesun Park

TABLE OF CONTENTS

I. INTRODUCTION

Adhesion is defined as the state in which two surfaces are held together by interfacial forces.[1] Adhesion is referred to as bioadhesion, if one or both of the adherends are of a biological nature. Thus a *bioadhesive* is defined as a substance that is capable of interacting with biological materials and being retained on them or holding them together for extended periods of time.[2] Bioadhesion can occur by virtue of electrostatic and dipolar interactions, hydrogen bonding, or by the adsorption and interpenetration of macromolecules.[3] According to the definition, adhesives derived from biological objects (biological adhesives[4]) are not necessarily bioadhesives, if they are applied to nonbiological adherends.

There are a variety of bioadhesion phenomena and bioadhesives that satisfy the above definitions. For convenience, bioadhesion and bioadhesive are classified into three types based on phenomenological observation, rather than on the mechanisms of bioadhesion.[2] Type I bioadhesion is characterized by adhesion occurring between biological objects without involvement of artificial materials. Cell fusion[5] and cell aggregation[6] are good examples of Type I bioadhesion. Type II bioadhesion refers to adhesion of biological materials to artificial substrates. Type II bioadhesion can be represented by cell adhesion onto culture dishes[7,8] or barnacle adhesion to a variety of substances including metals, woods, and other synthetic materials.[9] Finally, Type III bioadhesion described adhesion of artificial substances to biological substrates, such as adhesion of polymers to skin or other soft tissues. All three types of bioadhesion are equally important. We will focus, however, on Type III bioadhesion, which is in accordance with the objectives of this book.

Type III bioadhesives have been used for quite a long time under different names. Many chemical adhesives have been used, instead of or in addition to sutures, for joining and sealing of tissues under the names of tissue adhesives,[10,11] clinical adhesives, biological glue,[12] or medical polymer adhesives.[13] A number of synthetic and natural polymers have been used as skin adhesives,[14] dental adhesives,[15] and mucoadhesives.[16]

The goal of the development of bioadhesives is to duplicate, mimic, or improve biological adhesives, which are both durable where required and degradable where necessary, and nontoxic at all.[12] Developing a new bioadhesive and applying it for a particular use requires elucidation of the bioadhesion mechanisms. Understanding the bioadhesion mechanisms begins with evaluating bioadhesive performance of various candidate materials. Thus the evaluation of bioadhesive properties is fundamental for the development of new bioadhesives. This chapter describes currently known bioadhesion evaluation methods and parameters that are important to the testing and design of new bioadhesives.

II. EVALUATION OF BIOADHESIVE PROPERTIES

A. BIOADHESION EVALUATION METHODS

The first step in the selection of a bioadhesive for a particular application is to determine if its properties are suitable for the intended application. Testing is essential for the development, qualification, processing, and proper use of bioadhesives. Since there are a large number of bioadhesives in different physical forms and biological substrates of different nature, evaluation of bioadhesive properties is inherently complex and diverse. Bioadhesives, as well as nonbioadhesives, are usually tested as one component of a system of many parts. This means that a test of bioadhesives actually tests the properties of many components including the bioadhesive itself, the biological substrates, and other experimental conditions. Thus, evaluation and comparison of the properties of various bioadhesives can be obtained only if all the conditions of the test and the experimental procedures are kept constant. If the experiment is changed by varying a factor other than the bioadhesive, the test method can provide information about the contribution of the other component to the overall bioadhesive performance.[17]

It is not easy to extrapolate the behavior of a bioadhesive from a test to its performance in an actual *in vivo* application, since testing is generally made under a controlled environment that is far from the actual service condition. In addition, each test measures a particular aspect of bioadhesion and a particular property of a bioadhesive while the actual *in vivo* performance of a bioadhesive depends on various interdependent properties. It is extremely difficult to simulate the exact conditions that a bioadhesive may be subject to *in vivo*. Although it is expected that a certain test method will represent the actual *in vivo* performance of a bioadhesive better than others, it is not clear what parameter is most suitable for evaluating the *in vivo* bioadhesive performance. For this reason, various properties of a bioadhesive have to be measured, and the obtained parameters have to be compared with the actual *in vivo* performance of the bioadhesive.

B. STANDARD TEST METHODS

As described later in this chapter, a number of different test methods are used to measure the same property of a bioadhesive. There is a tendency for each investigator to use his or her own distinct test method. This is partly because there are no standard test methods specifically designed to measure a certain property of bioadhesives. The lack of standard test methods creates confusion among investigators, since data generated at different laboratories cannot be compared, and thus the real meaning of reported test values is not transferable. The standardization of test methods acceptable to everyone will improve the communication between researchers and allow them to speak a common language when comparing the test data and results.[18] Although there is a need for developing standard test methods designed for bioadhesives, fulfilling such a need will take time. Research on bioadhesives is still in its early stage, and more data will be necessary in order to have a consensus among investigators on standard test methods. Thus it appears that there is no alternative now other than trying various test methods to accumulate experimental data and improve our understanding of the bioadhesion phenomena. It is necessary, however, that investigators are aware of the need for establishing standard test methods.

C. QUANTIFICATION OF BIOADHESIVE PROPERTIES

The performance of a bioadhesive can be evaluated by various parameters, such as adhesion strength, adhesion number, or duration of adhesion. One is reminded that for measuring any given bioadhesive property, a small change in experimental variables, such as the initial loading pressure, the initial contact time, or the rate of removal of the adhesive, may result in significantly different values. Thus even the quantitative data may be considered to be subjective. In this regard, numerical values may have to be used on a comparative basis to establish adhesive properties measured by a certain specified procedure under specified conditions.

1. Adhesion Strength

Measuring mechanical properties of a bioadhesive may be the most direct way to quantify the bioadhesive performance. There are three basic types of stress that are most commonly used to measure the strength of adhesive joints. They are tensile, shear, and peel stress as shown in Figure 1. They are popular because they are relatively quick and simple to perform and enable poor candidates to be screened out.[19] In tensile loading, the forces are perpendicular to the plane of the joint. In shear loading, the stress is parallel to the plane of the joint. In both cases, the stress is distributed uniformly over the entire joint, and all of the adhesive is put to work at the same time.[20] In peel loading, the stress is limited to a very fine line at the edge of the joint.[20] Peel testing measures the ability to resist peeling forces, rather than mechanical properties of the adhesive.[17]

2. Adhesion Number

The measurement of adhesion strength using tensile, shear, or peel test will be very difficult, if a bioadhesive is in the form of small particles. In such a case, the adhesion number can be used to measure the adhesive properties. The adhesion number N_a is defined as the ratio between the number of particles N remaining after the application of a certain detachment force and the number of particles N_o originally present on the test surface.[21] The adhesion number is often expressed as a percentage.

$$N_a = (N/N_o)100 \tag{1}$$

The adhesive force can be evaluated from the adhesion number, since the detachment force is known, and it is numerically equal to but opposite in direction to the force of adhesion.[21] The use of an adhesion number, however, is good enough to evaluate and compare properties of various bioadhesive particles. Obviously, many variations of the adhesion number method can be used.

3. Durability

Probably the most important property of a bioadhesive is to maintain satisfactory performance in the actual service condition for a desired period of time. Thus the durability of a bioadhesive may be the ultimate parameter that should be used to compare various bioadhesives. Since the durability does not solely depend on the adhesive strength alone, other factors that affect it should be identified and examined. For structural adhesives, the durability of adhesive joints can be assessed by a number of methods, such as sustained load methods, the endurance limit method, cyclic stress testing, or fracture mechanics tests.[22] The durability of bioadhesives may be evaluated by changing experimental conditions for bioadhesive-tissue joints, such as changing pH, temperature, ionic strength, water content, etc. For example, Chen and Cyr[23] devised an apparatus that measured *in vitro* duration of adhesion of intraoral bandages (see Section III.A.1). The condition of the *in vitro* duration test was different in one significant respect from the actual condition in the oral cavity. Since the test system was completely submerged in water during *in vitro* testing, the excess water

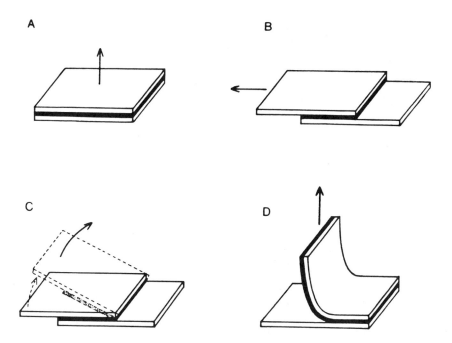

FIGURE 1. Testing of adhesive bonds by tensile (A), shear (B), and peel (C and D) tests. Peel tests with stiff detaching strip (C) are also known as cleavage tests[20] or bending tests.[23] Peel tests can be done at various peel angles. The white and black areas represent adherend and adhesive, respectively.

caused further and more rapid hydration of the hydrocolloid particles. As this additional water was absorbed, the adhesive bond was weakened due to the formation of a slippery mucilage. As a result, the *in vitro* test was considered to be an accelerated test for duration of adhesion in the actual service condition. The duration of adhesion for Orahesive® bandage ranged from 4 to 25 min in the *in vitro* tests, while the value ranged from 6 to 24 h under the actual clinical conditions.

III. *IN VIVO* AND *EX VIVO* EVALUATION OF BIOADHESION

This and the next two sections describe currently known *in vivo* and *in vitro* test methods. The test methods described here are neither the only test methods nor the standard test methods for particular bioadhesive-tissue systems. They can be modified for other applications. The test methods in this chapter are concerned only with Type III bioadhesion, i.e., adhesion of artificial substances to biological substrates such as gingiva, teeth, skin, or the gastrointestinal mucus layer.

A. QUALITATIVE EVALUATION
1. Intraoral Bandages

Chen and Cyr[23] designed a simple *in vivo* screening test for overall performance of intraoral bandages. Candidate hydrocolloid powders were mixed with polyisobutylene at a 6:4 ratio and pressed into disks about 1/16 in. thick. One side of the disk was covered with a thin polyethylene film of equal size. The exposed side was then pressed with a finger onto the anterior gingiva for 30 s. If the disk did not stick, pressure was continued for another 30 s. If a composition adhered to the gingiva under normal application pressure with the first 30 s and was difficult to dislodge, it was referred to as ''Excellent''. If a composition was easily dislodged, the performance was described as ''Satisfactory''. The composition designated as "Fair" required more pressure and/or time to adhere and was even more easily dislodged. If a sample required more than a few minutes to develop adhesiveness, it was referred to as "Poor".

From the above description, one can easily find a few uncertain experimental conditions. The applied pressure was not well characterized, and the dislodging procedure of the adhered disk was not clearly indicated. In the absence of specifications of such procedures, the test results tend to be subjective. Thus the comparison of data produced at different times in the same laboratory or in different laboratories may not be easy. In addition, the evaluation scale is not broad enough to accurately judge the bioadhesive property of the test samples. The advantage of this method, however, is that it measures the overall performance of bioadhesive-gingiva joints in the *in vivo* condition, which includes tongue action and disruptive contribution of saliva.[23]

2. Mucosal Adhesive Ointment

Bremecker et al.[24] formulated a nonirritating mucosal adhesive ointment based on poly(methyl methacrylate). The authors reported that the ointment was free of irritation and had good mucosal adhesion at pH 6.4 of the normal saliva. Although the ointment base was characterized by an excellent adhesion, test methods were not described.

B. QUANTITATIVE EVALUATION

1. Tensile Testing

a. Tissue Adhesives

Leonard et al.[25] measured tissue bond strengths of various cyanoacrylate esters using rats. Midline incisions 3 cm in length, extending into the subcutaneous tissues, were made over the lumbar region of the anesthetized rats and the incision sealed with two drops of various alkyl cyanoacrylate monomers. The edges were held in apposition for up to 2 min until polymerization occurred depending on the nature of the monomers. The adhered wounds were pulled apart 1 h following wound closure as shown in Figure 2, and the adhesive strength was measured using a table model Instron testing machine at a cross-head rate (pulling rate) of 0.5 in./min.

Margules and Harris[26] used tension tests to compare the adhesive property of medical grade cyanoacrylate and acrylic adhesives. Test buttons were made of polymethylmethacrylate in a cylinder of 6.35 mm length and 6.35 mm diameter with a hole in the middle for pin placement. The skin was shaved and prepared for adhesion with benzalkonium chloride swabbing followed by air drying. The buttons with adhesives were applied to both wet and dry skin. The wet skin was prepared by swabbing the entire shaved area with normal saline. Test buttons were pressed to both wet and dry skin for 30 s. A strain rate of 2 cm/s was applied for each tension test, and the maximum yield strength was measured using a manually operated Chatillion force gauge.

b. Denture Adhesives

Ow and Bearn[27] developed a method to evaluate denture adhesives under controlled conditions *in vivo*. The adhesiveness was measured using a custom made pressure-sensitive device. Orahesive® was used as a model denture adhesive.

2. Peel Testing

a. Intraoral Bandages

Chen and Cyr[23] used a Chatillon gauge to quantitatively measure the force required to separate the bandage from oral mucous membrane or from the teeth. The authors concluded that the *in vivo* peel adhesion tests agreed reasonably well with those obtained in the *in vitro* lap-shear tests (Figure 1B, Section IV.C.1), although the curvature of the gingiva was

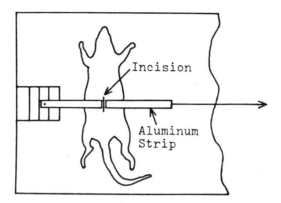

FIGURE 2. Test system for measuring wound strength. The aluminum strip was bonded to the skin surface of a rat using *n*-butyl α-cyanoacrylate. (From Leonard, F., Hodge, J. W., Jr., Houston, S., and Ousterhout, D. K., *J. Biomed. Mater. Res.*, 2, 173, 1968. With permission from John Wiley & Sons, Copyright © 1968.)

variable, manually applied pressure was not controllable, and the rate of pulling was also uncontrollable. The good agreement between results of *in vivo* and *in vitro* tests should be taken with caution, since the *in vitro* tests employed cellophane membranes instead of excised tissues. The issue of using artificial substrates in the evaluation of bioadhesives is briefly discussed in Section IV.C.

b. Prosthetic Skins

Skornik et al.[28] developed a quantitative technique to evaluate adherence of different types of prosthetic skins using a modified Keil tester. The rat's skin was excised from the dorsal surface and replaced with prosthetic material, which consisted of an adherent layer of nylon 66 velour and an outer barrier layer of polyurethane. Rats were selected at various days postapplication, anesthetized, and subjected to adhesion evaluation. The posterior end was freed from subcutaneous tissue and attached to the machine by means of a clamp. Pulling was maintained at a constant velocity (5 cm/s) in a posterior-to-anterior direction.

C. Indirect Evaluation

Lipatova described in his review[13] a method that was used to estimate the strength of adhesion joints under conditions approaching real ones. The effectiveness of closing the defected aortal wall or kidney wounds of animals by cyanoacrylate adhesives was investigated by measuring the maximum arterial pressure that broke the adhesion joints. The arterial pressure was raised by injecting adrenaline. The method achieved a maximum approximation to a real surgical situation and thus the results obtained from such study are of definite interest for clinical applications.

In the application of bioadhesives to controlled drug delivery systems, bioadhesives are used as platforms. Their major role is to secure dosage forms to a certain position of the body and thus to increase the overall drug absorption. As long as the desired bioavailability is achieved for a planned period of time using a particular bioadhesive, the actual adhesive strength of the bioadhesive to tissue surfaces may not be that important. Therefore, the bioadhesive performance may be inferred from measuring either the residence time at the target sites or bioavailability of drugs. For example, the gastric residence time or the gastric emptying pattern of bioadhesives can be noninvasively measured in a quantitative manner using gamma-scintigraphy.[29] Alternatively, pharmacokinetics can be used as a parameter indicating bioadhesive performance in the actual service environment. These indirect methods are, in fact, the ultimate test methods for the evaluation of bioadhesives.

IV. *IN VITRO* MEASUREMENT OF BIOADHESIVE STRENGTH

A. TENSILE TESTING
1. Tissue Adhesives

Wang and Forrester[30] measured the adhesion of hydrophobic polymers to parenchymal tissue of rats. Their study was done to find the amount of *p*-chlorobenzoyl chloride (an acylating agent) required to induce the maximum adhesion of hydrophobic polymers to tissue. Rats were anesthetized, and the surface of liver was exposed through a midline incision. The liver was covered with a piece of cellophane film with a hole (1 cm in diameter) in the center. A thin layer of the rubber or silicone adhesive solution containing various amounts of the acylating agent was applied with a spatula over the exposed portion of the liver. A regular laboratory cork (size 00) was also coated with a thin layer of the polymer adhesive and pressed gently to the previously coated area of the liver surface. After 30 min, a portion of the organ was excised, and placed immediately on the platform of a tension tester. The cork was pulled at a rate of 1.3 mm/s and the force for detachment was measured using a Chattillon motorized tension tester.

Matsumoto[10] devised a tension test that provided the evaluation of both speed of bonding and bond strength of various cyanoacrylate adhesives. Fresh samples of beef lung and muscle tissue were used as model adherends. They were cut into $1/2$ in. diameter cylindrical plugs and wiped free of excess water and blood. The cyanoacrylate adhesive was applied, and the tissue samples were pressed together for a few seconds. At regular intervals, the tensile strength of the bonds was measured.

2. Gastric Adhesives

Park and Robinson[31,32] measured the force required to separate a polymer specimen from freshly excised rabbit stomach tissue using a modified automatic surface tensiometer (Fisher Autotensiomat®). The isolated stomach was opened with scissors, washed with saline solution to remove its contents, and kept at 4°C saline solution until use. A section of the tissue was cut from the fundus and secured, mucosal side out, onto a tissue mounting device prepared in the laboratory using rubber stoppers and aluminum serum bottle seals with a hole (10 mm) in the center (Figure 3). Another section of the stomach was secured on the modified plunger of a 20 ml plastic syringe and suspended from the balance beam of the tensiometer. Test bioadhesives (acrylic hydrogels) were synthesized in a sheet form, cut into disks using a cutting mold, and placed over the upper tissue in the test solution. The contact between the disk and the lower tissue was maintained for 1 min with the initial weight of 1.8 g. After a predetermined time, usually 1 min, the force to separate two tissues was measured by lowering the bottom tissue mounting device at a constant rate of 0.2 in/s until the polymer layer became detached from the mucus layer.

When tissues are not available in large quantity, bioadhesive hydrogels can be secured onto other substrates. We have found that nitrocellulose membrane is an excellent substrate for securing acrylic hydrogels. Figure 4 shows interaction of cross-linked poly(acrylic acid), which was secured on the nitrocellulose membrane, with excised gastric tissue of rabbits in the arificial gastric juice. As the bioadhesive disk was separated from the tissue surface after contact for 1 min as described above, the mucus layer was pulled away from the tissue surface with the bioadhesive disk. Eventually, the breakup occurred in the mucus layer close to the disk instead of the interface between the disk and the mucus layer. A visual as well as microscopic inspection of the disk at the end of the experiment showed the mucus residues remaining on the disk.

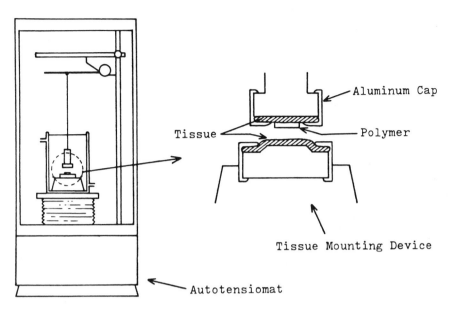

FIGURE 3. Test system for measuring the adhesive strength between acrylic hydrogels and the gastric tissues. Test hydrogel is placed between two tissue layers.

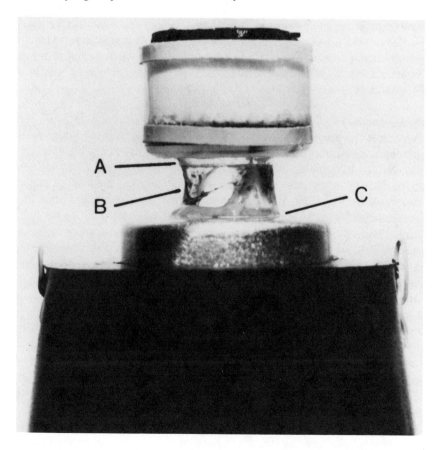

FIGURE 4. Measurement of adhesive strength between cross-linked poly(acrylic acid) (A) and the rabbit gastric tissue (C) using the system shown in Figure 3. The bioadhesive disk (A) was secured on the nitrocellulose membrane. The mucus residues are clearly seen at the bottom of the disk after the cohesion failure occurred in the mucus layer (B).

3. Intraocular Lenses

Reich et al.[33] constructed an instrument for measuring the force of adhesion between the plastic material and endothelium after contact. The device was designed to eliminate surface tension effects by keeping the contacting surface submerged in isotonic saline solution during testing. The cornea was held on a hemispherical ball made from transparent poly(methyl methacrylate). The excised corneas were inverted, placed endothelial surface up on the hemispherical ball, and secured at the limbus with a metal ring that was screwed into the ball. The polymer probe was a cylinder 3 mm high and 3.2 mm in diameter. The probe was machined on a lathe and pressed against the cornea for 30 s with constant weight of 16 g. After the loading, the cuvette was moved down manually with the help of the micrometer, and the force for detachment was measured.

4. Intraoral Tablets

Ponchel et al.[34] used a tensile apparatus (Instron®) to determine the bond strengths of poly(acrylic acid)-hydroxypropyl methylcellulose tablets to bovine sublingual tissue. The tissue was frozen at $-20°C$ immediately after sacrifice of the animal and kept at that temperature until use. The tissue was thawed to 4°C in an isotonic saline solution containing quaternary ammonium and formaldehyde. The tissue was fixed to a support using a cyanoacrylate adhesive. In a bioadhesion test, 15 μl of water was uniformly placed on the exposed side of the tablet, and the two surfaces were brought immediately in contact with an initial force of 0.5 N. The contact between tablet and mucus was maintained for 10 min. The tensile experiment was performed at 26°C, and the extension rate was 5 mm/min. After the experiment, selected samples were dried for 3 d at room temperature and studied in an electron microscope to examine surface changes due to partial adhesion of mucus on the tablet surface. The authors further examined the force-elongation behavior of mucus-mucus and tablet-tablet adhesive joints.

5. Dental Adhesives

Fusayama et al.[35] developed an apparatus for a nonpressure tensile adhesion test, which evaluated the adhesive properties of the restorative materials. Enamel and dentin surfaces were prepared flat by grinding the facial surface of the human teeth. The teeth were stored in water and dried with air immediately before use. Portions of the teeth were etched with 40% phosphoric acid for 60 s, washed, and then dried. A copper tube (5 mm in diameter and 4 mm in height) with a knife edge at its lower end was placed on the test surface, and the assembly was clamped with a specially designed frame and a rubber ring. Then the copper tube was filled with restorative resin with no substantial pressure being applied. A hooking wire loop was inserted into the resin before setting (Figure 5). Ten minutes after filling, the specimens were immersed in water at 37°C and stored for an extended time period ranging from 1 week to 3 months before they were subjected to the tensile test. Similar tension tests were used to evaluate adhesive properties of periodontal dressings,[36] and glass ionomer cement to dentin and enamel.[37,38]

B. SHEAR TESTING

1. Esophageal Adhesives

Marvola et al.[39] developed a method to study the tendency of dosage forms to adhere to the esophageal wall. The study was initiated by the fact that adherence of the drug products to the esophageal wall resulted in high local drug concentrations, which in turn caused drug-induced esophageal ulceration or stricture in humans. Thus their goal was to find less sticky dosage forms, instead of higher strength bioadhesive dosage forms.

The esophagi were removed from pigs and kept in Tyrode solution at 4°C until use.

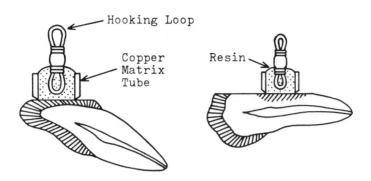

Enamel Surface   Carious Dentin Surface

FIGURE 5.   Schematic description of the specimens for testing the nonpressure adhesion of restorative resin. (From Fusayama, T., Nakamura, M., Kurosaki, N., and Iwaku, M., *J. Dent Res.*, 58, 1364, 1979. With permission.)

During experiments, the solution was aerated with pure oxygen and kept at 37°C. Segments 6 to 7 cm long were cut from the esophagus and mounted in an organ bath as shown in Figure 6. The lower end of the esophageal segment was tied off, and the upper end was attached around a glass tube (diameter of 15 mm). In another experiment, the lower end of the esophageal segment was also attached around a glass tube (diameter of 8 mm) to wash the mucosa. A hole (diameter of 1 mm) was drilled in the dosage forms to be tested. The product was attached to a copper wire (diameter of 0.25 mm) and placed in the esophageal preparation for a fixed time ranging from 10 s to 3 min. In most cases, the contact time was limited to 2 min because of disintegration of the dosage forms. The force required to detach the dosage form was measured using a modified prescription balance.

2. Mucoadhesives

Smart et al.[16,40] measured interaction of soluble polymers with mucus molecules by coating a glass plate with water-soluble polymers and measuring the force to remove it through a mucus solution using a tensiometer. Crude mucus samples obtained by scraping guinea pig intestines were mixed with the same volume of water and slowly stirred for 24 h at 4°C. The mixture was then centrifuged at 32,500g for 30 min, and the middle gel layer retained. The sample was stored frozen in 1 ml aliquots until use. The frozen mucin gel was thawed in a 5 ml glass vial placed in the water bath at 20°C. The vial was then transferred to a platform that could be mechanically lowered at a rate of 1 mm/min. Glass plates were coated with test polymer materials by dipping into a 1% polymer solution and oven drying at 60°C to constant weight. The polymer-coated glass plates, 11 mm wide, were suspended from a microforce balance. The platform was then raised until the plate was completely immersed in the mucus gel. The plate was left in contact with the mucin gel for 7 min, after which the platform was lowered at a rate of 1 mm/min. The maximum force necessary to detach the plate from the gel was recorded.

3. Gastric Adhesives

Leung and Robinson[41] measured the bioadhesive properties of copolymers of acrylic acid and methyl methacrylate using the tensiometer described in Section IV.A.2. The force to detach the bioadhesives from the gastric mucus layer of rabbits was measured by pulling the upper tissue in the direction parallel with the lower tissue.

4. Dental Adhesives

Jedrychowski et al.[42] compared the adhesive effects of various adhesion promoters

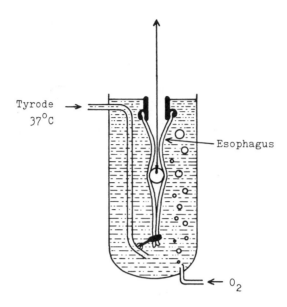

FIGURE 6.   Measurement system for the force necessary to
detach oral dosage form from esophagus. (From Marvola, M.,
Vahervuo, K., Sothmann, A., Marttila, E., and Rajaniemi, M.,
J. Pharm Sci., 71, 975, 1982. Reproduced with permission of
the copyright owner, the American Pharmaceutical Association.)

utilizing acid-etched human permanent teeth. Extracted, human, caries-free permanent man-
dibular incisors were embedded in acrylic bases, and surfaces of the teeth were cleaned with
a pumice slurry. The washed and dried teeth were etched with 50% phosphoric acid, rinsed,
and dried with compressed oil-free air. The tooth was covered with a template with three
holes of 0.01 in. diameter. The template insured that each resin sample tested would have
the same resin-enamel contact area. The adhesion promoters were applied with a cotton
pellet immediately before the testing resin was mixed and applied to the treatment area. The
resin was applied by tamping it into a 0.125 in. diameter plastic tube. The tube was placed
over the treatment area, and the resin was condensed against the enamel surface with a
wooden dowel. The sample was stored in 100% humidity for 24 h at 37°C. The bond
strengths were determined using an Instron® universal testing machine at a cross-head speed
of 0.05 in./min. The wire loop was placed around the tube to measure a pure shear force.
The loop was pulled in the direction parallel to the enamel surface.

C. *IN VITRO* BIOADHESION TESTS USING NONBIOLOGICAL SUBSTRATES

It is natural to expect that excised biological tissues are used for *in vitro* bioadhesion
experiments. However, if a large number of candidate bioadhesives are to be screened,
obtaining enough tissues by sacrificing many animals may be difficult and may not be
economical. In such cases, nonbiological substrates can be used in place of tissues. According
to the definition, then, the tests are not bioadhesion tests anymore. The only way to justify
the use of nonbiological substrates for *in vitro* bioadhesion tests is to find the correlation
between test results obtained using biological tissues and nonbiological substrates.

1. Intraoral Bandages

Chen and Cyr[23] used lap-shear and bending test methods (Figures 1B and 1C) to determine
the adhesive property of intraoral bandages. These methods provided a quantitative expression of wet adhesive strength by measuring the force necessary to separate a sample bandage
from a wet dialyzing cellophane representing gingiva. The preparation of the sample bandages

was described above in Section III.A.1. Both the thin polyethylene film of the bandage and the cellophane were cemented to a plastic slide by means of double-faced tape. The lap-shear measurements were made with the direction of the pull in line with the adhesive layer. Bending resistance was measured by placing the slides perpendicular to the base of the platform. In the bending resistance experiments, the value depends on the angle of pull. In both tests, the adhesion strength was measured either by using a strain gauge or manually increasing the force for separation.

The authors observed that the results of the lap-shear tests correlated with those of the *in vivo* screening tests (Section III.A.1) in many cases. This does not mean that the cellophane membrane is the perfect replacement for gingiva. As pointed out by the authors, the adhesive performance of an intraoral bandage may not be judged by one test alone, since the *in vivo* qualitative test measures total adhesive performance as affected by pushing, pulling, and angular lifting forces.

2. Gastric Adhesives

The bioadhesive property of cross-linked poly(acrylic acid) was measured using excised gastric mucus layer of rabbits as described in Section IV.A.2. As shown in Figure 4, the cross-linked poly(acrylic acid) disk was secured onto the nitrocellulose membrane. In the course of the experiments measuring bioadhesive properties of various polymers, it was observed that the cross-linked polyacrylamide did not interact with the nitrocellulose membrane as tenaciously as the cross-linked poly(acrylic acid).[43] It was further observed that the adhesive properties of the copolymers of acrylic acid and acrylamide to the nitrocellulose membrane were dependent on the contents of acrylic acid. The trend of interaction between the copolymers and the nitrocellulose membrane was the same as that between the copolymers and the gastric mucus layer,[32] although the exact adhesive strengths were different. Thus it may be said that the nitrocellulose membrane can be used instead of the gastric mucus layer to comparatively examine the bioadhesive strengths of acrylic hydrogels, at least copolymers of acrylic acid and acrylamide.

V. OTHER *IN VITRO* TEST METHODS OF BIOADHESION

A. ADHESION WEIGHT METHOD

Smart and Kellaway[40] developed a test system where suspensions of ion exchange resin particles flowed over the inner mucosal surface of a section of guinea pig intestine, and the weight of the adherent particles determined. Although the method was of limited value due to poor data reproducibility resulting from fairly rapid degeneration and biological variation of the tissue, it was possible for them to determine the effect of particle size and charge on the adhesion after 5 min contact with everted intestine. A sieve size fraction (63 to 178 µm) showed a significant increase in the weight of the intestine. No weight changes were observed with smaller sieve size fractions. This is a variation of the adhesion number method described in Section II.C.2.

B. FLUORESCENT PROBE METHOD

Park and Robinson[44] studied polymer interaction with the conjunctival epithelial cell membrane using fluorescent probes. The study was done in an attempt to understand structural requirements for bioadhesion in order to design improved bioadhesive polymers for oral use. The membrane lipid bilayer and membrane proteins were labeled with pyrene and fluorescein isothiocyanate, respectively. The cells were then mixed with candidate bioadhesives and the changes in fluorescence spectra were monitored. The fluorescence spectrum of pyrene in the cell membrane showed two distinct bands known as monomer and excimer bands. It was known that the ratio of excimer/monomer was dependent on the viscosity of the environment.[45] Thus the idea was to detect the change in membrane viscosity by measuring the excimer/monomer ratio. The fundamental assumption of this approach was that the change in membrane viscosity was directly related to the adhesive strength of the test polymer. Polymer binding to membrane proteins was examined using fluorescence depolarization.

This technique is useful to quantitatively compare interactions of various soluble polymers with the cell membrane. It, however, fails to measure the interaction of water-insoluble polymers to the cell membrane due to the interference of the insoluble polymers to fluorescence spectra. In addition, the size of the cell must be measured using an electrical particle counter to accurately interpret the data.

C. FLOW CHANNEL METHOD

Mikos and Peppas[46] have developed a flow channel method that utilizes a thin channel made of glass and filled with 2% (w/w) aqueous solution of bovine submaxillary mucin, thermostated at 37°C (Figure 7). Air was used as a model fluid (A in Figure 7) to test the adhesive characteristics of polymers for nasal application. A gas cylinder containing air was used for the gas flow. The gas stream was passed through a humidifier, where it was saturated at 37°C. The flow cell (C), consisting of two parallel plexiglass plates 15 cm long and 4 cm wide, was constructed with a jacket (E) connected to a water bath (F) and outside insulating fiberglass (G). The temperature of the cell was measured using a thermometer (L). A particle of a bioadhesive polymer (size in the range of 10 and 200 μm) was placed on the mucin gel (D), which had a depth of 0.5 cm through the top of the flow cell (H). Both the static and the dynamic bioadhesive behavior of the particle were determined by taking pictures of the motion of the particle at frequent intervals using a camera (I) and a light source (J). The velocity of the particle was measured using a permanently attached micrometer (K). The flow rate of the air was increased slowly and at a constant rate using a regulating valve with gauge (B), and the time corresponding to the particle detachment was recorded. As pointed out by the authors, this experiment can be done using freshly excised mucus layer or gastrointestinal tissue.

The bioadhesive force is equal to the hydrodynamic force necessary for the particle detachment, assuming no cohesion failure occurs. In the simplest case of a rigid particle interacting to a rigid surface, the hydrodynamic force (F) exerted on the sphere is

$$F = 6\pi fuvR \tag{2}$$

where $f = 1.7009$, u is the air viscosity, R is the particle radius, and v is a characteristic velocity.[47]

D. FALLING LIQUID FILM METHOD

Teng and Ho[48] developed a technique that used excised intestinal segment and micro-size particles (Figure 8). Polymer-coated latex particles were prepared by adding a known volume of 1% polymer solution to the cleaned latex particles (5×10^8 particles/ml) in water and stirring at least for 2 h. To further prepare the polymer coated particles in the buffer solutions varying in ionic strength, an aliquot of the polymer coated particles in water was directly transferred into a beaker containing the desired buffer solution to give about 5×10^6 particles/ml. The suspension was subsequently sonicated for 30 s and used 15 min later. The small intestine obtained from Sprague-Dawley rats was cut into segments of desired length, and the lumen was cleaned with normal saline. The intestinal segment was cut lengthwise with surgical scissors and immediately spread out on the flute prepared by cutting open the Tygon tubing (1 in. internal diameter). The Tygon flute was supported by a platform

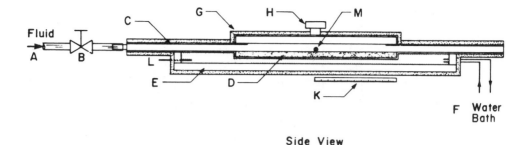

Side View

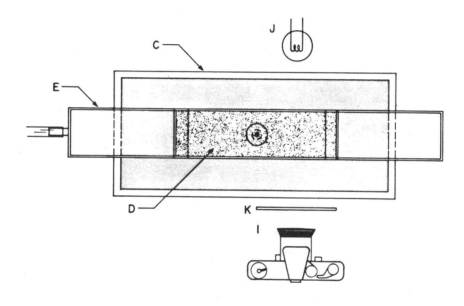

Top View

FIGURE 7. Flow channel device simulating the bioadhesive behavior of polymer particles in contact with mucus. See text for details. (From Mikos, A. G. and Peppas, N. A., *Proc. Int. Symp. Controlled Release Bioact. Mater.*, 13, 97, 1986. With permission.)

composed of a plastic foam board. The angle of inclination was adjusted by a laboratory jack to 78°. The prepared intestinal segment mounted on the Tygon flute was perfused using a perfusion pump and a sample syringe for 10 min with a buffer to remove any loosely held mucus. With the aid of the pump, a liquid film of the buffer solution was established on the intestinal segment. In the next 2 min, samples of the elluent solution were collected and used as a control solution for the particle counting. They observed a constant sloughing of an extraneous substance, presumably mucus, with time. To test the adhesion of polymer-coated particles to the intestinal surface by the perfusion of the particle suspension, 0.5 ml samples of the elluent particle solution were collected, and the number of particles remaining in the sample was counted using an electronic particle counter (Coulter). The fraction of particles adsorbed on the mucous layer (F_a) was measured using the following equation.

$$F_a = 1 - N_f/N_o \qquad (3)$$

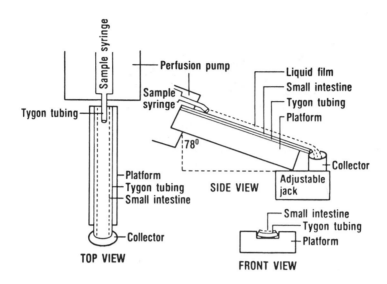

FIGURE 8.   Schematic diagram of the falling liquid film perfusion system. (From Teng, C. L. C. and Ho, N. F. L., *J. Controlled Release*, 6, 133, 1987. With permission.)

where N_o and N_l are the particle concentrations entering the intestinal segment from the dilute suspension reservoir and leaving the segment, respectively. By comparing the fraction of adsorbed particles, the authors were able to compare the adhesion of polymer coated particles to the intestinal mucous surface. This falling liquid film method is essentially the same as the adhesion number method (Section II.C.2).

E. COLLOIDAL GOLD-MUCIN CONJUGATE METHOD

Colloidal gold staining techniques have been used widely to study protein-protein or protein-polymer interactions.[49,50] Recently, the colloidal gold staining technique was applied to the study of bioadesion.[51] Colloidal gold particles with an average diameter of 18 nm were prepared by boiling $HAuCl_4$ in the presence of trisodium citrate.[50,52,53] The formation of the monodisperse colloidal gold particles was indicated by a color change from dark blue to red. The concentration of colloidal gold particles can be easily calculated by measuring the absorbance at 525 nm. The absorbance of 1.0 at 525 nm corresponds to 8.5×10^{11} particles per milliliter.[50] The colloidal solution was cooled and centrifuged. The colloidal gold particles were resuspended in the buffer solution of the desired pH. The buffer concentration was always less than 5 mM. To this solution was added bovine submaxillary mucin solution dialyzed against deionized distilled water. Mucin molecules adsorbed onto the gold particles and stabilized them. The total amount of the mucin necessay to stabilize the colloidal gold particles depends on the pH. We varied pH and the total amount of added mucin, and found that the conjugates were very stable if 0.2 ml of mucin (at least 0.112 mg/ml) was added to a 2 ml of the colloidal gold solution (7.7×10^{11} particles per milliliter or absorbance of 0.9 at 525 nm) at pH 1.3. The colloidal gold and mucin were gently mixed using a rotary mixer for 15 min at 10 rpm. The mixture was then centrifuged at 20,000g for 45 min to remove unadsorbed mucin molecules. The sedimented mucin-gold conjugates were resuspended in the desired buffer solution. Once conjugates are formed, they are very stable under all conditions so that the pH and ionic strength of the solution can be varied. The advantage of using the mucin-gold conjugates is that the red color is formed on the bioadhesive hydrogels as the hydrogels interact with the conjugates. Thus the adhesive interaction between them can be easily quantified either by measuring the intensity of the red color on the hydrogel surface or by measuring the decrease in the concentration of the conjugates from the absorbance change at 525 nm.

Figure 9 shows various hydrogels differing in the ratio of acrylic acid to acrylamide. Those hydrogels were allowed to react with mucin-gold conjugates at pH 1.3 for 1 h. It is clear from the figure that as the content of acrylic acid is increased, the interaction with mucin is also increased. Using this technique, we have also found that once mucin interacts with poly(acrylic acid) at pH 1.3, the mucin is not dissociated from the polymer by simply changing pH to 7. This suggests that the poly(acrylic acid) bioadhesives that interact with mucin molecules in the stomach will maintain the interaction even in the intestine. This technique can be used to screen a large number of potential bioadhesives quantitatively under a variety of conditions.

VI. FACTORS AFFECTING BIOADHESION

The results of any bioadhesion experiment are expected to depend on many variables. The lack of proper control of experimental variables will cause inconsistencies in the data. Some of the variables are extremely difficult to control. For example, when excised soft tissues are used for *in vitro* tests, it is not clear how much the tissues are undergoing changes under the experimental time period. It is also not clear whether tissues obtained from different animals are in the same condition. The effects of such uncontrollable variables may be minimized by using a large number of tissue samples. The factors in which we are interested here are those that can be controlled, but are often ignored in the bioadhesion experiments. Voyutskii discussed in detail in his excellent book the factors that affect autohesion and adhesion of nonbioadhesives.[54]

A. EXPERIMENTAL CONDITIONS
1. Initial Contact Time
In the evaluation of the bioadhesive performance, it is a normal procedure to allow bioadhesives and tissue surfaces to contact for a certain time period before adhesive strength is measured. The optimum initial contact time that results in the maximum adhesion strength depends on many variables, such as the nature of bioadhesives and tissues, the initial pressure, or water content.

In case of cyanoacrylate adhesives, the initial contact has to be maintained at least until polymerization occurs. Thus the optimum initial contact time depends on the nature of the monomer, since the polymerization time is different for different monomers[25,55] (Section III.B.1.a). If bioadhesive tablets are used[34,39] (Sections IV.A.4 and IV.B.1), the initial contact time as well as the amount of water applied onto the tablets will determine the bioadhesive strength by controlling the dissolution of the tablets. When dry or partially swollen hydrogels are used, the gels will continue swelling as long as the contact is maintained with the wet tissues. Continuous swelling of the bioadhesive hydrogels may have a profound effect on the overall bioadhesion. Even hydrogels swollen to equilibrium may have different bioadhesive properties depending on the initial contact time. As the contact time is increased, the interaction and mutual entanglement between bioadhesive polymer chains and the tissue glycoprotein molecules may be substantially increased.[31,32] When lens materials were in contact with the endothelial cell layer, the period of the initial loading (16 g) was limited to 30 s, since much longer times always completely damaged the endothelial cells (Section IV.A.3).[33] Obviously the contact time can be extended if lower pressure is applied or vice versa. For practical reasons, it is preferable to adjust other variables so that the optimum contact time is less than a minute.

2. Initial Pressure
It is a common experience that the manner of applying pressure to contact adhesives

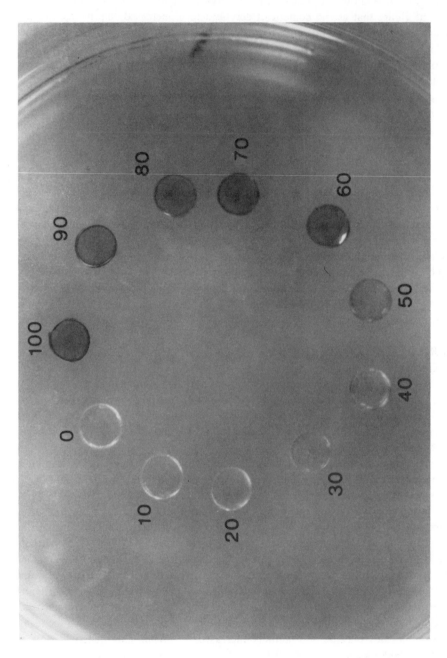

FIGURE 9. Interaction of colloidal gold-mucin conjugates with various hydrogels at pH 1.3. The hydrogels in disk shape are cross-linked copolymers of acrylic acid and acrylamide. The numbers describe percentages of acrylic acid in the copolymers. The colloidal gold-mucin conjugates begin interaction with the polymer disk of 50% acrylic acid. The interaction is indicated by the appearance of red color of the conjugates.

and tissues affects the measurement and results in inconsistent values.[31,35] Park and Robinson[31] examined the effect of the pressure applied to contact the gastric tissue layer and various hydrogels. They found that the adhesion strength was increased linearly as the applied force was increased up to a certain level. In the early stage of their research, however, the authors did not take such effect into account in measuring the adhesion strength. Thus the effect of pH on the bioadhesion of polycarbophil, which was measured in the absence of such consideration,[56] had to be corrected later.[31] Noticing the linear relationship between the tensile strength and the applied pressure, they were able to extrapolate back to the zero applied pressure and determine the intrinsic bioadhesiveness. One surprising, but very reasonable, result was that poly(hydroxyethyl methacrylate) had a negative adhesion with the gastric mucus layer. In other words, they did not adhere in the absence of the applied pressure. This kind of information is essential in the design of oral dosage forms, since the external pressure cannot be applied to them in the gastrointestinal tract (GIT). On the other hand, external pressure can be easily applied to the intraoral or skin bioadhesives.

3. Speed of Testing

The speed of testing is the relative rate of motion of test fixtures during the test.[18] In most cases, the speed of testing is maintained at a constant rate using a motor-driven device. The rate can be maintained manually also. The testing speed is generally chosen empirically to observe the largest difference between different bioadhesives. The speed of testing described in Sections III and IV ranges from 1 mm/min[16] to 5 cm/s.[28] It is necessary to fully examine the effects of the testing speed on the bioadhesives strength. According to Voyutskii,[54] the work of adhesion increases with the increase of the peeling rate of the adhesive from the substrate.

4. Temperature

In most bioadhesion experiments, the temperature may be fixed at either room temperature or 37°C. The study on the effect of temperature, however, is important in understanding the behavior of adhesives. As pointed out by Voyutskii,[54] there are two different effects of temperature on the adhesion strength. The effect of temperature at which the adhesive bond is formed should be distinguished from the effect of temperature at which the force for detachment is measured. In reality, it may be the case that the bioadhesive is applied at room temperature and detached at 37°C. The drastic changes in temperature at which adhesion force is measured may be useful in evaluating the durability of bioadhesives.

B. BIOLOGICAL FACTORS
1. Treatment of Tissues

The adhesion of cyanoacrylate and acrylate adhesives to skin depends on the content of water on the skin surface[26] (Section III.B.1.a). The acrylic adhesives do not adhere measurably to wet skin while the cyanoacrylates do not adhere to dry skin.[26] The bioadhesive properties of some polymers, such as polyurethane prepolymer or silicone elastomer,[30,57] depend on the hydrophobicity of the tissue surface. Thus it appears that the priming of the tissue surface with water or hydrophobic agents, whether intentional or not, has significant influence in the evaluation of bioadhesives. The adhesion of acrylic hydrogels to the gastric mucus layer is known to depend in part on the flexibility of mucin molecules.[31] Park and Robinson[31] observed that treating the gastric mucus layer with N-acetylcysteine increased the adhesion strength up to 40%, presumably due to the increased flexibility of the mucin molecules. On the other hand, treating with glutaraldehyde resulted in a 30% decrease in the adhesion strength.

2. Mucin Turnover

The natural turnover of the tissue surface should be considered for the *in vivo* application of bioadhesives. For example, mucoadhesives adherent to the gastric mucus layer may be removed from the surface regardless of their bioadhesive strength by the normal mucin turnover, which may be shorter than the desired time period for drug delivery. In such case, the difference between various mucoadhesives may not be observed. In addition, the natural mucin turnover in the GIT will result in a substantial amount of soluble mucin molecules. Teng and Ho[48] noticed that surface fouling by mucus was unavoidable despite the efforts made to wash out loosely bound mucus from the intestinal wall. Studies using mucus-coated particles showed the presence of an interfacial barrier between the particles and the intestinal mucus surface. Thus, in practice, mucus contamination of polymer coated particles could lead to unfavorable conditions for bioadhesion, even though the particle surfaces have been originally designed to promote adhesion to the intestinal mucus wall.[48] The exact turnover rate of the mucus layer remains to be determined. When strong gastric mucoadhesives such as poly(acrylic acid) are used, it is common to observe the cohesion failure at the mucus layer as shown in Figure 4. The rupture did not occur at the interface between polymer and mucus but rather inside the mucus.[34] Thus, once a bioadhesive is separated from the mucus layer, there is little chance that the contaminated bioadhesive will readhere to the mucus layer.

VII. SUMMARY

The studies on the Type III bioadhesion and bioadhesives are not new. Only recently, however, was the concept of using bioadhesives to controlled drug delivery established. Research on the evaluation of bioadhesives is still in its early stage. Poor understanding of biological tissue surfaces has resulted in the lack of universal test methods, which in turn results in poor understanding of bioadhesion mechanisms. Although a number of test methods are already available as described in this chapter, they are by no means perfect test methods. We need to continue modifying old test methods and developing new ones as they may be necessary.

REFERENCES

1. *Annual Book of ASTM Standards,* Vol. 15.06, Sect. 15, American Society for Testing and Materials, Philadelphia, PA, 1984.
2. **Park, K., Cooper, S. L., and Robinson, J. R.,** Bioadhesive hydrogels, in *Hydrogels in Medicine and Pharmacy,* Vol. 3, Peppas, N. A., Ed., CRC Press, Boca Raton, FL, 1987, chap. 8.
3. **Eirich, F. R.,** Bioadhesion as an interphase phenomenon, in *Biocompatibility of Implant Materials,* Williams, D., Ed., Sector Publishing, London, 1976, chap. 19.
4. **Wake, W. C.,** *Adhesion and the Formulation of Adhesives,* Applied Science, London, 1976, chap. 13.
5. **Sowers, A. E., Ed.,** *Cell Fusion,* Plenum Press, New York, 1987.
6. **Edwards, J. G.,** The biochemistry of cell-adhesion, *Prog. Surf. Sci.,* 13, 125, 1983.
7. **Grinnell, F.,** Cellular adhesiveness and extracellular substrata, *Int. Rev. Cytol.,* 53, 65, 1978.
8. **Taylor, A. C.,** Adhesion of cells to surfaces, in *Adhesion in Biological Systems,* Manly, R. S., Ed., Academic Press, New York, 1970, chap. 3.
9. **Hillman, R. E. and Nace, P. F.,** Histochemistry of barnacle cyprid adhesive formation, in *Adhesion in Biological Systems,* Manly, R. S., Ed., Academic Press, New York, 1970, chap. 6.
10. **Matsumoto, T.,** *Tissue Adhesives in Surgery,* Medical Examination, Flushing, NY, 1972, 195.
11. **Chu, C. C.,** Survey of clinically important wound closure biomaterials, in *Biocompatible Polymers, Metals, and Composites,* Szycher, M., Ed., Technomic Publishing, Lancaster, 1983, chap. 22.
12. **Gross, L. and Hoffman, R.,** Medical and biological adhesives, in *Handbook of Adhesives,* 2nd ed., Skeist, I., Ed.,Van Nostrand Reinhold, New York, 1977, 818.
13. **Lipatova, T. E.,** Medical polymer adhesives, *Adv. Polym. Sci.,* 79, 65, 1986.
14. **Cleary, G. W.,** Transdermal controlled release systems, in *Medical Applications of Controlled Release,* Vol. 1, Langer, R. S. and Wise, D. L., Eds., CRC Press, Boca Raton, FL, 1984, chap. 7.

15. **Brauer, G. M. and Huget, E. F.,** Dental adhesives, in *The Chemistry of Biosurfaces,* Vol. 2, Hair, M. L., Ed., Marcel Dekker, New York, 1972, chap. 16.

16. **Smart, J. D., Kellaway, I. W., and Worthington, H. E. C.,** An in-vitro investigation of mucosa-adhesive materials for use in controlled drug delivery, *J. Pharm. Pharmacol.,* 36, 295, 1984.

17. **Portelli, G. B.,** Testing, analysis, and design of structural adhesive joints, in *Structural Adhesives,* Hartshorn, S. R., Ed., Plenum Press, New York, 1986, 407.

18. **Shah, V.,** *Handbook of Plastics Testing Technology,* Wiley-Interscience, New York, 1984, 1.

19. **Hartshorn, S. R.,** Introduction, in *Structural Adhesives,* Hartshorn, S. R., Ed., Plenum Press, New York, 1986, 1.

20. **Been, J. L.,** Bonding, in *Encyclopedia of Polymer Science and Technology,* Vol. 1, Interscience, New York, 1964, 503.

21. **Zimon, A.D.,** *Adhesion of Dust and Powder,* 2nd ed., Consultant Bureau, New York, 1982, chap. 3.

22. **Hartshorn, S. R.,** The durability of structural adhesive jonts, in *Structural Adhesives,* Hartshorn, S. R., Ed., Plenum Press, New York, 1986, 347.

23. **Chen, J. L. and Cyr, G. N.,** Compositions producing adhesion through hydration, in *Adhesion in Biological Systems,* Manly, R. S., Ed., Academic Press, New York, 1970, chap. 10.

24. **Bremecker, K. D., Strempel, H., and Klein, G.,** Novel concept for a mucosal adhesive ointment, *J. Pharm. Sci.,* 73, 548, 1984.

25. **Leonard, F., Hodge, J. W., Jr., Houston, S., and Ousterhout, D. K.,** Alpha-cyanoacrylate adhesive bond strengths with proteinaceous and nonproteinaceous substrates, *J. Biomed. Mater. Res.,* 2, 173, 1968.

26. **Margules, G. S. and Harris, D. L.,** Adhesives for intact skin: a preliminary investigation, *Med. Biol. Eng. Comput.,* 18, 549, 1980.

27. **Ow, R. K. K. and Bearn, E. M.,** A method of studying the effect of adhesives on denture retention, *J. Prosthet. Dent.,* 50, 332, 1983.

28. **Skornik, W. A., Dressler, D. P., and Richard, J. K.,** Adherence of prosthetic skin, *J. Biomed. Mater. Res.,* 2, 447, 1968.

29. **Theodorakis, M. C., Digenis, G. A., Beihn, R. M., Shambhu, M. B., and DeLand, F. H.,** Rate and pattern of gastric emptying in humans using ^{99m}Tc-labeled triethylenetetraamine-polystyrene resin, *J. Pharm. Sci.,* 69, 568, 1980.

30. **Wang, P. Y. and Forrester, D. H.,** Conditions for the induced adhesion of hydrophobic polymers to soft tissue, *Trans. Am. Soc. Artif. Int. Organs,* 20, 504, 1974.

31. **Park, H. and Robinson, J. R.,** Physico-chemical properties of water insoluble polymers important to mucin/epithelial adhesion, *J. Controlled Release,* 2, 47, 1985.

32. **Park, H. and Robinson, J. R.,** Mechanisms of mucoadhesion of poly(carboxylic acid) hydrogels, *Pharm. Res.,* 4, 457, 1987.

33. **Reich, S., Levy, M., Meshorer, A., Blumental, M., Yalon, M., Sheets, J. W., and Goldberg, E. P.,** Intraocular-lens-endothelial interface: adhesive force measurement, *J. Biomed. Mater. Res.,* 18, 737, 1984.

34. **Ponchel, G., Touchard, F., Duchene, D., and Peppas, N. A.,** Bioahesive analysis of controlled release systems. I. Fracture and interpenetration analysis in poly(acrylic acid)-containing systems, *J. Controlled Release,* 5, 129, 1987.

35. **Fusayama, T., Nakamura, M., Kurosaki, N., and Iwaku, M.,** Non-pressure adhesion of a new adhesive restorative resin, *J. Dent. Res.,* 58, 1364, 1979.

36. **Haugen, E., Espevik, S., and Mjor, I. A.,** Adhesive properties of periodontal dressings — an in vitro study, *J. Periodontal Res.,* 14, 487, 1979.

37. **Powis, D. R., Folleras, T., Merson, S. A., and Wilson, A. D.,** Improved adhesion of a glass ionomer cement to dentin and enamel, *J. Dent. Res.,* 61, 1416, 1982.

38. **Goldman, M., DeVitre, R., and Pier, M.,** Effect of the dentin smeared layer on tensile strength of cemented posts, *J. Prosthet. Dent.,* 52, 485, 1984.

39. **Marvola, M., Vahervuo, K., Sothmann, A., Marttila, E., and Rajaniemi, M.,** Development of a method for study of the tendency of drug products to adhere to the esophagus, *J. Pharm. Sci.,* 71, 975, 1982.

40. **Smart, J. D. and Kellaway, I. W.,** In vitro techniques for measuring mucoadhesion, *J. Pharm. Pharmacol.,* 34, 70P, 1982.

41. **Leung, S. H. S. and Robinson, J. R.,** The contribution of anionic polymer structural features to mucoadhesion, *J. Controlled Release,* 5, 223, 1988.

42. **Jedrychowski, J. R., Caputo, A. A., and Foliart, R.,** Effects of adhesion promoters on resin-enamel retention, *J. Dent. Res.,* 58, 1371, 1979.

43. **Park, K. and Park, H.,** unpublished data, 1987.

44. **Park, K. and Robinson, J. R.,** Bioadhesive polymers as platforms for oral-controlled drug delivery: method to study bioadhesion, *Int. J. Pharm.,* 19, 107, 1984.

45. **Dembo, M., Glushko, V., Aberlin, M. E., and Sonenberg, M.,** A method for measuring membrane microviscosity using pyrene excimer formation. Application to human erythrocyte ghosts, *Biochim. Biophys. Acta,* 552, 201, 1979.

46. **Mikos, A. G. and Peppas, N. A.,** Comparison of experimental technique for the measurement of the bioadhesive forces of polymeric materials with soft tissues, *Proc. Int. Symp. Controlled Release Bioact. Mater.,* 13, 97, 1986.

47. **O'Neill, M. E.,** A sphere in contact with a plane wall in a slow linear shear flow, *Chem. Eng. Sci.,* 23, 1293, 1968.

48. **Teng, C. L. C. and Ho, N. F. L.,** Mechanistic studies in the simultaneous flow and adsorption of polymer-coated latex particles on intestinal mucus. I. Methods and physical model development, *J. Controlled Release,* 6, 133, 1987.

49. **Goodman, S. L., Hodges, G. M., and Livingstone, D. C.,** A review of the colloidal gold marker system, *Scanning Electron Microsc.,* 1980/II, 133, 1980.

50. **Park, K., Simmons, S. R., and Albrecht, R. M.,** Surface characterization of biomaterials by immunogold staining-quantitative analysis, *Scan. Microsc.* 1, 339, 1987.

51. **Park, K. and Park, H.,** A new approach to study mucoadhesion: colloidal gold staining, *J. Int. Pharm.,* in press.

52. **Frens, G.,** Controlled nucleation for the regulation of the particle size in monodisperse gold suspensions, *Nature London Phys. Sci.,* 241, 20, 1973.

53. **Horisberger, M.,** Evaluation of colloidal gold as a cytochemical marker for transmission and scanning electron microscopy, *Biol. Cellulaire,* 36, 253, 1979.

54. **Voyutskii, S. S.,** *Autohesion and adhesion of high polymers,* Interscience, New York 1963, chap. 6.

55. **Leonard, F.,** Hemostatic applications of alpha cyanoacrylates: bonding mechanism and physiological degradation of bonds, in *Adhesion in Biological Systems,* Manly, R. S., Ed., Academic Press, New York, 1970, chap. 11.

56. **Ch'ng, H. S., Park, H., Kelly, P., and Robinson, J. R.,** Bioadhesive polymers as platforms for oral controlled drug delivery. II. Synthesis and evaluation of some swelling, water-insoluble bioadhesive polymers, *J. Pharm. Sci.,* 74, 399, 1985.

57. **Wang, P. Y.,** Adhesion mechanism for polyurethane prepolymers bonding biological tissue, in *Biomedical Applications of Polymers,* Gregor, H. P., Ed., Plenum Press, New York, 1975, 111.

Chapter 4

BIOADHESIVES/MUCOADHESIVES IN DRUG DELIVERY TO THE GASTROINTESTINAL TRACT

Pardeep K. Gupta, Sau-Hung S. Leung, and Joseph R. Robinson

TABLE OF CONTENTS

I. INTRODUCTION

Bioadhesives in drug delivery systems have recently gained interest among pharmaceutical scientists as a means of promoting dosage form residence time as well as improving intimacy of contact with various absorptive membranes of the biological system.[1] Besides acting as platforms for sustained release dosage forms, bioadhesive polymers can themselves exert some control over the rate and amount of drug release, and thus contribute to the therapeutic advantage of such systems.

The use of bioadhesives in oral delivery systems makes a particularly attractive area of research. Oral controlled delivery systems are limited in their therapeutic performance by a variety of factors, chief among them is residence time of a dosage form at the site of action (for local effect) or absorption (for systemic effect) in the gastrointestinal tract (GIT). Bioadhesives, by virtue of their adhesiveness to biological membranes, including the lining of the GIT can help to prolong residence time and considerably improve drug bioavailability from oral delivery systems. If transit time through the gut can be controlled by such systems, a long standing goal of once-a-day dosing can be achieved. In addition, bioadhesive dosage forms make it possible to explore other areas of the digestive tract for drug delivery, such as the buccal cavity, which has traditionally been of limited value as a route of administration due to the difficulty of dosage form retention.

A. DEFINITIONS
1. Bioadhesives

Bioadhesives are materials that can bind to a biological membrane and are capable of being retained on that membrane for an extended period of time.[2,3] This binding, which usually takes place due to interfacial forces between two surfaces, can be directly to the membrane surface (cell layers), or to a coating on the membrane surface, such as the mucin layer. The bioadhesive material itself can be biological or nonbiological in nature and source, although in a drug delivery context, it is usually a nonbiological macromolecular or hydrocolloid material. The term ''mucoadhesive'' is commonly used for materials that bind to the mucin layer on a biological membrane, but throughout this chapter, the general term bioadhesive will be used. Section II outlines the concept of bioadhesion.

2. Oral Delivery Systems

The term oral will be used to include all areas of the digestive tract including the mouth, stomach, intestinal area, and rectum, although for purposes of discussion, individual areas will be dealt with separately. The basic concept of bioadhesion will be the same in these areas because the nature of the mucin layer on the membrane lining the entire digestive tract is similar, despite differences in chemical structure.

B. PAST WORK

A systematic study of the use of bioadhesives to overcome the relatively short GI transit time and achieve localization for controlled release drug delivery systems was initiated many years ago and has received renewed attention in the 1980s. Nagai and Machida[1] reported on a buccal bioadhesive system to successfully treat aphthous stomatitis. Peppas and Buri[4] reported on several aspects of the mechanism of bioadhesives, and Park and Robinson[5] studied a number of polymers, both natural and synthetic, for their bioadhesive potential and to obtain information on the structural requirements for bioadhesion. Their findings suggest that highly charged carboxylated polyanions are good candidates for use as bioadhesives in the GIT. Later work by Ch'ng et al.[6] reported various physicochemical properties and GI transit times of a series of cross-linked, swellable polymers in the rat. *In vitro* and *in vivo* methods were developed by a number of workers[4] to estimate the force of bioadhesion, and on the basis of the data obtained, it was concluded that the degree of swelling, pH, ionic-strength, and degree of cross-linking of polymers are all important parameters in bioadhesion. Gurney et al.[7] have attempted to delineate mechanism(s) of polymer attachment to the tissue. The above studies have been aimed not only at characterizing optimal conditions for bioadhesion but also at obtaining some meaningful information on the specificity of attachment. Specificity of attachment occurs when the adhesive and the substrate have a substrate-receptor interaction. Such information will be valuable in synthesizing polymers to attach to specific areas in the GIT for the purpose of drug localization.

One of the models for bioadhesion is the well-studied phenomenon of bacterial adhesion to various membranes and surfaces. A variety of infectious diseases of the oral cavity and the GIT in man involves attachment of disease causing microorganisms to surfaces of the mouth (e.g., teeth and gums) and epithelia of the intestine. In addition, the large intestine, in man and animals, contains a variety of normal flora attached to the epithelial or mucus surface.[8] Attachment of a filamentous Gram-positive organism to intestinal absorptive cells in rodent ileum has been the subject of recent studies.[9,10] This organism holds on to the apical membrane of the absorptive cell by a process of invagination. A study of the structural requirements for this kind of attachment can be very useful in designing certain macromolecules that will attach directly to the absorptive surface of the gut epithelium.

Another well studied model in this regard is the enterotoxigenic *Escherichia coli* (ETEC) group of microorganisms, which are responsible for various diarrheal diseases in man and animals. Their enterotoxicity comes from their ability to attach to the surface of intestinal epithelium through highly specialized surface antigens. This group of antigens is collectively known as colonization factor antigens (CFAs).[11] These antigens are lectins in nature and are believed to attach to epithelial surface carbohydrates. Cheney et al.[12,13] have implicated carbohydrates, both from the fuzzy coat that covers the intestinal epithelium and the mucus layer, as intestinal cell surface components in the binding process. Lectins, which are proteins or glycoproteins of nonimmune origin, and have the ability to combine specifically with particular carbohydrate residues, can serve as models for developing specific bioadhesive materials.

There have been a number of efforts to develop dosage forms based on the concept of bioadhesion during the past few years. Machida et al.[14,15] have reported encouraging clinical reports on an erodible bioadhesive system to treat carcinoma colli. A chlorthiazide formulation in albumin beads for sustained delivery has been shown to improve bioavailability by a factor of two in rats when administered as a physical mixture with the bioadhesive polycarbophil compared to when given alone.[16] The *in vitro* release profile of chlorthiazide from albumin beads was similar in the presence or absence of polycarbophil, indicating that improved bioavailability was due either to a longer retention of the formulation at the site of absorption or to a more intimate contact with the absorptive surface, due to presence of the bioadhesive. A mucosal adhesive ointment based partly on neutralized polymethacrylic acid methyl ester has been reported to show longer retention times on skin and oral mucosa without any irritation as compared to a conventional ointment.[17] The rehological behavior as well as adhesion on the mucosal membrane could be varied by the type and concentration of polymer and the base used for neutralization.

C. PROJECTED COVERAGE OF THE CHAPTER

The scientific framework necessary for a systematic study of the area of bioadhesives in oral drug delivery will consist of a basic understanding of a number of issues, among which are the structure-activity relationships of bioadhesive polymers, the nature and extent of interfacial interactions between the two surfaces, and various characteristics of the biological membrane to which the adhesive attaches. This chapter will address the above issues at a fundamental level. Emphasis will be on an effort to put together our current understanding of the bioadhesive phenomenon in terms of molecular events at the interface. On the biological side, some of the membrane characteristics including permeability and enzymatic activity will also be discussed. Since most bioadhesive material is envisaged as being macromolecular in nature, immunogenicity can become an important issue in their use, and consequently will be included in the discussion. Potential areas of the GIT for bioadhesion will be identified, and the variables associated with their use will be discussed in order to develop some strategies for formulation of bioadhesive oral delivery systems.

II. FUNDAMENTALS OF BIOADHESION

Formation of an adhesive bond between a polymer and a biological membrane or its coating can be visualized as a two step process: initial contact between the two surfaces, and formation of secondary bonds due to noncovalent interactions. This process of bond formation has contributions from three areas: surface (or surface coat) of the biological membrane, surface of the adhesive, and the interfacial layer between the two surfaces. Molecular events that take place in the interfacial layer depend on various characteristics of the polymer and membrane. In order to obtain an understanding of interfacial events and possible mechanisms of bioadhesion, a brief discussion of characteristics of the two surfaces will be presented.

A. BIOLOGICAL MEMBRANE

Membranes of the internal tracts of the body, including the GIT, buccal cavity, eye, ear, nose, vagina, and rectum are covered with a thick gel-like structure known as mucin. Therefore, all bioadhesives must interact with the mucin layer during the process of attachment. Mucus itself exhibits considerable binding property, and thus serves as a link between the adhesive and the membrane. Indeed, most polymers bind to mucin and never penetrate deep enough to form a bond with the underlying epithelial cells, and are consequently termed ''mucoadhesives.'' The process of binding between cells and the mucin layer itself presents a model of bioadhesion and offers an opportunity to understand this phenomenon.

Mucus is a network of mucin glycoproteins that form a continuous layer that covers the internal tracts of the body. Mucins are synthesized by goblet cells and special exocrine glands with mucus cell acini.[18] In the form that mucus is secreted, the glycoprotein constitutes less than 5% of the total weight of mucus.[19] There are about 160 to 200 oligosaccharide side-chains in the glycosylated region of the glycoprotein,[20] each oligosaccharide unit contains eight to ten monosaccharide residues.[21] The terminal end of these oligosaccharides is either sialic acid,[22,23] or L-fucose.[24,25] At physiological pH, the mucin network has a negative charge due to the presence of sialic acid, which has a pK_a of 2.6.[26] Similarly, the presence of sulfate residues also contributes to this negative charge, making the glycoprotein an anionic polyelectrolyte, Thus, from a bioadhesive standpoint, mucin consists of highly hydrated cross-linked, linear, flexible, and random coil glycoprotein molecules with a net negative charge.

The cell surface of membranes also has a net negative charge due to the presence of charged groups. Thus binding of mucin to cell surfaces, which is a result of interaction between two surfaces with the same net charge, indicates that adhesive forces dominate the electrostatic repulsive forces between the two surfaces. This is explained on the basis of electron transfer and dipole induction, and will be explained further under mucoadhesive mechanisms.

B. BIOADHESIVE POLYMERS

Mucoadhesive polymers are divided into two categories: (1) compounds that are water-soluble, linear, and random polymers, and (2) water-insoluble compounds that are swellable networks joined by cross-linking agents. Some of the polymer properties important to bioadhesion are as follows.

1. Molecular Weight, Chain Length, and Cross-Linking Density

Chen and Cyr[27] suggested that bioadhesive strength increases as molecular weight of the polymer increases above 100,000, and there seems to be a critical molecular weight requirement for significant bioadhesion. It was found that the molecular weight of sodium carboxymethyl cellulose (NaCMC) should exceecd 78,600 in order to have significant bioadhesion.[28] Thus molecular weight and chain length of the macromolecule are important parameters in the process of bioadhesion.

For all water-swellable insoluble polymers, the linear chains are connected via cross-linking agents, as in the case of polycarbophil, a well-known mucoadhesive, which is polyacrylic acid cross-linked with divinyl glycol.[29] Cross-linking density of polycarbophil is expected to influence mucoadhesion by influencing the effective number of polyacrylic acid chains in a given volume and their chain segment mobility. The strength of mucoadhesion has been found to decrease with an increase in concentration of the cross-linking agent, a partial explanation of which may lie in the fact that an increase in cross-linking density decreases the diffusion coefficient[30,31] and chain-segment flexibility and mobility, thereby reducing the extent of interpenetration.

2. Charges and Ionization

In a study of a series of anionic, cationic, and neutral polymers, using a cell culture-fluorescent probe technique,[4,32] it was found that the charge sign and density are important elements for bioadhesion. Polyanionic polymers are preferred over polycationic and neutral polymers when both bioadhesive strength and cellular toxicity are considered. Furthermore, polyanions with carboxyl groups appear to be better candidates than those with sulfate groups.

3. Hydrophilic Functional Groups and Hydration

Bioadhesive polymers are usually macromolecules with numerous hydrophilic functional groups that can form hydrogen-bonds, e.g., carboxyl, hydroxyl, amide, and sulfate groups.[27]

The presence of these fixed charges within the macromolecular network establishes a swelling force, or swelling pressure, or a net osmotic pressure,[33] which drives the solvent into the polymer gel from the more dilute external bulk solution. When counterions are added to the hydrating media, they bind to some of the fixed charged groups resulting in a screening effect. Thus the ionic strength and the amount of counterions in solution are important parameters that have to be considered in mucoadhesive studies.

The amount of water at the interface between the interacting adhesive and substrate surface is an important factor for bioadhesion. Sufficient water is needed to properly hydrate the mucoadhesive to expose the adhesive sites for secondary bond formation, expand the gel to create pores of sufficient size and mobilize all the flexible polymer chains for interpenetration.

4. Chain-Segment Mobility and Expanded Nature of the Network

The ability of the polymer and mucin chains to interpenetrate can be approximated by their ability to diffuse. Over a sufficiently restricted temperature range, the experimental diffusion coefficient, D, shows an exponential temperature dependence of the Arrhenius type[34]

$$D = D_o \exp(-E/RT) \tag{1}$$

where the pre-exponential factor D_o is a constant and is independent of temperature over a given temperature range, and E is the experimental activation energy for diffusion or for mobility of the segment chains. At a particular temperature, interdiffusion will increase with chain segment mobility. This chain segment mobility may be increased by an increased degree of hydration, expanded nature of network, and reduced cross-linking.

The effect of the expanded nature of the mucin and adhesive network on mucoadhesion has been shown to be one of the factors that controls the strength of mucoadhesion.[35]

Besides the above-mentioned structural features that contribute to mucoadhesion, another factor that influences mucoadhesive strength is the pressure applied to the interacting interface. The increase in applied pressure improves the intimacy of contact and contact area, which increases secondary bond formation and physical entanglement, resulting in a greater strength of mucoadhesion until secondary bond formation and physical entanglement are maximized.[36]

C. MECHANISM(S) OF MUCOADHESION

Based on the discussion to this point, it is clear that it is hard to define a single parameter or theory to explain the process of bioadhesion. Four theories have been proposed to explain events at the interface, and typically in bioadhesion, a combination of more than one of these theories is usually involved. A brief discussion of these theories follows.

1. Wetting Theory

The ability of the adhesive to spread spontaneously on mucin influences establishment of intimate contact between the mucoadhesive and mucin, and consequently influences mucoadhesive strength. The thermodynamic work of adhesion is a function of the surface tensions of the surfaces in contact, as well as the interfacial tension. A small value of interfacial tension would mean a more intimate contact between the two surfaces.

Interfacial tension has been predicted to be proportional to the square root of the polymer-polymer interaction parameter.[37-39] A low value of the polymer-polymer interaction parameter, which is the result of structural similarities of the two polymers, means a smaller interfacial tension, which results in greater contact between the adhesive and substrate.

2. Diffusion Theory

The diffusion theory describes interpenetration of the mucoadhesive (polymer) and substrate (mucin) to a sufficient depth and creation of a semipermanent adhesive-bond.[40] Although interdiffusion in compatible polymers has been demonstrated by radiometric studies,[41] the exact depth of penetration required to achieve adequate mucoadhesion is not known. However, the mean diffusional path length, s, can be approximated as[42]

$$s = (2tD)^{1/2} \tag{2}$$

where D is the diffusion coefficient. The diffusion coefficient was found to depend on the molecular weight of the polymer strand, and to decrease significantly with increasing cross-linking density,[43] indicating that flexibility and chain segment mobility of the mucoadhesive polymer and mucus glycoprotein molecules are important parameters that control interdiffusion.

3. Electronic Theory[44,45]

The mucoadhesive polymer and mucin glycoprotein have different electronic structures; therefore electron transfer is likely to occur when contact is made. The transfer of electrons will result in formation of an electrical double layer at the adhesive interface with subsequent adhesion. Therefore the adhesive/mucin interface can be treated as a capacitor, which is charged when the two surfaces are in close contact and discharged when they are separated.

4. Adsorption Theory

Adsorption theory describes the attachment of adhesives to biological tissues on the basis of a group of interactions known collectively as "secondary" forces.[46-49] The van der Waal's forces of attraction are the sum of all attractions between uncharged molecules. These attractive forces arise out of three effects: (1) polar or Keesom forces arising from the orientation of permanent dipoles in two molecules, (2) induction or Debye forces arising out of induced dipole and permanent dipole, and (3) dispersion or London forces that arise from changes in the charge distribution around nonpolar molecules. Hydrogen bonding can arise between two nonpolar groups due to the tendency of water molecules to exclude nonpolar molecules, or between ionized carboxyl groups or surfaces. These secondary forces are by far the strongest components of interactions contributing to bioadhesion.

D. BIOADHESION AT EXPOSED EPITHELIAL SURFACE

Bioadhesion at an epithelial surface can occur when continuity of the mucus layer is physically interrupted by abrasion or altered chemically by mucolytic agents. The use of bioadhesive polymers/copolymers to attach to these exposed epithelial surfaces can serve the following purposes: (1) maintain continuity of the mucus layer and minimize the exposed area; (2) replace the mucus layer and provide a protective covering for the underlying cell layers from physical and chemical insult; and (3) act as a platform for drug delivery to local tissues and facilitate recovery of the damaged or diseased cell layers.

The cell membrane is viewed as a two-dimension-oriented viscous lipid solution where proteins are free to move.[50] The membrane is known to be surrounded by exopolysaccarides, either on or in the periphery of all cells.[51,52] For animal cell membranes, the carbohydrates are bound covalently to proteins and lipids to form glycoproteins and glycolipids,[53] which are oriented asymmetrically in the plasma membrane with the carbohydrate chains projecting to the exterior of the cell.[53] All the polysaccharide-containing structures on the external surface of cells are collectively referred to as the glycocalyx.[54] The glycocalyx, which may be a dynamic component of the cell and is maintained and synthesized continuously by the underlying cell,[54] appears to be partly responsible for the adhesive property of the cell.

Sucralfate, a basic aluminum salt of sulfated sucrose, is advocated for use in peptic ulcer disease.[55] Sucralfate was found to adhere selectively to ulcerous and eroded surfaces of the stomach in animal studies.[56,57] Electrostatic attraction[58,59] was proposed to explain the adhesion of sucralfate to the exposed epithelial surfaces. Other possible mechanisms for cellular attachment of bioadhesives are charge distribution[60,61] and redistribution.[62]

E. NATURALLY OCCURRING BIOADHESIVES

There are some specialized macromolecules that are synthesized by cells and have potential to be utilized as mucoadhesives, e.g., fibronectin, which is a major glycoprotein constituent of plasma and other body fluids[63] and is present on epithelial cell surfaces; lectins that exist on the surface of a diversity of mammalian cells;[64] and several different cell adhesion molecules (CAMs) in a number of vertebrate species in different tissues[65] and glycocalyx.[52]

Fibronectin is a component of the extracellular matrix, and is synthesized by endothelial and glial cells.[66-68] It is an important adhesive protein that binds certain forms of collagen and glycosaminoglycans and mediates the adhesion and spreading of cells in culture.[69-74] Fibronectin is a dimer that consists of two subunits linked by disulfide bridges at the carboxy terminal ends,[63] and contains approximately 5% by weight of carbohydrate.[75] The adhesive property of fibronectin can be duplicated by small synthetic peptides,[74,76,77] and a synthetic peptide from fibronectin was found to inhibit experimental metastasis of murine melanoma cells.[78]

Lectins are carbohydrate-binding proteins and glycoproteins derived from both plants and animals[79] that have two important properties: (1) they have specificity for particular sugar residues and (2) they are bivalent or polyvalent.[80] Although a great number of plant and animal lectins have been found and purified, only a few of them have been reported to be specific for sialic acids, e.g., limulin,[81,82] carcinoscorpin,[83] *Limax flavus*,[84] and achatinin.[85] Lectins belong to two categories: (1) integrated lectins, which integrate into membranes and require detergents for solubilization and bind glycoconjugates to membranes at the cell surface or within vesicles, thus localizing the glycoconjugates at particular membrane sites,[86] and (2) soluble lectins, which move freely in the aqueous compartments intra- and extracellularly and interact with complementary glycoconjugates on and around the cells that release them.[80] Since the surface of virtually all cells have a number of glycosylated moieties, lectins have potential as bioadhesives in areas of exposed epithelial cell surfaces.

F. MODULATION OF MUCOADHESION

Since the process of mucoadhesion involves intimate contact of mucoadhesives and the mucin layer, any factor that influences the chemical and/or physical characteristics of the mucin or mucoadhesive layer will have an effect on the extent of interaction and strength of mucoadhesion.

A number of substances interact with mucin and are known as mucus thickening/thinning agents, e.g., tetraborate, tetracyclines,[87] and progesterone.[88] Aggregation may be caused by formation of bridges or by reduction of electrostatic charges of the mucin molecules with a simultaneous change in conformation of the mucin network.[89] Calcium is known to precipitate mucin, and when used to adjust media tonicity, it reduces shear stress.[90,91] Increasing the ionic strength of the media also decreases the degree of hydration of the mucoadhesive (polycarbophil), with a subsequent decrease in tensile stress.[92] This can be explained by reduction of the expanded nature of the mucin network in the presence of calcium ion or by an increase in ionic strength, with a subsequent decrease in the process of interpenetration.[35]

The network of mucin can be altered by a number of mucolytic agents, which may reduce the viscosity of mucus by altering the molecular composition of mucus via rupture of disulfide bonds or by the proteolytic action of enzymes.[93] Disulfide bond-breaking agents, e.g., acetylcysteine, carbocysteine, and dithiothreitol, act directly to split the disulfide bridges connecting different glycoprotein molecules,[94] whereas proteolytic enzymes, e.g., deoxyribonuclease, trypsin, elastase, papain, protease, chymotrypsin, and leucine aminopeptidase exert their activity only by gaining access to protein regions that are not glycosylated.[94] The result of breaking disulfide bonds and the protein backbone is depolymerization of mucin molecules, breaking of the mucin network, and a marked decrease in mucus viscosity.[93] Under these conditions, maintenence of an intact interacting interfacial region becomes questionable, and mucoadhesive strength may be reduced. Structural breakdown of the mucus was also observed by addition of sodium deoxycholate, sodium taurodeoxycholate, sodium glycocholate, and lysophosphatidylcholine. Duodenogastric reflux has been shown to disrupt the structure of the mucin network and subsequently cause gastric ulcer.[95]

Integrity of the mucin layer is also disrupted in some disease states, e.g., ulceration and inflammation of the intestine resulting in a thinning of the mucin layer, while thickening of the layer may lead to obstruction of bronchi, as in cystic fibrosis.[96] Intestinal mucin in cystic fibrosis is denser, more highly glycosylated, and probably contains more sulfate groups than normal intestinal mucin.[97] The thick secretion of mucus in cystic fibrosis may be explained by the obligatory reabsorption of water as a result of an intracellular calcium-stimulated increase in sodium reabsorption,[98] and an excess secretion of calcium from exocrine glands.[99] Furthermore, in normal human enteric microflora, bacterial enzymes are present,[100] which can degrade the mucin oligosaccharide side-chains extensively and the mucin polypeptide core to a lesser extent.[101,102] Thus, in developing mucoadhesive dosage forms, the presence or absence of a local disease state and location of application need to be considered.

III. PERTINENT BIOLOGICAL PARAMETERS

To set the stage for subsequent discussion of strategies for use of bioadhesives in oral drug delivery, basic physiological characteristics of the digestive tract will be presented. In this respect, permeability, enzymatic activity, and immunogenicity of the oral cavity, stomach, intestines, and rectal areas need to be considered. Enzymatic metabolism will be considered only in relation to peptides and proteins, due to their vulnerability to extensive enzymatic degradation, which results in the loss of most of the drug before or during the course of its transmembrane passage. This problem of degradation, although observed in membranes of all routes studied so far, is especially acute in the GIT where the peptide, in addition to mucosal activity, is also subject to luminal enzymatic activity.

A. ORAL CAVITY

The oral cavity forms a convenient and easily accessible site for delivery of drugs. Drugs can be absorbed from any of the mucosal tissues in the oral cavity; the sublingual (beneath the tongue) and buccal (between the cheek and gingiva) regions have been the most often used. The buccal route, apart from having the possibility of a lower enzymatic barrier to peptides, offers the advantages of avoiding hepatic first-pass metabolism and local intestinal enzymes and secretions. Insertion of dosage forms in the buccal area is convenient, allowing self-administration and a higher level of patient compliance than parenteral or rectal dosage forms. In addition, the microenvironment of the buccal cavity lends itself to modifications.

Substantial progress has been made in understanding structural features of the oral mucosa in recent years. The oral mucosa consists principally of two components, an epithelium and an underlying connective tissue. The epithelium of the human oral mucosa shows two distinct patterns of maturation, nonkeratinized and keratinized. Keratinized epithelium is a part of the mucosae of the hard palate and in parts of the dorsum of tongue and gingiva. Nonkeratinized epithelium forms the surface of the distensible lining of the soft palate, ventral surface of the tongue, floor of the mouth, alveolar mucosa, vestibule, lips, and cheek.[103] In the region of primary interest, the buccal area, the tissue is nonkeratinized epithelium.

1. Permeability of the Buccal Mucosa

Most buccal permeability studies suggest that the epithelium and its basal lamina constitute the major resistance barrier and that the lamina propria contributes little resistance to penetration.[104] Substances can cross the buccal epithelial membrane by the mechanisms of simple diffusion, carrier-mediated diffusion, active transport, and pinocytosis, although neither active transport nor pinocytosis have been demonstrated in the oral epithelium. Most permeability studies point towards simple diffusion, although evidence is accumulating that can be interpreted as demonstrating that carrier-mediated transport may also be a mechanism for transfer of solutes across the oral epithelium.

There is also evidence suggesting that there may be multiple barriers to diffusion of relatively large, hydrophilic substances, which are believed to traverse the oral epithelium through an intercellular pathway. The basal lamina may act as a barrier to the passage of insulin[105] and endotoxins.[106] A second barrier to penetration of large water-soluble molecules is believed to be extrusion into the intercellular region of membrane-coating granules.[107] Penetration of horseradish peroxidase has been demonstrated to be limited to the level of extrusion of the membrane-coating granules.[108] Its penetration was less limited when applied to epithelial cell cultures in which membrane coating granules are not formed.[109,110] Tolo and Jonsen[111] studied *in vitro* buccal permeation of dextrans of different molecular weights (16,000 to 250,000) in rabbits at 37°C. Their results show that dextrans up to a molecular weight of 70,000 or less can permeate the nonkeratinized oral mucosa of the rabbit within 2 h, although the amounts permeating were low.

More important, from a practical point of view, is the relative permeability of human skin, oral mucosa, and GIT, for all are important routes of drug administration. There is considerable evidence that for a number of drugs, absorption from the GIT is more rapid than absorption from either the skin or the oral mucosa.[112] Despite assertions that the oral mucosa is more permeable than skin, there appears to be little supporting evidence, and permeability of the oral mucosa to water and small ions has been shown to be the same as that of hydrated skin.[113,114] However, experimental conditions, type of buccal tissue, and animal model all influence buccal tissue permeability, and thus the above generalization is considered suspect.

2. Buccal Delivery of Peptides

A systematic study to explore the potential of the oral mucosa for delivery of peptides is yet to be reported. Some work is available in this regard and much of this centers around buccal delivery of insulin. Success in delivering insulin by this route has been variable, depending upon conditions used to deliver the peptide. Buccal absorption of insulin, with and without absorption enhancers, has been reported in healthy beagles.[114] In this study, an adhesive drug delivery system was developed for insulin delivery to the buccal mucosa, and blood glucose and plasma insulin levels were determined over a period of 6 h. It was found that by coadministration of sodium glycocholate, an absorption enhancer, a 40% reduction in blood glucose levels and a substantial increase in plasma insulin concentration were obtained, even though the plasma concentration of insulin achieved was only 0.5% of that obtained after i.m. injection. Use of insulin-containing liposomes in the buccal cavity of normal rats has been shown to produce a hypoglycemic effect.[115]

Sublingual delivery of insulin has been attempted with limited success.[116] The ratio of sublingual to subcutaneous dose to produce the same hypoglycemic effect in the dog has been reported to be about 15, while some workers have reported no hypoglycemic effect after a 20-fold sublingual dose of insulin compared to subcutaneous administration.[117] Thus the claims about delivery of insulin via the oral mucosa are variable and contradictory at this point. It has to be kept in mind that insulin, being a protein, exhibits unfavorable lipid solubility, and this can contribute to its limited absorption characteristics. Indeed it has been suggested that the poor therapeutic response elicited by insulin administered either perorally or by other routes is primarily due to poor absorption rather than degradation in the GIT or the liver,[118] although intuitively it is hard to believe that a protein-like insulin would survive the hostile environment of the gut lumen.

Other proteins, for which buccal delivery has been attempted, include papain, trypsin, alpha amylase, and oxytocin.[119] Success in all of the above cases has been limited. Among the factors likely to influence buccal delivery of peptides are the presence of mucosal secretions, immunological reactions, and activity of neutrophils, macrophages, and lymphocytes. As is evident from the existing literature, most efforts to deliver peptides/proteins via the oral mucosa have been directed towards large molecules. Taking into consideration buccal permeability, and the potential for enhancing this permeability, delivery of smaller peptides (2 to 10 amino acid residues) should be more promising.

3. Peptidase Activity in the Oral Mucosa

Unlike the intestinal mucosa, the oral mucosa has not been a subject of extensive investigation for proteolytic activity. Initial interest in this area came from physiologists and dentists and has been restricted for the most part to proteolytic activity in saliva, gingiva, and dental plaque.[120] In saliva, proteolytic activity is directly related to the content of epithelial cells.[121] Considering that most buccal delivery systems can be expected to be buccal patches, the oral lumen protease activity may not be of significance in relation to drug delivery.

Recently, there has been some work to characterize peptidase activity in the oral mucosa of rabbit. In these studies, aminopeptidases, a class of exopeptidases that cleave peptides/proteins at their N-terminus, have been the subject of considerable attention. Amino-peptidases have been shown to be widely distributed in various types of tissues, have broad substrate specificities, and have a primary role in terminating the activity of several neuropeptides.[119] Using 4-methoxy-2-naphthyl amides of leucine and alanine as substrates, Stratford and Lee have shown that the buccal mucosal activity of aminopeptidases is comparable to that of the ileal and duodenal aminopeptidases in albino rabbits.[122] This has also been demonstrated using enkephalin analogs.[123] On the other hand, when insulin and proinsulins were used as substrates, buccal protease activity was found to be four times less compared to the gut.[124] However, in all these studies, no effort was made to distinguish between extracellular and intracellular activities of the mucosa. While claiming from these studies that the bioavailability of certain peptides like enkephalins and insulin from the buccal mucosa is low because of peptidase activity, the authors have overlooked the fact that permeability studies of these peptides have not been conducted, and the observed low bioavailability may be attributed to slow absorption instead of metabolic degradation. In addition, since gut aminopeptidase activity has been used as the standard to measure activity from other tissues, caution must be exercised because the albino rabbit is being used as the animal model, which may not make a representative model for intestinal or buccal peptidase activity in man. None of the studies reported thus far have made any attempt towards separating cytosol and membrane bound peptidase activity in buccal tissue.

B. STOMACH AND INTESTINES

Oral dosage forms have been the most commonly used forms of drug delivery. Still, most formulations, intended to be swallowed, are based only on an empirical knowledge of the biology of the GIT. Recently, there have been efforts to better understand some of the key biological aspects of this route, e.g., transit. Movement of dosage forms through the stomach and intestines, which expose them to a variety of harsh conditions, such as pH, mucin content, variable permeability, enzymatic activity, and potential immunogenicity, makes this route complex for drug delivery.

1. Gastrointestinal Motility

An important factor to consider when contemplating the use of bioadhesives in the GIT is shear forces due to movement of the gut. This motility pattern, which is a characteristic feature of the GIT, can hinder initial attachment of polymer to the membrane or dislocate it after it has attached, either of which will defeat the purpose of the bioadhesive. Thus for bioadhesives to function as a delivery system in the GIT, a basic understanding of GI motility is required.

It is now well documented that there are two modes of GI motility patterns in man and animals, which consume food on a discrete basis: the digestive (fed) mode and the inter-digestive (fasted) mode. The characteristic of fasting GI motility is a cyclic pattern, which has been fully characterized in dog and man.[125,126] This cyclic pattern of motility, which originates in the foregut and propagates to the terminal ileum, can be divided into four distinctive phases: Phase I — representing a quiescent period with no electrical activity and no contractions; Phase II — the period of random spike activity or intermittent contractions; Phase III — the period of regular spike bursts or regular contractions at the maximal frequency that migrate distally; and Phase IV — the transition period between Phases III and I.[136] The average length of one complete cycle, commonly known as the interdigestive migrating motor complex (IMMC), ranges from 90 to 120 min in man. Certain disease conditions like bacterial overgrowth,[127] mental stress,[128] and diurnal variations,[129] or a combination of more than one of the above factors can affect the length of the total cycle or its individual phases. Phase III — also known as the housekeeper wave, — serves to clear the digestive tract of all indigestible materials from the stomach and small intestine. Nondigestible solids when administered during Phase I are emptied from the dog stomach only during Phase III.[130] Shear forces involved during this phase can pose a problem for bioadhesive systems in the GIT, consequently any system that is made to stay during the fasted mode must adhere to the membrane strongly enough to withstand the force of the housekeeper wave.

A characteristic feature of cyclic motor activity is its association with the secretory GI component. Gastric, pancreatic, and biliary secretory component of MMC in the human duodenum indicates that the migratory motor and secretory activity constitutes two aspects of the same periodicity.

The gastric, pancreatic, and biliary secretory components of MMC in the human duodenum indicates that migratory motor and secretory activity constitutes two aspects of the same periodic activity phenomenon.[126] It may be concluded that under fasting conditions, both motor and secretory activities of the stomach, gut, pancreas, and liver change period-ically to provide both mechanical and chemical means of intestinal housekeeping.

Feeding results in interruption of the interdigestive motility cycle of the GIT and in appearance of a continuous pattern of spike potentials and contractions, called postprandial motility. A minimum amount of gastric content appears to be necessary in order to change motility from an MMC to postprandial. Gupta and Robinson[131] have shown that oral admin-istration of 150 ml water during Phase I changes the fasted motor activity to a fed-like pattern in dogs. A normal meal changes the motility pattern to a fed state for up to 8 h depending upon caloric content of the food.[132]

2. Intestinal Permeability

Absorption in the GIT takes place predominantly in the small intestine because of a large surface area and high permeability of the lining membrane. The apical membrane of the absorptive cell microvilli in the small intestine lies under a mucin layer, whereas the absorptive cell basolateral membrane rests directly on the lamina propria. Since the epithelium of the intestinal membrane consists of only a single layer of loosely packed cells, permeability of this membrane is high. A variety of routes exist for drug and nutrient passage through this membrane. Drugs can pass directly through the cell membranes into the underlying blood vessels (transcellular) or permeate through the spaces between the cells (paracellular). Attempts have been made to correlate various physicochemical properties of molecules to determine their rate and predominant route of passage through intestinal tissue. For relatively lipophilic drugs, which permeate predominantly via the transcellular route, the pH partition hypothesis and the three aqueous compartment model generally explain the absorption characteristics, unless some active transport mechanism exists in the system. Small hydrophilic compounds are apparently absorbed through aqueous pores or channels formed by protein components in the membrane. There can be segmental differences in absorption of different kinds of drugs in the intestine, but most absorption takes place in the first half of the small intestine. One of these specialized areas of absorption, Peyer's patches, will be discussed in detail in Section IV.

3. Protein Absorption and Metabolism in the GI Mucosa

Intestinal degradation and absorption of peptides and proteins from the GIT has been the subject of intense investigation during the last three decades. It is now well established that the intestine is capable of absorbing intact small peptides from the gut lumen and can metabolize these peptides before delivering them to the blood or lymph. Initial studes in this area suggested that the size of peptides, which can be absorbed by the intestine, is restricted to two to three amino acid residues only,[133] but some recent studies have suggested that peptides with as many as six amino acid residues can be taken up by the microvillus membrane of the intestine.[134] This microvillus membrane contains several peptidases, among them aminopeptidases N and A, which have been extensively studied,[145] and are the only exopeptidases capable of hydrolyzing tetrapeptides, pentapeptides, and hexapeptides. By contrast, the cytoplasm of enterocytes lacks such enzymes, and is, therefore, capable of metabolizing only dipeptides and tripeptides. An active transport system for uptake of dipeptides and tripeptides by the brush border membrane of enterocytes has been discovered by some workers and outlined in a number of reviews.[114] Thus peptides consisting of up to six amino acid residues are taken up by the microvillus membrane of the intestine and degraded to di- and tripeptides, which are then subsequently taken up by enterocytes, metabolized to free amino acids and finally find their way to the portal blood. Some observations suggest that peptides are quantitatively a more important substrate for absorption sites in the intestine than are amino acids.[135] The hydrolysis of oligopeptides to amino acids requires aminopeptidases, which are present predominantly in the intestinal epithelium, and only in trace amounts in pancreatic secretions and the jejunal lumen. The intestinal epithelium, therefore, appears to be the principal site for terminal digestion of luminal peptides. Nevertheless, it is now well known by investigations in man and animals that a few small peptides that are unusually resistant to hydrolysis are capable of crossing the intestinal wall intact, especially when present in the intestinal lumen in high concentrations. Such peptides include gly-gly, peptides of proline and hydroxyproline, and dipeptides containing D-amino acids.[136]

The ability of the small intestine to absorb large intact proteins has been studied and reported. Molecules such as insulin, horseradish peroxidase,[137] and bovine serum albumin[138] have been shown to traverse the small intestine and appear in the portal blood, but only in trace amounts. Presumably the mechanism of absorption involves pinocytosis or uptake by specialized cells like Peyer's patches.

Peptidases of the intestine fall into two distinct groups: those of the cytosol and those of the brush border. About 90% of the total activity against dipeptides is found in the cytosol, and only about 10% in the brush border membrane, whereas, with some tripeptides, a larger proportion of the activity (up to 60%) is found in the brush border.[139] It is well established that there are morphological and functional differences between the jejunal and ileal segments of the small intestine and that the activity of the intestinal microvillus membrane peptidase is higher in jejunal than in ileal segments.[140] In contrast to peptidases of the brush border, those of the cytosol have been reported to have little or no activity against peptides of more than three amino acid residues.[141] Enzymes in both the brush border and cytosol are not very specific in their action, i.e., they are isozymes with overlapping specificities. The brush border amino-oligopeptidases that have been solubilized, purified, and characterized have been shown to be integral transmembrane glycoproteins.[142]

C. RECTAL AREA
1. Permeability of the Rectal Mucosa

Permeability characteristics of the colorectal area to drugs are quite different from both the oral cavity and small intestine. The primary function of the rectum is absorption of water. Most drugs and nutrients given orally are normally absorbed by the time the GI contents reach the rectal area. Also high viscosity of fecal matter can interfere with absorption of drugs and introduces considerable variability in bioavailability. Unlike the intestine, where a multitude of drug absorption mechanisms, including active transport for a number of drug categories, exist, rectal absorption is primarily a simple diffusion process through the lipid membrane, with no evidence yet of any carrier-mediated system.[143] Consequently, of the entire intestine, absorption via the rectal mucous membrane is most consistent with the pH partition theory.[144] It is, therefore, conceivable and usually observed that the absorption rates of most drugs increase with increasing solubility and release rate by vehicles.

One advantage of the rectal membrane is the degree to which it lends itself to be modulated by membrane-acting adjuvants to promote drug absorption. These adjuvants are more effective in promoting permeability through the rectal mucous membrane than in the upper GIT. A number of adjuvants acting on the membrane in various ways have been described[154] and will be discussed in detail in Section IV.

Due to relatively easy access to the absorptive membrane of the rectum, and the possibility of using membrane permeability enhancers, the potential of delivering drugs by the lymphatic route through this organ seem more promising than in the intestine. In the small intestine, most compounds, with the exception of cholesterol and a few other compounds, are absorbed primarily via blood. However, the distribution of drug to plasma and lymph from the rectal area has not been thoroughly explored. In one such study, the blood-lymph permselectivity to different molecular weight FITC (fluorescein isothiocyanate)-labeled dextrans (FD) was studied.[145] While the lymph vessels appeared to be independent of molecular weight, plasma levels of FD decreased with an increase in molecular weight, so that the lymph/plasma concentration ratio was more than unity for molecular weights higher than 10,000. This threshold for permselectivity was found to be about 17,000 in the intestine. Thus with the use of adjuvants, high molecular weight drugs may be delivered selectively into the lymphatic system via the rectal route.

2. Rectal Delivery of Peptides

Since the predominant mechanism of drug permeation through the rectal mucosa has been found to be by a transcellular route through the lipid membrane, peptides and proteins, due to their hydrophilic nature are expected to be absorbed only to a limited extent from the rectum. Studies have been carried out to investigate the possibility of delivering peptides via the rectal route. Once again, insulin has been the peptide studied. In most cases, some kind of adjuvant was necessary to achieve therapeutically significant concentrations of insulin in the plasma. Touiton et al.[146] reported a hypoglycemic effect in rats by administering insulin via the rectal route, in a dosage form containing surface active agents and polyethylene glycol. The effect of pH on the extent of insulin absorption, with or without adjuvants has been studied in diabetic rabbits.[147] Up to a 60% reduction in blood glucose level was observed from 100 U/Kg insulin suppositories without the presence of adjuvants. This hypoglycemic effect was observed under all pH conditions except at pH close to the isoelectric point of insulin. Of the various membrane permeability enhancers used as adjuvants in additional studies, an optimal effect was observed with the addition of 1% polyoxyethylene (9) lauryl alcohol ether, which gave plasma immunoreactive insulin levels comparable to those from i.v. and i.m. use. Other peptides studied for rectal delivery include pentagastrin and gastrin.[148] As before, systemic bioavailability was increased up to five times by sodium 5-methoxy-salicylate, a permeability enhancer.

There have been reports of the use of peptides/proteins as absorption promotors for drugs that are poorly absorbed from the rectum. Yata et al.[149] have reported enhanced blood levels of sodium ampicillin, following rectal administration in the presence of N-acyl derivatives of collagen.

3. Peptidase Activity of the Rectum

There has not been a systematic study to assess peptidase activity in the rectum. Since most protein from the diet is broken down and absorbed before it reaches the colorectal region, peptidase activity in the rectal lumen may be lower compared to that in the intestine. There have been some studies in rabbits where tissue homogenates of the rectum were compared with those of the intestine for peptidase activity in rabbits.[122,123] It was concluded that peptidase activity in the rectal mucosa is comparable to that in the small intestine. However, in all these studies, tissue homogenates were used, without any distinction between membrane-bound and cytosolic enzymes. Since most peptides/proteins may be absorbed primarily via the paracellular route, cytosolic activity may not play an important role in degradation. Therefore, if meaningful information is to be obtained about peptidase activity in the rectum, a distinction must be made between cytosolic and membrane-bound enzymatic activity.

D. IMMUNOLOGY OF THE GIT

The entire GIT is exposed to an immense and diverse range of potentially antigenic material, primarily from food, but also from a number of pathogenic and nonpathogenic microorganisms. In response to this antigenic challenge, the GIT is populated by an abundance of immunological elements, both as individual lymphoid cells and as organized lymphoid tissue.[150,151] Organized lymphoid aggregates have been collectively termed gut-associated lymphoid tissue (GALT). GALT are present primarily at two locations: near the basement of epithelial cells, where they are known as intraepithelial lymphocytes, and in loose connective tissue of the lamina propria. Rudzik et al.[152] have proposed that lymphoid tissue from all mucosal surfaces, i.e, the intestine, respiratory, and urinogenital tracts, together constitute a common mucosal system, in which IgA precurser cells originating from antigenic stimulation within mucosal tissue circulate and lodge. When challenged by an antigen, these cells produce IgA antibodies, which by virtue of their secretory component are able to traverse the epithelial layer and appear at the epithelial surface and in the lumen of the GIT. In mouse and rat, only IgA antibodies have been detected in gut; in man, plasma cells are mostly IgA, but there are some IgM and IgG cells. IgA antibodies are primarily responsible for providing an immunological barrier against mucosal penetration of antigens encountered by the GI tract.

1. Oral Cavity

GI immunology begins in the oral cavity. Interest in immunology of the oral cavity has come mainly from dental research. The lamina propria of oral mucosa contains a variety of immunological cells, including mast cells, macrophages, lymphocytes, and plasma cells.[153] While mast cells and macrophages are permanent residents of the oral mucosa, lymphocytes and plasma cells are transient visitors, arriving via the bloodstream. The presence of mast cells in the oral mucosa is important for a buccal patch delivery system, since any reaction to dosage form material can cause inflammation and irritation, resulting in involvement of plasma cells and subsequent immunological reaction.

2. Stomach and Intestines

It has been suggested that the stomach mucosa is involved in local specific immune responses.[154] However, there are no studies available on antigen absorption from this organ. In terms of nonspecific immune reactions, production of acid and pepsin is thought to denature most ingested antigens and bacteria and thus relieve the stomach of the necessity to have an active immune system.

The intestinal tract, consisting of the small intestine, cecum, and large intestine, has a well developed immune system that is both specific and nonspecific. A detailed discussion of this system is beyond the scope of this chapter, but two aspects of intestinal immunity are important in the context of drug delivery: the amount of IgA antibody in the gut lumen and epithelial surface, and antigen uptake mechanisms in intestine, and both will be discussed briefly.

IgA antibody in lamina propria of the intestinal mucosal layer as well as in the gut lumen is particularly suited to the role of a nonspecific immune element due to its relative stability towards proteolytic enzymes, its ability to bind to four antigens at the same time, and its tendency to bind to mucus. The mechanism by which IgA works is of a dual nature: it can bind to soluble antigen that has traversed the epithelial layer, and with the help of its secretory abilities, transport back antigenic molecules into the gut lumen, or it can bind and prevent absorption of antigens from the epithelial surface. This process of preventing absorption of antigen can be accomplished by agglutination with antigen, preventing the adherence, or associating it with mucin. In this respect, it acts to prevent entry of a macromolecule into the circulatory system.

Antigen uptake from various parts of the intestine is important not only from an immunological point of view, but also in the context of drug delivery, because it provides an opportunity to deliver large molecules, including peptides and proteins, provided they can be protected from degradation in the intestine and localized at the site of uptake. Two compartments through which antigen absorption might occur are the villous mucosa and Peyer's patches.[154] Peyer's patches will be discussed as potential sites for drug delivery in Section IV. Through the formation of pinocytotic vesicles at the base of the microvilli, the villous mucosa is able to absorb molecules as large as horseradish peroxidase and ferritin.[154] This process has also been implicated in maternal immunoglobin uptake by the neonate. However, the amounts absorbed are generally very small.

IV. STRATEGIES FOR DRUG DELIVERY

A. BUCCAL PATCH

The buccal route has been one of the areas studied as part of the effort to explore alternative administration routes that might be deficient in enzymatic degradation, particularly for peptides, and yet show acceptable permeability characteristics. Mention has already been made of studies to deliver peptides like insulin and oxytocin.[114,115,119] Schurr et al.[155] have reported the use of a self-adhesive patch containing 10 mg of thyrotropin-releasing hormone (TRH), which can be attached to buccal mucosa. A more prolonged TRH effect was observed after buccal administration compared to nasal and bolus injection, achieving plateau levels after 120 to 180 min. Although success has been claimed in delivering various peptides through the buccal mucosa, none of the blood concentrations achieved, from reasonable doses, have been close to therapeutically required levels. The reasons for the observed low bioavailability could be due either to low permeability of the tissue to peptides or high enzymatic activity. Both possible reasons for low bioavailability, i.e., tissue permeability and enzymatic activity, however, can be modified. Use of membrane permeability enhancers can not only facilitate the rate of drug penetration, but also may serve to protect it from degradation by reducing the exposure time to degrading enzymes in the membrane or providing an alternate route of penetration.

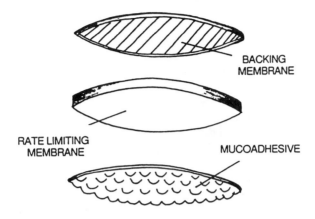

FIGURE 1. Proposed design of a unidirectional buccal patch.

1. Concept of a Unidirectional Patch

A successful bioadhesive buccal delivery system consists of a thin patch, which can be conveniently attached to the mucus membrane for extended periods of time. Since it will be designed to release the drug for absorption through the buccal membrane, it has to be unidirectional in its delivery, delivering the drug only from the side attached to the buccal membrane. One such patch has been reported by Veillard et al.[156] The patch is unidirectional consisting of three membranes: (1) a mucoadhesive basement membrane consisting of a bioadhesive polymer polycarbophil, (2) a rate-limiting center membrane containing the drug, and (3) an impermeable membrane facing the oral cavity. A schematic diagram of the patch is shown in Figure 1. This patch has been shown to stay on dog buccal mucosa for up to 17 h without any obvious discomfort, irrespective of food or drink consumed, and similar findings have been reported in humans. Adjuvants for inhibiting enzyme activity, suppressing immune reaction, or increasing membrane permeability can be incorporated into the center membrane. The polymer, due to swelling, will make a flexible network through which drug diffusion can occur.

2. Candidate Drug Criteria

One of the drug properties required for a practical buccal patch formulation will be high pharmacological activity or a low dose requirement. There is a limit to the size and thickness of the drug containing center layer, and only a limited amount of drug can be incorporated. In general, any drug with a daily requirement of 25 mg or less would make a good candidate. Other than dose considerations, the following properties will make a drug a suitable candidate for a buccal patch:

1. Relatively short biological half-life — Drugs with biological half-lives of 2 to 8 h will in general be good candidates for sustained release dosage forms.
2. Limited solubility/absorption from stomach or intestines — Drugs that are soluble, or able to permeate through the GI membrane, at a slow rate will be assured a constant concentration and membrane intimacy in the buccal patch. Adjuvants can also be used both to enhance solubility of the drug or to increase permeability of the membrane.
3. Drugs susceptible to degradation — Drugs susceptible to degradation either by the stomach/intestinal enzymes or by first pass liver metabolism will be assured protection in the buccal patch.

B. STOMACH AND INTESTINES

1. Stomach Adhesive

If a once-a-day oral dosage form for any drug is to be developed, it will be necessary for it to attach either in the stomach or in the intestine. A bioadhesive delivery system that adheres in the stomach will be able to provide a continuous dose of drug into the intestine for absorption for extended periods of time. However, there are a number of problems, as listed below, associated with development of an adhesive for the stomach.

1. Gastric motility will be a dislocating force for the adhesive. This motility is particularly strong during Phase III of the fasted state. During the fed state also, the stomach is in a state of continuous motility, with substantial retropulsive forces, particularly in the antral area. Only bioadhesives that bind strongly enough to withstand these shear forces will be practical.

2. Most of the adhesive polymers studied so far actually attach to the mucin layer on the mucosal membrane. In the stomach, the mucin turnover rate is substantial, both in the fed as well as in the fasted state. Thus the adhesive will attach to the mucus, and be detached along with the mucus when it is released from the membrane. Further attachment of polymer may not be possible because all active binding sites on it will be covered with mucin.

3. pH of stomach, which normally ranges between 1.5 and 3.0, may not be suitable for bioadhesion. This is not the case for the poly acid polymers such as cross-linked polyacrylic acid, where the predominant mechanism of bioadhesion is through hydrogen bond formation.

However, all of these problems can be overcome either by designing suitable polymers or by incorporating certain ingredients in the dosage form, which will modify conditions in the immediate vicinity of the dosage form to maximize bioadhesion. One approach would be to develop adhesive polymers that attach to the epithelial membrane, instead of mucin. Incorporation of a mucolytic agent in the formulation may create a mucosal free surface and attach to it, although it will raise the question of causing physical insult to the membrane or making it more susceptible to acid and enzymes in the stomach.

Similar problems can be anticipated in the intestine, but the pH may be more acceptable in this region. The key to success of a bioadhesive polymer in these areas seems to lie in an understanding of the adhesive phenomenon at a molecular level, to a degree that suitable adhesives can be designed to attach to specific areas in the GIT. This area of research is ongoing and needs to be pursued vigorously.

2. Peyer's Patches

Peyer's patches are organized mucosal lymphoid tissues of the gut and play an important function in regulating the immune response to orally presented antigens. They are generally larger and more numerous in the distal than in the proximal small intestine and are usually present on the antimesenteric circumference of the intestinal wall. Their size and number varies from species to species, being 18 to 26 in rat intestine[157] and up to 100 in man.[158] Peyer's patches consists of a collection of lymphoid follicles that occupy the full thickness of the small intestinal mucosa.

It is well documented that Peyer's patches are able to internalize particulate matter,[159] bacteria,[160] and marker proteins.[161] The general agreement is that soluble and colloidal substances enter Peyer's patches by vesicular transport through specialized epithelial cells. Some of the cells covering Peyer's patches have microfolds and have been called microfold or "M" cells. These cells have been demonstrated to be involved in antigen uptake[161] and serve as a satisfactory explanation for uptake of high molecular weight soluble and colloidal proteins.

Due to their capability of absorbing large molecules, Peyer's patches present a potential for delivery of macromolecules. The exact nature of the surface characteristics of these patches has not been fully understood yet, but if adhesive systems are to be devised to attach to or around them, a successful delivery system for large molecules may emerge.

3. Vaccines

Vaccines consist either of attenuated virus or bacteria particles, or some of their component proteins, being high molecular weight in either case. The proteinaceous nature of vaccines makes it very difficult for them to be administered orally since they stand little chance of escaping degrading enzymes of the GIT. However, if the potential of Peyer's patch to absorb high molecular weight compounds can be exploited, and suitable protection provided to vaccine components from intestinal enzymes, oral vaccine formulations can be successfully produced.

C. RECTAL DELIVERY

Bioadhesives in rectal dosage forms will be aimed at achieving better bioavailability by two strategies.

1. Maintenance in the Lower Third of the Rectum

The rationale for this approach comes from evidence suggesting that systematic availability of rectally administered drugs, particularly those that show significant first-pass metabolism, is dependent upon the site of absorption within the rectum, being maximal when the dosage form is close to the anus.[162] Therefore, despite substantial interindividual variability and differences between high clearance drugs, drugs should be administered and localized as close as possible to the anus in order to achieve maximal benefit of first-pass avoidance. This observation is usually explained in terms of venous blood drainage within the rectum; in the lower rectum, blood drains directly into the general circulation, whereas for the upper and middle rectal areas blood drains into the portal system and thus susceptible drugs undergo first-pass hepatic metabolism. Another advantage of keeping the dosage form in the lower third of the rectum is the possibility of avoiding interference from fecal matter.

Normally, a rectal suppository after insertion tends to gradually move higher and rest in the middle or upper third of the rectum. Bioadhesives can help attach the suppository to the mucin layer of the lower rectal area immediately after insertion and prevent its movement into the upper area. Such a formulation will consist of the suppository containing the drug, coated with a layer of bioadhesive on the outside. The bioadhesive can draw water from the mucin layer and the membrane and form a kind of a swollen matrix in which the drug can be trapped either as a single unit or multiunit particles.

Hosny has reported one such system for ketoprofen using polycarbophil as bioadhesive.[163] A less variable blood level appears to result when polycarbophil was added to sustained-release beads of ketoprofen in polyvinylacetate. One explanation for this observation can be that polycarbophil causes the particles to remain together with less dispersion in the rectal vault so that the surface area exposed to the rectal fluid is kept relatively constant. Thus an essentially constant rate of drug release occurs, which may be due to the fact that polycarbophil, as it attaches itself to the rectal tissue, serves as a diffusion barrier and helps modulate drug release. In addition, polycarbophil improves therapy by increasing the duration of action and bioavailability of the drug due to an increase in contact time and intimacy of contact of drug with the absorbing membrane. Figures 2 and 3 compare the plasma ketoprofen levels in humans from a commercial suppository and a sustained-release formulation containing 7% polycarbophil, each with 100 mg drug. An excellent *in vitro/in vivo* correlation was also obtained for this bioadhesive system (Figure 4).

2. Penetration Enhancement

A variety of penetration enhancers have been used as adjuvants in rectal suppositories

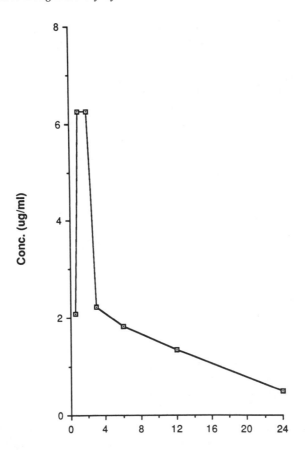

FIGURE 2.   Plasma ketoprofen levels in humans from a commercial suppository (100 mg). (From Hosny, E. A., Rectal Drug Delivery Using a Bioadhesive Containing Dosage Form, Ph.D. thesis, University of Wisconsin, Madison, 1988.)

to enhance membrane permeability. The adjuvants appear to significantly increase permeability of the barrier membrane to those solute species that tend to be hydrophilic.[164] The effect of these absorption promoters appears to be particularly evident for polar and/or macromolecular substances, indicating that they act primarily by enhancing the paracellular pathway.[164] This makes the use of these enhancers particularly attractive for delivering compounds of high molecular weight, e.g., proteins.

One class of adjuvants is the micelle-forming surfactant. A nonionic surfactant such as polysorbate is generally a mild, effective adjuvant that does not disrupt the rectal membrane. Another class of adjuvants is salicylates. Bioavailability of insulin has been reported to have been considerably improved by the use of sodium salicylate and 5-methoxysalicylate in dogs.[165] The rectal area is known to have a well-developed lymphatic system. One of the mechanisms of observed enhancement of macromolecular penetration could involve the uptake of these compounds by lymph, after they have been able to cross the epithelium. Thus the use of adjuvants can open another pathway for delivery of drugs by the rectal route.

Potential problems associated with the use of adjuvants are physical injury to the membrane, and other local or systemic side effects of such compounds. Since bioadhesives can improve the intimacy of a dosage form with the membrane, they can help reduce the concentration of adjuvants required for improving drug absorption. This improved contact

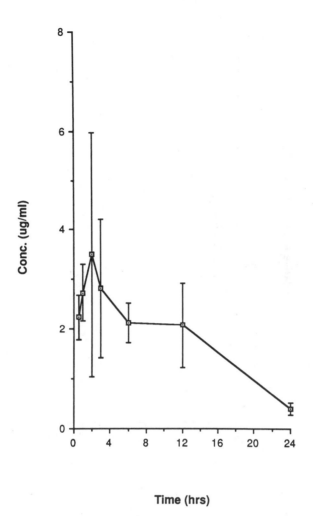

FIGURE 3. Plasma ketoprofen levels in humans from a sustained-release suppository containing 7% polycarbophil. (From Hosny, E. A., Rectal Drug Delivery Using a Bioadhesive Containing Dosage Form, Ph.D. thesis, University of Wisconsin, Madison, 1988.)

due to bioadhesives can work in two ways: increase the contact of adjuvant with membrane and increase the contact of drug to be absorbed, thus increasing the absorption rate.

V. SUMMARY

Bioadhesive oral dosage forms are desirable due to four main advantages over conventional dosage forms: (1) a longer GI transit time that may be sufficient to obtain once-a-day dosing; (2) ability to localize the dosage form in a particular area of the GIT, for drugs that show an absorption window, or to exploit some specialized areas of the small intestine, e.g., Peyer's patches for delivery of high molecular weight compounds, including proteins; (3) increase the intimacy of contact of the formulation with the absorptive membrane to improve bioavailability; and (4) develop dosage forms for use in the buccal and rectal areas where the potential for use of membrane modifiers also exists. Systematic studies have been under way for the last few years to understand three fundamental aspects of bioadhesives: (1) physicochemical properties and structure-activity correlations of bioadhesive polymers,

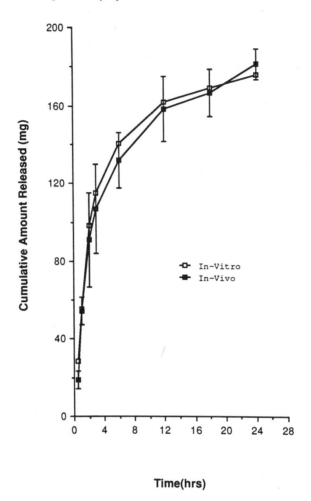

FIGURE 4.   Cumulative amount of ketoprofen released from a
sustained-release suppository containing 7% polycarbophil *in vitro*
and *in vivo* after rectal application during 24 h. (From Hosny,
E. A., Rectal Drug Delivery Using a Bioadhesive Containing Dosage Form, Ph.D. thesis, University of Wisconsin, Madison, 1988.)

(2) nature of bioadhesion in terms of molecular events at the interface between the bioadhesive
and the membrane, and (3) characterization of the biological membrane for various parameters including permeability, nature of the mucin layer covering the membrane, immunogenicity, and enzymatic activity. An understanding of these concepts will be helpful in
developing strategies for bioadhesive formulations for use in various parts of the GIT.

REFERENCES

1. **Nagai, T. and Machida, Y.,** Advances in drug delivery: mucosal adhesive dosage forms, *Pharm. Int.,* 6,
   196, 1985.
2. **Park, K., Cooper, S. L., and Robinson, J. R.,** Bioadhesive hydrogels, in, *Hydrogels in Medicine and
   Pharmacy,* Peppas, N. A., Ed., CRC Press, Boca Raton, FL, 1986.

3. **Park, H. and Robinson, J. R.,** Physico chemical properties of water insoluble polymers important to mucin/epithelial adhesion, *J. Controlled Release,* 2, 47, 1985.

4. **Peppas, N. A. and Buri, P. A.,** Surface, interfacial and molecular aspects of polymer bioadhesion on soft tissues, *J. Controlled Release,* 2, 257, 1985.

5. **Park, K. and Robinson, J. R.,** Bioadhesive polymers as platforms for oral-controlled drug delivery; method to study bioadhesion, *Int. J. Pharm.,* 19, 107, 1984.

6. **Ch'ng, H. S., Park, H., Kelly, P., and Robinson, J. R.,** Bioadhesive polymers as platforms for oral controlled drug delivery. II. Synthesis and evaluation of some swelling, water-insoluble bioadhesive polymers, *J. Pharm. Sci.,* 74, 399, 1985.

7. **Gurny, R., Meyer, J. M., and Peppas, N. A.,** Bioadhesive intraoral release systems: design, testing and analysis, *Biomaterials,* 5, 36, 1984.

8. **Boedeker, E. C., Ed.,** *Attachment of Organisms to the Gut Mucosa,* Vol. 1, CRC Press, Boca Raton, FL, 1984

9. **Savage, D. C.,** Localization of certain indigenous microorganism on the ileal villi of rats, *J. Bacteriol.,* 97, 1505, 1969.

10. **Hampton, J. C. and Rosario, B.,** The attachment of microorganisms to epithelial cells in the distal ileum of the mouse, *Lab. Invest.,* 14, 1464, 1965.

11. **Boedeker, E. C., Ed.,** *Attachment of Organisms to the Gut* Mucosa, Vol. 2, CRC Press, Boca Raton, FL, 1984.

12. **Cheney, C. P., Boedeker, E. G., and Formal, S. B.,** Quantitation of the adherence of an enteropathogenic *Escherichia coli* to isolated rabbit brush borders, *Infect. Innumol.,* 26, 736, 1979.

13. **Cheney, C. P., Schad, P. A., Formal, S. B., and Boedeker, E. C.,** Species specificity of *in-vitro Escherichia coli* adherence to host intestinal cell membranes and its correlation with *in-vivo* colonization and infectivity, *Infect. Immunol.,* 28, 1019, 1980.

14. **Machida, Y., Masuda, H., Fujiyama, N., Ito, S., Iwata, M., and Nagai, T.,** Preparation and Phase II clinical examination of topical dosage form for treatment of carcinoma colli containing bleomycin with hydroxypropyl cellulose, *Chem. Pharm. Bull.,* 27, 93, 1979.

15. **Machida, Y., Masuda, H., Fujuyama, N., Iwata, M., and Nagai, T.,** Preparation and Phase II clinical examination of topical dosage form for treatment of carcinoma colli containing bleomycin, carboquone, or 5-fluorouracil with hydroxypropyl cellulose, *Chem. Pharm. Bull.,* 28, 1125, 1980.

16. **Longer, M. A., Ch'ng, H. S., and Robinson, J. R.,** Bioadhesive polymers as platforms for oral controlled drug delivery. III. Oral delivery of chlorthiazide using a bioadhesive polymer, *J. Pharm. Sci.,* 74, 406, 1985.

17. **Bremecker, K.-D., Stempel, H., and Klein, G.,** Novel concept for a mucosal adhesive ointment, *J. Pharm. Sci.,* 73, 548, 1984.

18. **Schachter, H. and Williams, D.,** Biosynthesis of mucus glycoproteins, *Adv. Exp. Med. Biol.,* 144, 3, 1982.

19. **Allen, A. and Garner, A.,** Progress report: mucus and bicarbonate secretion in the stomach and their possible role in mucosal protection, *Gut,* 21, 249, 1980.

20. **Silberberg, A. and Meyer, F. A.,** Mucus in health and disease. II, in *Advances in Experimental Medicine and Biology,* Chantler, E. N., Elder, J. B., and Elstein, M., Eds., Plenum Press, New York, 1982, 53.

21. **Schmid, K.,** Isolation, characterization, and polymorphism of glycoproteins, in *Biochemistry of Glycoproteins and Related Substances, Part II,* Rossi, E. and Stoll, E., Eds., S. Karger, Basel, 1966.

22. **Gottschalk, A.,** Mucoproteins, mucopolysaccharides, and mucopolysaccharide-peptides: historical and general aspects, in *The Chemistry and Biology of Sialic Acid and Related Substances,* Cambridge University Press, London, 1960.

23. **Jeanloz, R. W.,** α-1 Acid glycoprotein, in *Glycoproteins, their Composition, Structure and Function,* Gottschalk, A., Ed., Elsevier, Amsterdam, 1972.

24. **Chantler, E. N. and Scudder, P. R.,** Terminal glycosylation in hyman cervical mucin, in *Mucus and Mucosa, Ciba Found. Symp.* 109, Pitman, London, 1984, 180.

25. **Beyer, T. A., Rearick, J. J., Paulson, J. C., Prieels, J. P., Sadler, J. E., and Hill, R. L.,** Biosynthesis of mammalian glycoproteins. Glycosylation pathways in the synthesis of the non-reducing terminal sequences, *J. Biol. Chem.,* 254, 12532, 1979.

26. **Johnson, P. M. and Rainsford, K. D.,** The physical properties of mucins, preliminary observations on the sedimentation behavior of porcine gastric mucin, *Biochim. Biophys. Acta,* 286, 72, 1972.

27. **Chen, J. L. and Cyr, G. N.,** Compositions producing adhesion through hydration, in *Adhesive Biological Systems,* Manly, R. S., Ed., Academic Press, New York, 1970, chap. 10.

28. **Smart, J. D., Kellaway, I. W., and Worthington, H. E. C.,** An in-vitro investigation of mucosa-adhesive materials for use in controlled drug delivery, *J. Pharm. Pharmacol.,* 36, 295, 1984.

29. U.S. Patent 3,202,577, Aug. 24, 1965.

30. **Park, H.,** On the Mechanism of Bioadhesion, Ph.D. thesis, University of Wisconsin, Madison, 1986.

31. **Barrer, R. M., Barrie, J. A., and Wong, P. S. L.,** The diffusion and solution of gases in highly crosslinked copolymers, *Polymer,* 9, 609, 1968.

32. **Park, K., Ch'ng, H. S., and Robinson, J. R.,** Alternative approaches to oral controlled drug delivery: bioadhesives and in-situ systems, in *Recent Advances in Drug Delivery Systems,* Anderson, J. M. and Kim, S. W., Eds., Plenum Press, 1984, 163.

33. **Flory, P. J.,** *Principles of Polymer Chemistry,* Cornell University Press, Ithaca, New York, 1953, 541.

34. **Peppas, N. A. and Reinhart, C. T.,** Solute diffusion in swollen membranes. I. A new theory, *J. Membr. Sci.,* 15, 275, 1983.

35. **Leung, S. H. S. and Robinson, J. R.,** The contribution of anionic polymer structural features to mucoadhesion, accepted by *J. Controlled Release,* 1987.

36. **Leung, S. H. S., Gu, J. M., and Robinson, J. R.,** Binding of polymer to mucin/epithelial surfaces: structure-property relationship, *CRC Crit. Rev. Ther. Drug Carrier Syst.,* 5, 21, 1988.

37. **Helfand, E. and Tagami, Y.,** Theory of the interface between immiscible polymers, *Polym. Lett.,* 9, 741, 1971.

38. **Helfand, E. and Tagami, Y.,** Theory of the interface between immiscible polymers. II, *J. Chem. Phys.,* 56, 3592, 1972.

39. **Helfand, E. and Tagami, Y.,** Theory of the interface between immisicible polymers, *J. Chem. Phys.,* 57, 1812, 1972.

40. **Voyutskii, S. S.,** *Autoadhesion and Adhesion of High Polymers,* John Wiley & Sons, New York, 1963.

41. **Bueche, F., Cashin, W. M., and Debye, P.,** The measurement of self-diffusion on solid polymers, *J. Chem. Phys.,* 20, p.1956, 1952.

42. **Campion, R. P.,** The influence of structure on autohesion (self-tack) and other forms of diffusion into polymers, *J. Adhes.,* 7, 1, 1974.

43. **Reinhart, C. T. and Peppas, N. A.,** Solute diffusion in swollen membranes. II. Influence of crosslinking on diffusion properties, *J. Membr. Sci.,* 18, 227, 1984.

44. **Deryaguin, B. V. and Smilga, V. P.,** *Adhesion: Fundamentals and Practice,* McLarer and Son, London, 1969, 152.

45. **Deryaguin, B. V., Toporov, Y. P., Mueler, V. M., and Aleinikova, I. N.,** On the relationship between the electrostatic and molecular components of the adhesion of elastic particles to a solid surface, *J. Colloid Interface Sci.,* 58, 528, 1977.

46. **Kinloch, A. J.,** The science of adhesion. I. Surface and interfacial aspects, *J. Mater. Sci.,* 15, 2141, 1980.

47. **Huntsberger, J. R.,** Mechanisms of adhesions, *J. Paint Technol.,* 39, 199, 1967.

48. **Good, R. J.,** Surface free energy of solids and liquids: thermodynamics, molecular forces and structure, *J. Colloid Interface Sci.,* 58, 398, 1977.

49. **Tabor, D.,** Surface forces and surface interactions, *J. Colloid Interface Sci.,* 58, 2, 1977.

50. **Singer, S. J. and Nicolson, G. L.,** The fluid mosaic model of the structure of cell membranes, *Science,* 175, 720, 1972.

51. **Gristina, A. G., Oga, M., Webb, L. X., and Hobgood, C. D.,** Adherent bacterial colonization in the pathogenesis of osteomyelitis, *Science,* 228, 990, 1983.

52. **Ito, I.,** Structure and function of the glycocalyx, *Fed. Proc.,* 28, 12, 1969.

53. **Rauvala, H.,** Cell surface carbohydrates and cell adhesion, *Trends Biochem. Sci.,* 323, 1983.

54. **Jones, G. W.,** The attachment of bacteria to the surface of animal cells, in *Microbial Interaction,* Reissig, J. L., Ed., Chapman & Hall, London, 1977, 139.

55. **Brogden, R. N., Heel, R. C., Speight, T. M., and Avery, G. S.,** Sucralfate: a review of its pharmacodynamic properties and therapeutic use in peptic ulcer disease, *Drugs,* 27, 194, 1984.

56. **Nagashima, R. and Hirano, T.,** Selective binding of sucralfate to ulcer lesion. I. Experiments in rats with acetic acid-induced gastric ulcer receiving unlabelled sucralfate, *Arzneim. Forsch./Drug Res.,* 30, 80, 1980.

57. **Steiner, K., Buhring, K. U., Faro, H. P., Garbe, A., and Nowak, H.,** Sucralfate: pharmacokinetics, metabolism and selective binding to experimental gastric and duodenal ulcers in animals, *Arzneim. Forsch./ Drug Res.,* 32, 512, 1982.

58. **Nagashima, R.,** Development and characteristics of sucralfate, *J. Clin. Gastroenterol.,* 3, 103, 1981.

59. **Nagashima, R. and Yoshida, N.,** Sucralfate, a basic aluminum salt of sucrose sulfate. I. Behavior in gastroduodenal pH, *Arzneim. Forsch.,* 29, 1668, 1979.

60. **Wright, T. C., Smith, B., Ware, B. R., and Karnovsky, M. J.,** The role of negative charge in spontaneous aggregation of transformed and untransformed cell lines, *J. Cell Sci.,* 45, 49, 1980.

61. **Deman, J. J. and Bruyneel, E. A.,** Intercellular adhesiveness and neuraminidase effect following release from density inhibition of cell growth, *Biochem. Biophys. Res. Commun.,* 62, 895, 1975.

62. **Massa, S. and Bosmann, H. B.,** Cellular adhesion: description, methodology and drug perturbation, *Pharmacol. Ther.,* 21, 101, 1983.

63. **Snyder, E. L. and Luban, N. L. C.,** Fibronectin: application to clinical medicine, *CRC Crit. Rev., Clin. Lab. Sci.,* 23, 15, 1986.

64. **Massa, S. and Bosmann, H. B.**, Cellular adhesion: description, methodology and drug perturbation, *Pharmacol. Ther.*, 21, 101, 1983.

65. **Edelman, G. M.**, Cell adhesion molecules, *Science*, 219, 450, 1983.

66. **Hedman, K., Vaheri, A., and Wartiovaara, J.**, External fibronectin of cultured human fibroblasts is predominantly matrix protein, *J. Cell Biol.*, 67, 748, 1978.

67. **Vaheri, A. and Mosher, D. F.**, High molecular weight, cell surface associated glycoprotein (fibronectin) lost in malignant transformation, *Biochem. Biophys. Acta*, 516, 1, 1978.

68. **Yamada, K. M. and Olden, K.**, Fibronectins: adhesive glycoproteins of cell surface and blood, *Nature*, 275, 179, 1978.

69. **Dessau, W., Jilek, F., Adelman, B. C., and Hormann, H.**, Similarity of antigelatin factor and cold insoluble globulin, *Biochim. Biophys. Acta*, 533, 227, 1978.

70. **Engvall, E. and Ruoslahti, E.**, Binding of soluble form of fibroblast surface protein, fibronectin, to collagen, *Int. J. Cancer*, 20, 1, 1977.

71. **Stathakis, N. E. and Mosesson, M. W.**, Interaction among heparin, cold insoluble globulin, and fibrinogen in formation of the heparin-precipitate fraction of plasma, *J. Clin. Invest.*, 60, 855, 1977.

72. **Grinell, F.**, Cellular adhesiveness and extracellular substrata, *Int. Rev. Cytol.*, 58, 65, 1978.

73. **Hughes, R. C., Pena, S. D. J., Clark, J., and Dourmashskin, R. R.**, Molecular requirements for the adhesion and spreading of hamster fibroblasts, *Exp. Cell Res.*, 121, 307, 1979.

74. **Ruoslahti, E., Pierschbacher, M. D., Oldberg, A., and Hayman, E. G.**, Synthetic peptides causing cellular adhesion to surfaces, *Biotechniques*, 2, 38, 1984.

75. **Mosher, D. F.**, Physiology of fibronectin, *Annu. Rev. Med.*, 35, 561, 1984.

76. **Pierschbacher, M., Hayman, E. G., and Ruoslahti, E.**, Synthetic peptide with cell attachment activity of fibronectin, *Proc. Natl. Acad. Sci. U.S.A.*, 80, 1224, 1983.

77. **Pierschbacher, M. D. and Ruoslahti, E.**, Cell attachment activity of fibronectin can be duplicated by small synthetic fragments of the molecule, *Nature*, 309, 30, 1984.

78. **Humphries, M. J., Olden, K., and Yamada, K. M.**, A synthetic peptide from fibronectin inhibits experimental metastasis of murine melanoma cells, *Science*, 233, 467, 1986.

79. **McCoy, J. P., Jr.**, Contemporary laboratory applications of lectins, *Biotechniques*, 4, 252, 1986.

80. **Barondes, S. H.**, Soluble lectins: a new class of extracèllular proteins, *Science*, 223, 1259, 1984.

81. **Marchalonis, J. J. and Edelman, G. M.**, Isolation and characterization of a hemagglutinin from Limulus polyphemus, *J. Molec. Biol.*, 32, 453, 1968.

82. **Nowak, T. P. and Barondes, S. H.**, Agglutinin from Limulus polyphemus, purification with formalinized horse erythrocytes as the affinity adsorbent, *Biochim. Biophys. Acta*, 393, 115, 1975.

83. **Bishayee, S. and Dorai, D. T.**, Isolation and characterization of a sialic acid-binding lectin (carcinoscoporin) from indian horseshoe crab Carcinoscoporus rotunda cauda, *Biochim. Biophys. Acta*, 623, 89, 1980.

84. **Miller, R. L., Colawn, J. F., Jr., and Fish, W. W.**, Purification and macromolecular properties of a sialic acid-specific lectin from the slug Limax flavus, *J. Biol. Chem.*, 257, 7574, 1982.

85. **Iguchi, S. M. M., Momoi, T., Egawa, K., and Matsumoto, J. J.**, An N-acetylneuraminic acid-specific lectin from the body surface mucus of african giant snail, *Comp. Biochem. Physiol.*, 81B, 897, 1985.

86. **Neufeld, E. F. and Ashwell, G.**, in *The Biochemistry of Glycoproteins and Proteoglycans*, Lennarz, W. J., Ed., Plenum, New York, 1980, 241.

87. **Marriott, C., Shih, C. K., and Litt, M.**, Changes in the gel properties of tracheal mucus induced by divalent cations, *Biorheology*, 16, 331, 1979.

88. **Martin, G. P., Marriott, C., and Kellaway, I. W.**, The interaction of steroidal hormones with mucus glycoproteins, *J. Pharm. Pharmacol.*, 30(Suppl.), 10P, 1978.

89. **Bettelheim, F. A.**, On the aggregation of a calcium precipitate glycoprotein from human submaxillary saliva, *Biochim. Biophys. Acta*, 236, 702, 1971.

90. **Boat, T. F., Wiesman, U. N., and Pallavicini, J. C.**, Purification and properties of the calcium-precipitable protein in submaxillary saliva of normal and cystic fibrosis subjects, *Pediatr. Res.*, 8, 531, 1974.

91. **Forstner, J. F. and Forstner, G. G.**, Calcium binding to intestinal goblet cell mucin, *Biochim. Biophys. Acta*, 386, 283, 1975.

92. **Leung, S. H. S. and Robinson, J. R.**, unpublished data.

93. **Barbieri, E. J.**, Mucolytics, *AFP Clin. Pharmacol.* 28, 175, 1983.

94. **Marriott, C.**, The effect of drugs on the structure and secretion of mucus, *Pharm. Int.*, 4, 320, 1983.

95. **Martin, G. P., Marriott, C., and Kellaway, I. W.**, Direct effect of bile salts and phospholipids on the physical properties of mucus, *Gut*, 19, 103, 1978.

96. **Forstner, G., Sturgess, J., and Forstner, J.**, Malfunction of intestinal mucus and mucus production, *Adv. Exp. Med. Biol.*, 89, 349, 1977.

97. **Wesley, A., Forstner, J., Qureshi, R., Mantle, M., and Forstner, G.**, Human intestinal mucin in cystic fibrosis, *Pediatr. Res.*, 17, 65, 1983.

98. **Jorscher, E. J. and Breslow, J. L.**, Cystic fibrosis: a disorder of calcium-stimulated secretion and transepithelial sodium transport?, *Lancet*, p. 368, February 13, 1982.

99. **Gibson, L. E., Matthew, W. J., Jr., Minihan, P. T., and Patti, J. A.**, Relating mucus, calcium, and sweat in a new concept of cystic fibrosis, *Pediatrics*, 48, 695, 1971.

100. **Miller, R. S. and Hoskins, L. C.**, Mucin degradation in human colon ecosystems. Fecal population densities of mucin-degrading bacteria estimated by a "most probable number" method, *Gastroenterology*, 81, 759, 1981.

101. **Hoskins, L. C. and Zamcheck, N.**, Bacterial degradation of gastrointestinal mucins. I. Comparison of mucus constituents in the stools of germ-free and conventional rats, *Gastroenterology*, 54, 210, 1968.

102. **Variyam, E. P. and Hoskins, L. C.**, Mucin degradation in human colon ecosystems. Degradation of hog gastric mucin by fecal extracts and fecal cultures, *Gastroenterology*, 81, 751, 1981.

103. **Bennett, H. S.**, Morphological aspects of extracellular polysaccharides, *J. Histochem. Cytochem.*, 11, 14, 1963.

104. **Siegel, I. A.**, Permeability of the oral mucosa, in *The Structure and Function of Oral Mucosa*, Meyer, J., Squier, C. A., and Gerson, S. J., Eds., Pergamon Press, Oxford, 1984.

105. **Alfano, M. C., Chasens, A. I., and Masi, C. W.**, Autoradiographic study of the penetration of rediolabeled dextrans and insulin through non-keratinized oral mucosa *in-vitro*, *J. Periodont. Res.*, 12, 368, 1977.

106. **Alfano, M. C., Drummond, J. F., and Miller, S. A.**, Techniques for studying the dynamics of oral mucosal permeability *in-vitro*, *J. Dent. Res.*, 54, 1143, 1975.

107. **Squier, C. A.**, Membrane coating granules in non-keratinizing oral epithelium, *J. Ultrastruct. Res.*, 60, 212, 1977.

108. **Hill, M. W. and Squier, C. A.**, The permeability of rat palatal mucosa maintained in organ culture, *J. Anat.*, 128, 169, 1979.

109. **Squier, C. A., Fejerskov, O., and Jepsen, A.**, The permeability of a keratinizing squamus epithelium in culture, *J. Anat.*, 126, 103, 1978.

110. **Fejerskov, O., Theildale, J., and Jepsen, A.**, Ultrastructure of rat oral epithelium in long term cell culture, *Scand. J. Dent. Res.*, 82, 212, 1974.

111. **Tolo, K. and Jonsen, J.**, *In-vitro* penetration of tritiated dextrans through rabbit oral mucosa, *Arch. Oral. Biol.*, 20, 419, 1975.

112. **Squier, C. A. and Johnson, N. W.**, Permeability of oral mucosa, *Br. Med. Bull.*, 31, 169, 1975.

113. **Keaber, S.**, The permeability and barrier functions of the oral mucosa with respect to water and electrolytes (thesis), *Acta. Odontol. Scand.*, Suppl. 66, 1974.

114. **Mathews, D. M. and Adibi, S. A.**, Peptide absorption, *Gastroenterology*, 71, 151, 1976.

115. **Weingarten, C., Moufti, A., Desjuex, J. F., Luong, T. T., Durand, G., Devisagguet, J. P., and Puisieux, F.**, Oral ingestion of insulin liposomes: effect of the administration route, *Life Sci.*, 28, 2747, 1981.

116. **Mofat, A. C.**, Absorption of drugs through the oral mucosa, in *Absorption Phenomenon*, Vol. 4, Robinowitz, J. L. and Meyerson, R. M., Eds., John Wiley & Sons, New York, 1971, 1.

117. **McCullogh, E. P. and Lewis, L. A.**, Comparison of effectiveness of various methods of administration of insulin, *J. Clin. Endocrinol.*, 2, 435, 1942.

118. **Gibaldi, M. and Kanig, K. L.**, Absorption of drugs through the oral mucosa, *J. Oral Ther. Pharmacol.*, 1, 440, 1965.

119. **Lee, V. H. L.**, Peptide and protein drug delivery: opportunities and challenges, *Pharm. Int.*, 7, 208, 1986.

120. **Soder, P. O.**, Proteolytic activity in the oral cavity: protelytic enzymes from human saliva and dental plaque material, *J. Dent. Res.*, 51, 389, 1972.

121. **Watanabe, T., Ohato, N., Morishita, M., and Iwamoto, Y.**, Correlation between the protease activities and the number of epithelial cells in human saliva, *J. Dent. Res.*, 60, 1039, 1981.

122. **Stratford, R. E. and Lee, V. H. L.**, Aminopeptidase activity in homogenates of various absorptive mucosae in the albino rabbit: implications in peptide delivery, *Int. J. Pharm.*, 30, 73, 1986.

123. **Kashi, S. D. and Lee, V. H. L.**, Enkephalin hydrolysis in homogenates of various absorptive mucosae of the albino rabbit: similarity in rates and involvement of aminopeptidases, *Life Sci.*, 38, 2019, 1986.

124. **Hayakawa, E. J., Chien, D. S., and Lee, V. H. L.**, Mucosal peptide delivery: susceptibility of insulin and proinsulin to proteolysis and protection from proteolysis by glycocholate, Poster PD-148, American Association of Pharmaceutical Scientists Meeting, Boston, 1987.

125. **Szurszewski, J. H.**, A migrating electric complex of the canine small intestine, *Am. J. Physiol.*, 217, 1757, 1969.

126. **Konturek, S. J.**, Gastrointestinal hormones and intestinal motility: characteristics of gut hormonal peptides affecting intestinal motility, in *Gastrointestinal Motility: Proc. 9th Int. Symp. Gastrointestinal Motility*, Roman, C., Ed., MTP Press, Boston, 1984, 593.

127. **Grivel, M.-L. and Ruckebusch, Y.**, The propagation of segmental contractions along the small intestine, *J. Physiol.*, 227, 611, 1972.

128. **McCree, S., Younger, K., Thompson, D. G., and Wingate, D. L.,** Sustained mental stress alters human jejunal motor activity, *Gut,* 23, 404, 1982.

129. **Ritchie, H. D., Thompson, D. G., and Wingate, D. L.,** Diurnal variation in human jejunal fasting motor activity, *Proc. Physiol. Soc.,* 1980, 54.

130. **Gruber, P., Rubinstein, A., Li, V. H. K., Bass, P., and Robinson, J. R.,** Gastric emptying of non-digestible solids in the fasted dog, *J. Pharm. Sci.,* 76, 117, 1987.

131. **Gupta, P. K. and Robinson, J. R.,** Gastric emptying of liquids in the fasted dog, *Int. J. Pharm.,* 43, 45, 1988.

132. **Kerlin, P. and Phillips, S.,** Variability of motility of the ileum and jejunum in healthy humans, *Gastroenterology,* 82, 694, 1982.

133. **Adibi, S. A. and Phillips, E.,** Evidence for greater absorption of amino acids from peptides than from free form in human intestine, *Clin. Res.,* 16, 446, 1968.

134. **Semeriva, M., Varesi, L., and Gratecos, D.,** Studies on transport of amino acids from peptides by rat small intestine *in-vitro* synthesis, properties and uptake of a photosensitive tetrapeptide, *Eur. J. Biochem.,* 122, 619, 1982.

135. **Adibi, S. A. and Mercer, D. W.,** Protein digestion in human intestine as reflected in luminal, mucosal, and plasma amino acid concentrations after meals, *J. Clin. Invest.,* 52, 1586, 1973.

136. **Newey, H. and Smyth, D. H.,** The intestinal absorption of some dipeptides, *J. Physiol.,* 145, 48, 1959.

137. **Walker, W. A., Cornell, R., and Davenport, L. M.,** Macromolecular absorption: mechanism of horse-radish peroxidase uptake and transport in adult and neonatal rat intestine, *J. Cell Biol.,* 54, 195, 1975.

138. **Warshaw, A. L., Walker, W. A., and Isselbacher, K. J.,** Protein uptake by the intestine: evidence for absorption of intact macromolecules, *Gastroenterology,* 66, 987, 1974.

139. **Peter, T. J.,** The subcellular localization of di- and tri-peptide hydrolase activity in guinea pig small intestine, *Biochem. J.,* 120, 195, 1970.

140. **Peter, T. J., Donlon, J., and Fottrell, P. F.,** The subcellular localization and specificity intestinal peptide hydrolases, in *Transport Across the Intestine,* Burland, W. L. and Samuel, P. D., Eds., Churchill Livingstone, Edinburgh, 1972, 153.

141. **Asatoor, A. M., Chadha, A., and Milne, M. D.,** Intestinal absorption of stereosiomers of dipeptides in the rat, *Clin. Sci. Mol. Med.,* 45, 199, 1973.

142. **Harrison, D. D. and Webster, H. L.,** Proximal to distal variations in enzymes of rat intestine, *Biochim. Biophys. Acta,* 244, 432, 1971.

143. **Binder, H. J.,** Amino acid absorption in the mammalian colon, *Biochim. Biophys. Acta,* 219, 503, 1970.

144. **Muranishi, S.,** Characteristics of drug absorption via the rectal route, *Methods Findings Exp. Clin. Pharmacol.,* 6, 763, 1984.

145. **Yoshikawa, H., Muranishi, S., and Sazeki, H.,** Development of bifunctional delivery system for selective transfer of drug into lymphatics via enteral route and transfer mechanism, *J. Pharmacobio. Dyn.,* 5, 569, 1982.

146. **Touiton, E., Donbrow, M., and Azaz, E.,** New hydrophilic vehicle enabling rectal and vaginal absorption of insulin, heparin, phenol red and gentamicin, *J. Pharm. Pharmacol.,* 30, 662, 1978.

147. **Icidawa, K., Ohata, I., Mitomi, M., Kawamura, S., Maeno, H., and Kawata, H.,** Rectal absorption of insulin suppositories in rabbits, *J. Pharm. Pharmacol.,* 32, 314, 1980.

148. **Yoshioka, S., Caldwell, L., and Huguchi, T.,** Enhanced rectal bioavailability of polypeptides using sodium 5-methoxysalicylate as an absorption promoter, *J. Pharm. Sci.,* 71, 593, 1982.

149. **Yata, N., Wu, W. M., Yamajo, R., Murkami, T., Higashi, Y., and Higuchi, T.,** Enhanced rectal absorption of sodium ampicillin by N-acyl derivatives of collagen peptide in rabbits and rats, *J. Pharm. Sci.,* 74, 1058, 1985.

150. **Guy-Grand, D.,** Gut associated lymphoid system, in *Immunology,* Bach, J.-F., Ed., John Wiley & Sons, New York, 1982, 31.

151. **Kagnoff, M. F.,** Immunology of the digestive system, in *Physiology of the Gastrointestinal Tract,* Johnson, L. R., Ed., Raven Press, New York, 1982, 1337.

152. **Rudzik, O., Clancy, R. L., Perey, D. Y. E., and Day, R. P., and Bienenstock, J.,** Repopulation with IgA-containing cells of bronchial and intestinal lamina propria after transfer of homologous Peyer's patch and bronchial lymphocytes, *J. Immunol.,* 114, 1599, 1975.

153. **Willoughby, S. G.,** Mast cells, macrophages and mononuclear inflammatory cells, in *The Structure and Function of Oral Mucosa,* Meyer, J., Squier, C. A., and Gerson, S. J., Eds., Pergamon Press, New York, 1984, 179.

154. **Mayrhofer, G.,** Physiology of the intestinal immune system, in *Local Immune Responses of the Gut,* Newby, T. J. and Stokes, C. R., Eds., CRC Press, Boca Raton, FL, 1984, 1.

155. **Schurr, W., Knoll, B., Ziegler, R., Anders, R., and Merkle, H. P.,** Comparative study of intravenous, nasal, oral and buccal TRH administration among healthy subjects, *J. Endocrinol. Invest.,* 8, 41, 1985.

156. **Veillard, M. M., Longer, M. A., Martens, T. W., and Robinson, J. R.,** Preliminary studies of oral mucosal delivery of peptide drugs, paper presented at the 3rd Int. Symp. Recent Advances in Drug Delivery Systems, Salt Lake City, February 24 to 27, 1987.

157. **Hummel, K. P.,** The structure and development of the lymphatic tissue in the intestine of the albino rat, *Am. J. Anat.,* 57, 351, 1935.

158. **Good, R. A. and Finstad, J.,** The phylogenetic development of the immune responses and the germinal center system, in *Germinal Centers in Immune Response,* Cottier, H., Odartchenko, N., Schindler, R., and Congdon, C. C., Eds., Springer-Verlag, Berlin, 1967, 4.

159. **Bockman, D. E. and Cooper, M. D.,** Pinocytosis by epithelium associated with lymphoid follicles in the bursa of fabricus, appendix and Peyer's patches. An electron microscopic study, *Am. J. Anat.,* 136, 455, 1973.

160. **Shimizu, Y. and Andrew, W.,** Studies on the rabbit appendix. I. Lymphocytoepithelial relations and the transport of bacteria from lumen to lymphoid nodule, *J. Morphol.,* 123, 231, 1967.

161. **Owen, R. L.,** Sequential uptake of horseradish peroxidase by lymphoid follicle epithelium of Peyer's patches in the normal unobstructed mouse intestine: an ultrastructural study, *Gastroenterology,* 72, 440, 1977.

162. **De Leede, L. G. J., DeBoer, A. G., Roozen, C. P. J. M., and Breimer, D. P.,** Avoidance of first-pass elimination of rectally administered lidocaine in relation to the site of absorption in rats, *J. Pharmacol. Exp. Ther.,* 225, 181, 1983.

163. **Hosny, E. A.,** Rectal Drug Delivery Using a Bioadhesive Containing Dosage Form, Ph.D. thesis, University of Wisconsin, Madison, 1988.

164. **Kamada, A., Nishihata, T., Kim, S., Yamamoto, M., and Yata, N.,** Effect of enamine derivatives of phenylglycine on the rectal absorption of insulin, *Chem. Pharm. Bull.,* 29, 2012, 1981.

165. **Nishihata, T., Rutting, J. H., Kamada, A., Huguchi, T., Routh, M., and Caldwell, L.,** Enhancement of rectal absorption of insulin using salicylates in dogs, *J. Pharm. Pharmacol.,* 35, 148, 1983.

Chapter 5

NANOPARTICLES AS A GASTROADHESIVE DRUG DELIVERY SYSTEM

V. Lenaerts, P. Couvreur, L. Grislain, and Ph. Maincent

TABLE OF CONTENTS

I. INTRODUCTION

Previous studies, many of which are reported in this volume, show that important efforts have been made in developing efficient bioadhesive peroral dosage forms.

The main interest in such dosage forms results from their ability to enhance the bioavailability of drugs impaired by a narrow absorption window in the upper intestinal tract.

Indeed, these drugs usually enter the duodenum in a high concentration and move along the intestinal tract in such a short transit time that an important part of the drug remains in the intestinal lumen beyond the absorption window and thus loses any chance to cross the wall and enter the blood compartment. This problem is even more dramatic when the drug displays poor water solubility for, in this case, part of the administered dose might even move along the duodenum and jejunum in a nondissolved state.

Obviously, for these compounds, the best chances of improvement in the bioavailability would come from a dosage form allowing a slow release of the drug in the upper gastrointestinal tract (GIT) so that low concentrations of the drug would be allowed to move along the duodenum over a prolonged period of time.

It is also preferable that such dosage forms be specifically adhesive to the stomach, since a prolongation of the residence time in the intestine could result in discomfort for the patient.

Such a specificity can be achieved, i.e., through the difference in the pH of the encountered fluids.

For this reason, most of the studies devoted to the development of gastroadhesive dosage forms start by a selection of the polymer on the basis of its mucoadhesive properties, which, ideally, should be as elevated as possible in acidic conditions and much lower in a neutral medium so that the intestinal transit would not be impaired.

The proper pharmacotechnological work — consisting mainly of evaluating the influence of the characteristics of the different dosage forms obtainable with the selected polymer on such variables as mucoadhesive behavior, drug release kinetics, toxicity of the system, compliance of the patients — is often given less attention and considered as relatively secondary.

In this chapter a somewhat different approach is reported.

Indeed, the bioadhesive material used has been primarily developed as a colloidal drug-targeting system and has, therefore, been extensively studied regarding morphology, drug adsorption potential, drug release kinetics, degradation pathway, body-distribution and elimination, toxicity, and other factors, and has shown a realistic potential as a controlled-release drug dosage form.

The rationale for evaluating this drug carrier — polyalkylcyanoacrylate nanoparticles — as a mucoadhesive system results from the somewhat theoretical consideration that a polymer possessing a cyano-group on the side has a good probability of developing bonds with a mucin gel. Furthermore, owing to their colloidal nature, it was very unlikely that nanoparticles adhering to the stomach mucus would be unevenly dispersed and would concentrate in specific spots.

Possible problems associated with the prolonged residence of elevated quantities of a potentially deleterious drug in a precise area of the stomach wall would then obviously be avoided.

II. POLYALKYLCYANOACRYLATE NANOPARTICLES

The nanoparticles are prepared by polymerization of alkylcyanoacrylate monomers emulsified in an acidic aqueous medium containing protective polymers such as dextran (mol wt. 70,000) aimed at avoiding adhesion between the particles.[1]

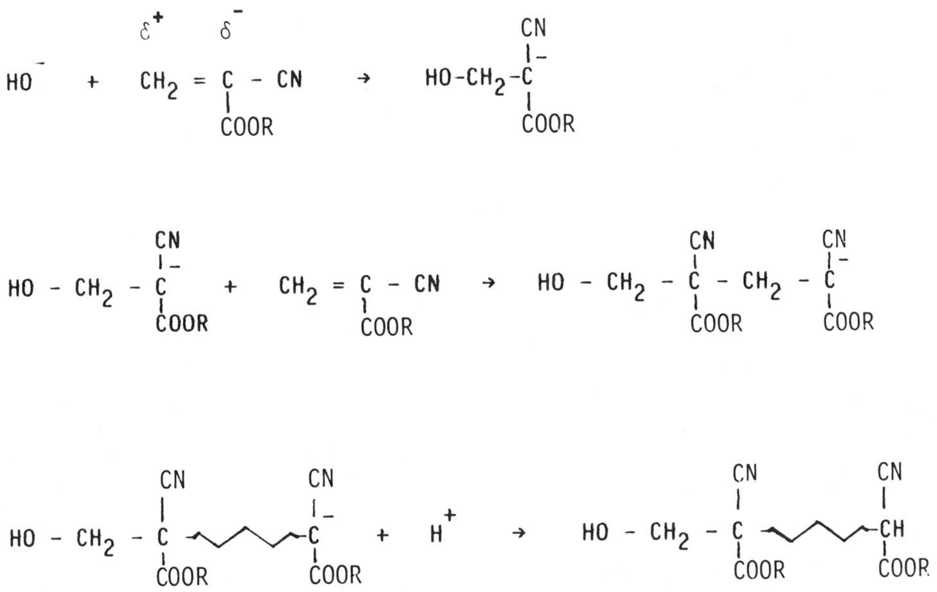

$$\overset{\delta^+}{\varepsilon} \quad \overset{\delta^-}{}$$

$$HO^- \ + \ CH_2 = \underset{\underset{COOR}{|}}{C} - CN \ \rightarrow \ HO-CH_2-\underset{\underset{COOR}{|}}{\overset{\overset{CN}{|}}{C}}^-$$

$$HO - CH_2 - \underset{\underset{COOR}{|}}{\overset{\overset{CN}{|}}{C}}^- \ + \ CH_2 = \underset{\underset{COOR}{|}}{C} - CN \ \rightarrow \ HO - CH_2 - \underset{\underset{COOR}{|}}{\overset{\overset{CN}{|}}{C}} - CH_2 - \underset{\underset{COOR}{|}}{\overset{\overset{CN}{|}}{C}}^-$$

$$HO - CH_2 - \underset{\underset{COOR}{|}}{\overset{\overset{CN}{|}}{C}} \sim\sim \underset{\underset{COOR}{|}}{\overset{\overset{CN}{|}}{C}}^- \ + \ H^+ \ \rightarrow \ HO - CH_2 - \underset{\underset{COOR}{|}}{\overset{\overset{CN}{|}}{C}} \sim\sim \underset{\underset{COOR}{|}}{\overset{\overset{CN}{|}}{C}}H$$

FIGURE 1. Anionic polymerization of alkylcyanoacrylates in aqueous media.

The polymerization reaction is initiated by the hydroxyl anions and probably terminated by fixation of a proton (Figure 1). The propagation requires no special conditions and is carried out at room temperature and under atmospheric pressure.

Increasing the acidity of the polymerization medium results in a reduction of the overall reaction speed and of the molecular weight (500 to 1500) of the formed polymer, because of the low concentration in initiating agent and the high level of terminating ions.[2]

The obtained particles are spherical with a diameter varying between 100 and 350 nm and a narrow size distribution (Figure 2). Their internal structure appears plain but porous, as seen in a transmission-electron micrograph of a freeze-fracture replica of nanoparticles (Figure 3).

The extremely high specific area displayed by nanoparticle suspension (between 0.1 and 0.3 m²/ml) explains their ability to adsorb drugs at elevated yields.[3]

In biological fluids, the polymer undergoes an enzymatic disruption of the ester functions. The progressive disappearance of its esters increases the hydrophilicity of the polymer, which, eventually, becomes water soluble and is released from the particle[4] (Figure 4).

Drugs added to the medium prior to the polymerization can be partly trapped inside the particles and partly adsorbed on the surface of these particles. It has further been shown that the kinetics of drug release from nanoparticles can in some cases parallel their degradation as estimated by the release of dissolved polymer[4] (Figure 5).

For the same reasons as hypothesized in Chapter 11 — namely the possibility that nanoparticles could adhere to the mucus through the formation of bonds between the macromolecules present in the latter and the cyano-group of the polyalkylcyanoacrylate — the bioadhesive properties of nanoparticles to the stomach have been investigated *in vivo*.

III. GASTROADHESION OF NANOPARTICLES

A. PREPARATION OF RADIOLABELED NANOPARTICLES

In order to avoid misinterpretation of the results due to radiomarker leakage, the labeling was realized by synthesizing a monomer using ¹⁴C-cyanoacetate in a Knoevenaegel reaction as summarized in Figure 6.

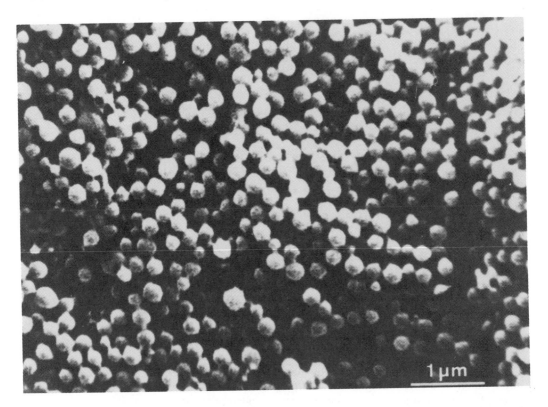

FIGURE 2.   Scanning electron micrograph of polyisobutylcyanoacrylate nanoparticles (From Lenaerts, V., Nagelkerke, J. F., Van Berkel, T. J. C., Couvreur, P., Grislain, L., Roland, M., and Speiser, P., in *Sinusoidal Liver Cells,* Wisse, E. and Knook, D. L., Eds., Elsevier Science, Amsterdam, 1982. With permission.)

The above-described polymerization reaction will, in this case, yield a labeling of the backbone of the polymer.

Nanoparticles were then prepared by addition of a radiolabeled monomer (10 mg/ml) to a polymerization medium consisting of an aqueous solution of citric acid (0.1%), dextran mol wt. 70,000 (1%) and glucose (5%).

After 3 h polymerization under mechanical stirring, the nanoparticle suspension was adjusted to a pH value of 7.0 using a 0.1 N sodium hydroxide solution.

The mean size of the radiolabeled poly *n*-hexylcyanoacrylate nanoparticles, estimated using a metering device based on the scattering of a laser beam, was 235 nm.

B. MATERIALS AND METHOD

1. *In Vivo* Procedure

Male NMRI mice weighing approximately 20 g were given an oral dosage of 0.2 ml of the radiolabeled nanoparticles suspension and were separated in three groups of five animals.

The different groups of animals were sacrificed by diethylether inhalation 30, 120, and 240 min after nanoparticle administration.

2. Whole-Body Autoradiography

In each group, one mouse was used for a whole-body autoradiography study according to the following technique: immediately after sacrifice, the animal was placed in liquid nitrogen in order to freeze as quickly as possible. The frozen body was placed in a 2% carboxymethylcellulose solution that, in turn, was frozen very quickly by immersion into liquid nitrogen. The block containing the animal was then secured to a chilled plate ($-30°C$) and cut in 40 μm thick sagittal sections using a refrigerated cryotome ($-30°C$).

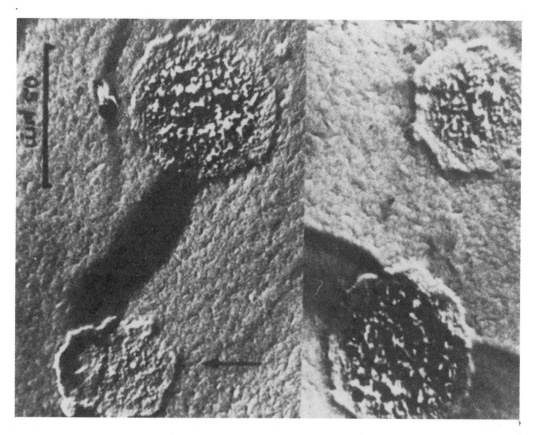

FIGURE 3. Transmission-electron micrograph of a freeze-fracture replica of polyisobutylcyanoacrylate nanoparticles. (From Lenaerts, V., Nagelkerke, J. F., Van Berkel, T. J. C., Couvreur, P., Grislain, L., Roland, M., and Speiser, P., in *Sinusoidal Liver Cells,* Wisse, E. and Knook, D. L., Eds., Elsevier Science, Amsterdam, 1982. With permission.)

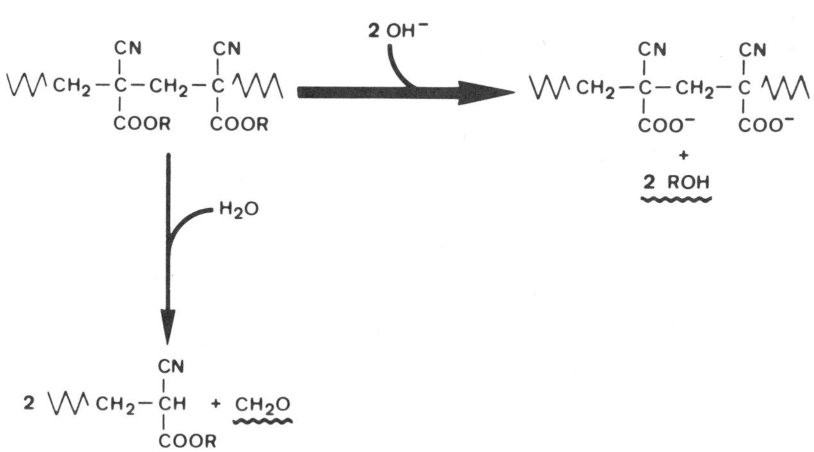

FIGURE 4. Main (ester hydrolysis) and secondary (chain scission) degradation pathways of polyalkylcyanoacrylate nanoparticles.

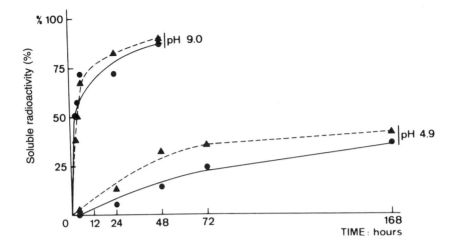

FIGURE 5. Release of dissolved ^{14}C-labeled polymer and of ^{3}H-labeled actinomycin D from polyisobutylcyanoacrylate nanoparticles incubated in nonbiological media of different pH values. (From Lenaerts, V., Couvreur, P., Christiaens–Leyh, D., Joiris, E., Roland, M., Rollman, B., and Speiser, P., *Biomaterials*, 5, 65, 1984. By permission of the publishers, Butterworth & Co. (Publishers) Ltd.)

$$CH_2O + CN - C^*H_2 - COOR \rightarrow CH_2 = \overset{\displaystyle CN}{\underset{\displaystyle COOR}{\overset{|}{\underset{|}{C^*}}}} + H_2O$$

FIGURE 6. Synthesis of radiolabeled *n*-hexylcyanoacrylate by the Knoevanaegel reaction.

This process was carried out in a low-humidity room in order to avoid water condensation on the slices. Sections were collected on adhesive tapes and allowed to dry for a period of 2 d in a dessicator at −25°C. A radiosensitive film was then pressed against the sections and maintained for 30 d at −25°C, after which the negative film was processed, and positive images were obtained using conventional photography techniques.

3. Liver and Kidney Uptake

The four other animals of each group were used for a quantitative estimation of the uptake of nanoparticles by the liver and the kidney.

The liver was selected since it is known that i.v. injected nanoparticles are taken up at an important extent and following rapid kinetics by the Kupffer cells.[5] It was thus thought that a transepithelial passage of the nanoparticles from the GI lumen to the bloodstream would most certainly have resulted in an accumulation of the radioactivity in the liver.

It has been shown that, after i.v. administration, the nanoparticles stored in the liver were metabolized and that their degradation products were transported by the plasma and eliminated mainly by glomerular filtration.[6]

However, the total accumulation of radioactive material in the kidney remained in this case relatively lower than in the liver.

Since upon peroral administration a processing of nanoparticles could take place inside the GIT, degradation products could gain access to the central compartment and be eventually filtered by the kidney, and thus contribute to the radiolabel accumulation in this organ.

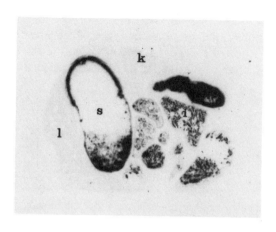

FIGURE 7. Whole-body autoradiograph of ^{14}C-polyhexylcyanoac-rylate nanoparticles administered perorally to mice sacrificed 240 min after administration (s = stomach, i = intestine, k = kidney, l = liver). (From Grislain, L., Etude de la Distribution Corporelle des Nanoparticles de Polycyanoacrylate d'Alkyle et des Molécules Associées, Ph.D. thesis, Université Catholique de Louvain, Belgium, 1984.)

Therefore, the radioactivity of the kidneys was also determined in this study, and the relative accumulation of radioactivity in the kidneys vs. the liver was compared to the data obtained upon i.v. administration in order to discriminate whether or not some processing of the nanoparticles could take place in the GIT.

Both organs were removed, and samples of the tissues were taken out and oxidized at high temperature. The radioactivity was recovered in the form of ^{14}C dioxide dissolved in water, to which scintillation liquid was added. The radioactivity of these tissues was determined using a liquid scintillation counter and expressed as percentage of the administered dose per organ weight unit.

C. AUTORADIOGRAPHIC STUDIES

From the autoradiograph shown in Figure 7, it clearly appears that most of the orally administered nanoparticles remained in the GIT and that their systemic absorption was limited, even 4 h after administration (autoradiographs taken at 30 and 120 min intervals were exactly similar to Figure 7 and were, therefore, not reproduced here).

Furthermore, while the radioactivity encountered in the intestinal loops was clearly associated with the luminal content, in the stomach, on the contrary, it is obvious that most of the nanoparticles were adhering to the wall.

This specificity might be explained either by a change in the polymer physicochemistry due to the different pH conditions or by the different compositions of gastric and intestinal mucuses.

The latter explanation seems more likely, since at the pH values encountered in the GIT, a shift in the polymer properties such that the nanoparticle-mucus interactions would suddenly disappear is most unlikely.

It has, indeed, been shown that in acidic and neutral conditions, the polymer undergoes no hydrolysis of whatever nature, and its physicochemical characteristics should, therefore, remain unchanged throughout the GIT.[7]

Although enzymatic degradation processes have also been described,[7] it is not probable that such mechanisms would induce a shift of the polymer characteristics in such a short time as that necessary for suspended nanoparticles to move across the pyloric sphincters.

Significant amounts of radioactivity can be seen in the stomach wall area for the whole

TABLE 1

Ratios of Radiolabeled Nanoparticle Concentration (in Percent Injected Dose per Gram of Organ) in the Kidneys Over the Liver as a Function of Administration Route and Time

| | Administration route | |
Time	Peroral	Intravenous
30 min	2.1	0.4
4 h	1.2	0.1

duration of the experiment — 240 min — showing that the bioadhesion of nanoparticles to stomach mucus can last for relatively long periods of time and could, therefore, find valuable applications for the controlled release of drugs in the stomach.

Quantitative evaluations of the uptake of radiolabeled material by the liver and kidneys are summarized in Table 1.

The liver uptake is relatively low as compared to the extremely elevated yields observed after an i.v. administration.[6] However, when nanoparticles were administered i.v., the time interval corresponding to the maximum level concentration of radiolabeled material was as short as 5 min after injection, and the subsequent decay was explained by the elimination of degradation products mainly to the plasma.

After oral administration, on the contrary, the concentration of radiolabeled material in the liver shows a slow increase over the time period (240 min) studied. Since, as mentioned earlier, degradation products are expelled relatively quickly from the liver, it can be hypothesized that the observed hepatic uptake is contributed to mainly by the slow absorption of intact nanoparticles from the GIT towards the plasma.

As explained earlier, the uptake of radioactivity by the kidney is most probably accounted for by the glomerular filtration of soluble degradation products. This degradation could take place not only in the liver cells where absorbed intact nanoparticles tend to accumulate, but also in the GIT.

In the case of an i.v. administration, on the contrary, since most of the carrier is taken up by the liver very quickly,[8] the degradation products filtered by the kidney are mainly originated from the liver.

The ratios of radiolabel concentration in the kidney to the liver is presented in Table 1 for both peroral and i.v. administration routes. The results show beyond a doubt that after peroral delivery, nanoparticles undergo a relatively important degradation inside the GIT followed by absorption of the degradation products. It is also a possible explanation that intact nanoparticles could be taken up by the enterocytes and processed inside these cells. This hypothesis is consistent with the slight but persistent staining of the gut walls observed in the autoradiogram (Figure 7) and with prior observations by Aprahamian et al.[9] and Damge et al.[10] who showed that after intraluminal injection, a nanoencapsulated radiotracer accumulated significantly more into the enterocytes — as well as into the intestinal mucus and lamina propria — than the same compound administered in a conventional emulsion. The relative contribution of each of these phenomena to the filtration of radiolabeled degradation compounds by the kidney has, however, not been investigated.

IV. VINCAMINE BIOAVAILABILITY

Owing to its low water solubility and the existence of a relatively narrow absorption window in the upper intestine, vincamine has proved poorly bioavailable.

It has been assumed that achieving a prolonged release of the drug from a device remaining in the stomach over a long period of time would probably be the best way to increase this bioavailability.

The potential of nanoparticles in reaching this purpose has been evaluated.

A. ADSORPTION OF VINCAMINE TO NANOPARTICLES

Poly-*n*-hexylcyanoacrylate nanoparticles were prepared by the addition and subsequent stirring for 4 d of 1 ml of monomer to 100 ml of an aqueous medium containing 0.5% dextran (average mol wt = 70,000), and 1.7 m M/L phosphoric acid (pH = 2.3).

After polymerization, 200 mg of vincamine were added to the suspension, and the drug was allotted an adsorption period of 2 h.

The percentage of adsorption of vincamine on nanoparticles was determined at pH 2.3 and after adjustment at pH 5.8 by addition of 0.1 N NaOH (above this value vincamine base would precipitate).

A 5 ml sample of the suspension was centrifuged at 40,000g and 4°C for 90 min, and the supernatant was separated from the sediment. This latter was dissolved in 5 ml dimethylformamide.

Drug concentration was determined in both supernatant (free drug) and sediment (drug-nanoparticles complex) by emission spectrofluorodensitometry after extraction and purification.

The samples' standard and blanks (0.5 ml) were extracted twice by 4 ml benzene under alkaline conditions. The collected organic extracts were evaporated under nitrogen, and the residue was dissolved in 0.5 ml chloroform:methanol (8:2).

After a second evaporation, the residue was redissolved in 40 µl chloroform:methanol (8:2) and transferred on a thin-layer chromatography plate. The plate was allowed to stand in a chloroform:ethylacetate:methanol (6:3:2) mixture, and subsequently dried in a hot air stream, treated with a ceric sulfate (0.03 N) solution in phosphoric acid (10 *M*) and heated at 100°C for 15 min. The vincamine spot fluorescence was quantitized on the plate.

Percentages of adsorption on nanoparticles in media of pH 2.3 and 5.8 were, respectively, 25 and 42% of the initially present drug (2 mg/ml), representing 5 and 8.4 mg drug per 100 milligrams of polymer.

B. PHARMACOKINETICS OF FREE VS. NANOPARTICLES-BOUND VINCAMINE

In order to compare the absolute bioavailability of free vs. nanoparticle-bound vincamine, both preparations were administered i.v. and perorally to male New Zealand rabbits. The injected dose was 2 mg/kg i.v. and 10 mg/kg p.o. For the i.v. administration, a pH 5.8 suspension was used, while for the peroral administration the pH 2.3 suspension was given to the rabbits. Blood samples were collected from the marginal ear vein of the preheparinized rabbits (5000 IU heparin per kilogram), and the plasma was processed in the same way as described above for the assay of vincamine in the polymerization media.

Values were fitted according to a two-compartment model hypothesis using equation:

$$C = Ae^{-\alpha t} + Be^{-\beta t} \tag{1}$$

where α and β are first-order rate constants, and A and B are concentration constants. The central compartment volume (Vc) was estimated by:

$$Vc = dose/Co = dose/(A + B) \tag{2}$$

The total body clearance was given by:

$$CL_t = dose/\left(\int_0^\infty C \cdot dt\right) \tag{3}$$

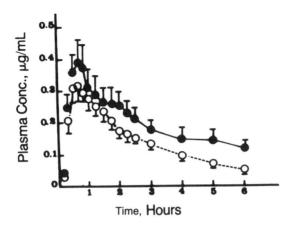

FIGURE 8.   Vincamine plasma concentration vs. time profiles after peroral administration of 10 mg/kg to rabbits (n = 10) as an aqueous solution (○) or in a suspension of nanoparticles containing 25% of the drug adsorbed on the polymer and 75% free (●). (From Maincent, Ph., Leverge, R., Sado, P., Couvreur, P., and Devissaguet, J. P., *J. Pharm. Sci.*, 75, 955, 1986. Reproduced with permission of the copyright owner, the American Pharmaceutical Association.)

Where $\int_0^\infty$ C·dt represents the total area under the curve (AUC) as estimated by the trapezoidal rule. The area under the curve from the last experimental point to infinite time was estimated by dividing the last concentration determined experimentally by β.

The distribution volume was obtained by:

$$Vd = \frac{CL_t}{\beta} \tag{4}$$

and the biological half-life $t_{1/2}$ was calculated using:

$$t_{1/2} = \frac{0.693}{\beta} \tag{5}$$

Absolute and relative bioavailabilities were calculated using the following equations:

Absolute bioavailability: $AUC_{po} \cdot AUC_{iv}^{-1} \cdot Dose_{po}^{-1} \cdot Dose_{iv}$ $\qquad$ (6)

Relative bioavailability: $AUC\text{-}NP_{po} \cdot AUC\text{-}F_{po}^{-1} \cdot Dose\text{-}NP_{po}^{-1} \cdot Dose\text{-}F_{po}$ $\qquad$ (7)

where F means free and NP nanoparticle-bound vincamine.

The plasma concentration vs. time profiles after peroral administration of free and nanoparticle-bound vincamine are shown in Figure 8.

The pharmacokinetic data obtained for the i.v. administration (Table 2) show that the clearance is not modified by adsorption onto nanoparticles. Bioavailability calculations using AUC are, therefore, considered as valid.

After peroral administration, the data (Table 3) show that the bioavailability of free vincamine was relatively poor (22 ± 1%) while nanoparticle-bound vincamine showed a slight superiority with a bioavailability of 36 ± 2% and a relative bioavailability of 162%.

TABLE 2
Disposition Kinetic Parameters of Free and
Nanoparticle-Loaded Vincamine

Parameters	Aqueous solution	Nanoparticle suspension
CL_t(ml/min/kg)	43 $\pm$ 3	43 $\pm$ 3
V_c(l/kg)	1.6 $\pm$ 0.1	1.9 $\pm$ 0.3
V_d(l/kg)	4.3 $\pm$ 0.3	8.3 $\pm$ 0.4
$t_{1/2}$ (min)	75 $\pm$ 9	151 $\pm$ 17

From Maincent, Ph., Leverge, R., Sado, P., Couvreur, P., and Devissaguet, J. P., *J. Pharm. Sci.*, 75, 955, 1986. With permission.

TABLE 3
Bioavailability Parameters after Oral Administration of
Free or Nanoparticle-Bound Vincamine

Parameters	Aqueous solution	Nanoparticle suspension
C_{max} (ng/ml)	370 $\pm$ 45	414 $\pm$ 69
t_{max} (min)	49 $\pm$ 6	35 $\pm$ 3
Absolute bioavailability (%; reference: i.v. route)	22 $\pm$ 1	36 $\pm$ 2
Relative bioavailability (%; oral route)	100	162 $\pm$ 20

From Maincent, Ph., Leverge, R., Sado, P., Couvreur, P., and Devissaguet, J. P., *J. Pharm. Sci.*, 75, 955, 1986. With permission.

However, since only 25% of the perorally administered vincamine was actually adsorbed on the nanoparticles, it can be calculated that the absolute bioavailability for the particle-associated vincamine was 78%, representing a threefold increase in comparison to the free drug.

Autoradiographic semiquantitative evaluation studies have shown that only a very minor percentage of the nanoparticles could gain access to the central compartment after peroral administration.

The observed increase in the bioavailability of vincamine is thus only explainable by a combination of bioadhesion of the nanoparticles on the stomach mucus and slow release of the vincamine from its carrier.

V. CONCLUSION

Polyalkylcyanoacrylate nanoparticles have been developed in the last decade as a drug targeting device. As such, their pharmaceutical properties have been studied and have proven theoretically suitable for other types of applications including the controlled release of perorally administered drugs.

For this reason, the body distribution of perorally administered radiolabeled nanoparticles was evaluated by autoradiography. This study evidenced the bioadhesive behavior of nanoparticles to the stomach mucus, further showing very little intestinal retention and a limited systemic absorption. The combination of both these characteristics — controlled release and gastroadhesion — bore great promise for the use of nanoparticles as a mean of enhancing the bioavailability of drugs, such as vincamine, with a narrow absorption window in the upper GIT.

In a pharmacokinetic study, vincamine adsorbed on nanoparticles showed a threefold increase in bioavailability as compared to a vincamine solution.

These results allow a more realistic look at the somewhat theoretical promises of nanoparticles as a gastric mucoadhesive drug delivery system.

Applications of this system could be extended to other therapeutic classes, including the cytoprotective agents used as locally acting antiulcers.

REFERENCES

1. **Couvreur, P., Lenaerts, V., Leyh, D., Guiot, P., and Roland, M.,** Design of biodegradable polyalkylcyanoacrylate nanoparticles, in *Microspheres and Drug Therapy: Pharmaceutical, Immunological and Medical Aspects,* Davis, S. S., Illum, L., McVie, J. G., and Tomlinson, E., Eds., Elsevier Science, Amsterdam, 1984.

2. **Vansnick, L., Couvreur, P., Christiaens-Leyh, D., and Roland, M.,** Molecular weights of free and drug-loaded nanoparticles, *Pharm. Res.,* 1, 36, 1985.

3. **Couvreur, P., Kante, B., and Roland, M.,** Les vecteurs lysosomotropes, *J. Pharm. Belg.,* 35, 51, 1980.

4. **Lenaerts, V., Couvreur, P., Christiaens-Leyh, D., Joiris, E., Roland, M., Rollman, B., and Speiser, P.,** Degradation of polyisobutylcyanoacrylate nanoparticles, *Biomaterials,* 5, 65, 1983.

5. **Lenaerts, V., Nagelkerke, J. F., Vanberkel, T. J. C., Couvreur, P., Grislain, L., Roland, M., and Speiser, P.,** In vivo uptake of polyisobutylcyanoacrylate nanoparticles by rat liver Kupffer, endothelial and parenchymal cells, *J. Pharm. Sci.,* 73, 980, 1984.

6. **Couvreur, P., Grislain, L., Lenaerts, V., Brasseur, F., Guiot, P., and Biernacki, A.,** Biodegradable polymeric nanoparticles as drug carrier for anti-tumor agents, in *Polymeric Nanoparticles and Microspheres,* Guiot, P. and Couvreur, P., Eds., CRC Press, Boca Raton, FL, 1986.

7. **Leyh, D., Couvreur, P., Lenaerts, V., Roland, M., and Speiser, P.,** Etude du mécanisme de dégradation des nanoparticles de polycyanoacrylate d'alkyle, *Labo Pharma Probl. Tech.,* 32, 100, 1984.

8. **Grislain, L., Couvreur, P., Lenaerts, V., Roland, M., Deprez-Decampeneere, D., and Speiser, P.,** Pharmacokinetics and distribution of a biodegradable drug-carrier, *Int. J. Pharm.,* 15, 335, 1983.

9. **Aprahamian, R., Damge, C., Humbert, W., Balboni, G., Andrieu, V., and Devissaguet, J. P.,** Les vecteurs colloidaux polymériques franchissent-ils la barrière intestinale?, *Proc. 4th Int. Conf. Pharm. Technol.,* Vol. 4, Association de Pharmacie Galénique et Industrielle, Paris, 1986, 175.

10. **Damge, C., Aprahamian, M., Balboni, G., Hoeltzel, A., Andrieu, V., and Devissaguet, J.-P.,** Intérêt des vecteurs polymériques (nanocapsules) dans l'absorption intestinale. Etude expérimentale d'un traceur iodé chez le chien, *Proc. 4th Int. Conf. Pharm. Technol.,* Vol. 4, Association de Pharmacie Galénique et Industrielle, Paris, June 1986, 239.

11. **Lenaerts, V., Nagelkerke, J. F., Van Berkel, T. J. C., Couvreur, P., Grislain, L., Roland, R., and Speiser, P.,** In vivo uptake and cellular distribution of biodegradable polymeric nanoparticles, in *Sinusoidal Liver Cells,* Wisse, E. and Knook, D. L., Eds., Elsevier Science, Amsterdam, 1982.

12. **Maincent, Ph., Leverge, R., Sado, P., Couvreur, P., and Devissaguet, J. P.,** Disposition kinetics and oral bioavailability of vincamine-loaded polyalkylcyanoacrylate nanoparticles, *J. Pharm. Sci.,* 75, 955, 1986.

13. **Grislain, L.,** Etude de la Distribution Corporelle des Nanoparticules de Polycyanoacrylate d'Alkyle et des Molécules Associées, Ph.D. thesis, Université Catholique de Louvain, Belgium, 1984.

Chapter 6

MUCOADHESIVE BUCCAL PATCHES FOR PEPTIDE DELIVERY

Hans P. Merkle, Reinhold Anders, and Aloys Wermerskirchen

TABLE OF CONTENTS

I. INTRODUCTION

Due to an increasing supply of potent peptide and protein drugs, the biopharmaceutical sciences are presently faced with an urgent need to develop alternative dosage forms for nonparenteral absorption. Among the nonparenteral sites suitable for administering peptides and proteins are the mucosae of the nasal, buccal, vaginal, rectal, and even ocular routes. The currently most popular site is the nasal pathway. According to various reports, e.g., reviewed by Su and Campanale[1] and Su et al.,[2] it represents the route of choice, mainly because of its superior permeability to peptides as compared to the other mucosal sites.

However, the nasal site does have distinct limitations. Upon long-term treatment, there might be a risk for pathologic changes of the nasal mucosa;[2] the drug or a preservative added to the preparation might interfere with the ciliary activity of the membrane, as shown by Van de Donk and co-workers.[3] Moreover, there is a debate on the consequences of vast individual variations in mucus secretion and turnover on the extent and rate of nasal absorption; in addition, proteases and peptidases present in the mucus or associated with the nasal membrane may act as a dense enzymatic barrier to peptide absorption.[4,5] It may thus be concluded that in spite of many promising aspects the nasal route may have its shortcomings and not be the only answer to peptide absorption problems.

Information on the buccal absorption of peptides is still rather scarce, except for a broad body of knowledge on the buccal absorption of oxytocin, e.g., by Wespi and Rehsteiner,[6] Bergsjö and Jenssen,[7] and Sjöstedt,[8] dating back to the 1960s. Moreover, for many conventional drugs, the oral mucosa has been an established absorption site. Recently more peptides were investigated, and it was shown that the buccal mucosa might provide a useful absorption site, mainly restricted to small peptides.[9-14] Data are also available for vasopressin analogs and insulin.[15-17] However, as compared to other alternative peptide absorption sites, such as the rectal, nasal, and vaginal mucosa, much less information is available for the oral mucosa.

In terms of permeability, in addition to the nasal mucosa, even the rectal and the vaginal mucosae seem to be preferable to the buccal site. On the other hand, what makes the oral mucosa, mainly the buccal, the labial, and the sublingual sites rather attractive for peptide delivery is the combination of several aspects:

*   Excellent accessibility
*   High patient acceptance and compliance
*   Significant robustness of mucosa

Because of the excellent accessibility of the oral mucosa, appropriate dosage forms can be easily attached and removed at any time, if necessary. Moreover, application is usually painless and without significant discomfort whatsoever. Since patients are well adapted to the oral administration of drugs in general, the acceptance of buccal or sublingual dosage forms should be good, and there should be a high compliance as well. According to its natural function, the oral mucosa is routinely exposed to a multitude of different foreign compounds and, therefore, is supposed to be rather robust and less prone to irreversible irritation or damage by the drug, the dosage form, or the additives, e.g., absorption promotors, used therein. In addition, there is no sex-specificity involved as with the vaginal absorption. Moreover, nasal and vaginal secretions and mucus flow are subject to rather pronounced variations, both in qualitative as well as quantitative terms. On the other hand, with respect to proteolytic enzymes present in the mucosal membrane or fluid there is no principal difference or advantage of the oral mucosa in comparison to the other sites.

Therefore, in spite of the undoubtedly higher natural permeability of the rectal, the vaginal, and especially the nasal mucosa, the buccal route appears to be a rather attractive one, but appropriate dosage forms have to be provided, and efficient absorption promotors should be found to increase its permeability.

II. RELEVANT ANATOMY AND PHYSIOLOGY OF THE ORAL MUCOSA

The oral cavity is lined by a relatively thick, dense, and multilayered mucous membrane of a highly-vascularized nature. Drug penetrating into the membrane can find access to the systemic circulation via nets of capillaries and arteries. The arterial flow is supplied by branches of the external carotid artery. The venous backflow goes via capillaries and a venous net is finally taken up by the jugular veins. The equally well developed lymphatic drainage runs more or less parallel to the venous vascularization and ends up in the jugular ducts.

As compared to the relatively thin nasal mucosa with only a few cell layers to be penetrated before uptake by the systemic circulation takes place, the oral mucosa with its multilayered structure appears to be much more resistant against penetration of drugs.

The epithelium of the oral cavity is in principle similar to that of the skin, with interesting differences regarding keratinization and the protective and lubricant mucus spread across its surface. The total area is about 100 cm.[2,18] The buccal part with about one third of the total surface is lined with an epithelium of about 0.5 mm thickness, and the rest by one of 0.25 mm thickness.[19] The multilayered structure of the oral mucosa is formed by cell divisions, which occur mainly in the basal layer. As reviewed by Jarrett,[20] the mucosa of the oral cavity can be divided into three functional zones. First, the mucus-secreting regions (consisting of the soft palate, the floor of the mouth, the under-surface of the tongue, and the labial and buccal mucosa) have a normally nonkeratinized epithelium. These regions are supposed to represent the major absorption sites in the oral cavity. Second, the hard palate and the gingiva are the regions of the masticatory mucosa and have a normally keratinized epidermis. Third, specialized zones are the borders of the lips and the dorsal surface of the tongue with its highly selective keratinization.

An important feature of the oral mucosa as a mucous membrane is the turnover of the cells, which is definitely greater — ranging from 3 up to 8 days for a complete turnover — than that of the skin epidermis (ca. 30 days). This is because of the constant replacement of the nonkeratinized or partly keratinized cells, which is necessary to stabilize function and integrity of the mucosa. A reduction of the mucosal mitotic activity would result in a loss of epithelial continuity.[20]

Keratinization and average size of the epithelial cells seem to have an inverse relationship. The mean cross-sectional area of the cells of the cheek is about 263 μm^2, while it is about

133 μm^2 for the cells of the keratinized palate. The basal cells of the hard palate are not markedly different from the basal cells producing the nonkeratinized buccal epithelium. But as the cells move towards the surface, increasing differences become apparent: palatal cells show a greater concentration of fibrillar and keratohyalin granular structures, while the buccal mucosa shows more glycogen granules and numerous ribosomes.[20]

Another important feature of the buccal membrane is the presence of numerous elastic fibers in the dermis, which provide its typical elastic and robust behavior. These fibers represent another effective barrier against the diffusion of drug molecules into the circulation system.

The nature of the junction between epidermis and dermis is different in the region of the hard palate from that in the region of the buccal and labial mucosa. Whereas the hard palate is a acanthotic-type epidermis with a large contact area between dermis and epidermis, the buccal mucosa has a much flatter dermo-epidermal junction and, therefore, a much smaller contact area. The collagen fibers of the buccal mucosa are relatively unpolymerized and less dense as compared to those of the hard palate dermis.

The surface of the mucous membrane is constantly washed by a stream of about 0.5 up to 2 l saliva daily, produced by the salivary glands. The main glands are the three pairs of the parotid, the submaxillary, and the sublingual glands. The first are located under and in front of each ear, with ducts opening to the inner surface of the cheek. The submaxillary glands lie below the lower jaw releasing saliva through one duct on each side. Finally, the sublingual glands are located below the tongue with its ducts opening to the floor of the mouth under the tongue. In addition to these main glands, there is a variety of small glands dispersed on the tongue and the buccal and sublingual mucosa. Minor salivary glands are situated in the buccal, palatal, and retromolar regions of the oral cavity. There are major differences with respect to the type of mucins, mucin content, and secretion.

The surface of the oral cavity is the site of a complex microbial flora. Its composition is widely different depending on the local type of surface. Large differences exist between the surface of the teeth, the gingiva, the tongue, and the buccal mucosa, etc. In order to retain health and appearance of the mucosae, each local bacterial composition has to be preserved in its balanced equilibrium containing a variety of site-specific species.

Transport of drugs through the oral mucosa is most likely to occur mainly through the nonkeratinized sections. The first efficient barrier against penetration, however, is the mucin layer covering the oral epithelium. It consists of glycoproteins produced by the nonkeratinized oral mucosae. According to the moist environment, all epithelial cells are fully hydrated offering a maximum of permeability. Two transport routes seem to operate: i.e., (1) by crossing the cell membranes and (2) by using the intercellular space. The latter is supposed to form the ordinary passage for ions and very small molecules.[20,21] The main route for regular drug molecules is by partitioning into the lipid bilayer of the cells and from there into the cells, etc. Hydrophilic medium and large molecules such as peptides, however, are not likely to cross the lipid bilayers of the cells to a great extent. Nevertheless, passage might occur through more polar fenestrations in the lipid bilayer. It still remains an open question how the junctions between the cells can be sufficiently opened to allow ready absorption of larger molecules. There is some evidence[20,22,23] that even large molecules may penetrate the oral mucosa to some extent.

A yet widely unknown influence on peptide absorption may be played by peptidase activity located in the saliva and the mucus layer, which is produced by the mucus secretions of the salivary glands, the mucosal surface, and the microbial flora. Peptidase activity is also supposed to be present in and between the cells and may affect peptide penetration through the mucosa. Further research on absorption promotors will, therefore, have to look into peptidase activity inhibition in the oral mucosa as a possible tool to enhance peptide absorption.[24]

III. DOSAGE FORM DESIGN FOR ORAL MUCOSAL APPLICATION

A. CONVENTIONAL DOSAGE FORMS

Delivery of a peptide drug to the oral mucosa by conventional means is limited to solutions or conventional buccal or sublingual tablets and capsules. Solutions in small quantities (less than about 1 ml) may be filled into capsules with the liquid being released upon chewing. More common dosage forms are erodible buccal or sublingual tablets or capsules, respectively. Their manufacture is based on well-known techniques using appropriate excipients and binders.

Due to (1) involuntary swallowing of the dosage form itself or parts of it, and due to (2) the continuous salivary dilution of the suspended or dissolved drug after disintegration of the dosage form, there is a high risk that a major part of the drug of such dosage forms may not be available for absorption. Moreover, administration of conventional buccal and sublingual tablets and capsules does not allow drinking and eating and is, at least, a handicap for speaking, so any administration is restricted to rather limited periods of time and controlled release is not within the scope of such formulations.

B. ADHESIVE DOSAGE FORMS

1. Adhesive Polymers

The use of adhesive polymers plays a dominant role in the development of adhesive mucosal dosage forms. Close attachment of a dosage form to the buccal, sublingual, or gingival mucosa will retain the dosage form in the oral cavity and will establish an intimate contact with the absorption site. Relevant dosage forms are adhesive tablets, adhesive gels, and adhesive patches, which will be covered in detail below. Table 1 gives an overview on some of the polymers useful for this purpose.[9,13,17,25-37]

Adhesion between polymer and mucosa is established by the thermodynamics and kinetics of the interaction and the intercalation of the polymer chains and the glycoprotein coat of the mucosa. Depending on the functional groups of both components, chemical as well as physical interactions may take place. A comprehensive review on the nature of mucosal interactions with polymers, its mechanisms, experimental methods to evaluate adhesion, and a survey of adhesive polymers is given by Peppas and Buri.[37] Fundamental aspects of adhesion to mucus glycoproteins are outlined by Park and Robinson.[36] Basic information on adhesion is presented by Manly[38] and by Anderson et al.[39]

2. Adhesive Tablets

Adhesive tablets for buccal or sublingual administration were suggested, for instance, on the basis of eroding hydrocolloid/filler tablets. An example is given by Davis et al.[40] and Schor et al.[41] Hydroxypropyl cellulose (Synchron®) and lactose as excipients were mixed with the drug, and the mix was compressed to tablets. As shown by a scintigraphic marker technique, the preparation remained in place for about 3 h. This was due to the adhesion of the gradually eroding polymer to the buccal mucosa. Erb[42] evaluated adhesive buccal nitroglycerin tablets, as before on the basis of hydroxypropyl cellulose, and found pharmacodynamic effects for up to 5 h. In principle, a multitude of other polymers also seems to be useful for this purpose. A small portion of the patent literature was reviewed by Chien,[43] and a thorough review on bioadhesive polymers was given by Peppas and Buri.[37] Unlike conventional tablets, adhesive tablets allow drinking and speaking without major discomfort.

3. Adhesive Gels

Viscous adhesive gels as an oral mucosal dosage form may be used to deliver drugs to the buccal, sublingual, or gingival mucosa. Examples for local therapy have been given by

TABLE 1
Mucosal Adhesive Polymers

Mucosal adhesive polymer	Ref.
Hydroxypropycellulose	25
Combination of hydroxy propylcellulose and	26
polyacrylic acid	17
	27
Polyacrylic acid	28
Polymethylmethacrylate	29
	30
	31
Na carboxymethylcellulose	32
Methylcellulose, methylhydroxyethylcellu-lose, hydroxyethylcellulose, hydroxypropyl cellulose, polyvinylpyrrolidone, polyvinyl-alcohol, agarose	9,13,33,34
Combination of hydroxy propyl cellulose and polyacrylic acid, or polyethylenglycol, review	35
Insoluble cross-linked polyacrylic acid poly-mers (polycarbophil type polymers), review	36
Review on potentially bioadhesive polymers of all above mentioned classes and others	37

Ishida et al.[27,28,44] and by Bremecker and co-workers,[29-31] using polyacrylic acid and poly-methylmethacrylate, respectively, as gel-forming polymers. Systemic therapy with peptides has not yet been reported, but appears feasible. As compared to solutions, gels can significantly prolong residence on the oral mucosa that may improve absorption and/or allow for some degree of sustained release of the active principle.

4. Adhesive Patches

Adhesive patches pose a relatively new technology to pharmacy. Design and manufacture may be partly derived from polymer technologies. The formulation of adhesive patches may take a number of different approaches: a collection of four different setups is given in Figure 1. It shows that such patches may range from simple adhesive disks to laminated systems.[13,17,27,33,34,45-47] The adhesive polymer may work as the drug carrier itself (Case a and d); on the other hand, it may act as an adhesive link between a drug loaded layer and the mucosa (Case c). Also a drug-containing disk may be fixed to the mucosa by using an adhesive shield (Case b). The polymers used as adhesives are in principle the same as for adhesive tablets and gels, with the principal types given in Table 1.

An important difference may be seen with respect to the directions open for drug release. Cases a and c allow for a bidirectional release of the drug, i.e., the drug is not only delivered to the mucosa, but also to the oral cavity, or the saliva, respectively. This may lead, however, as we have seen, to a substantial loss of the drug due to involuntary swallowing of saliva. On the other hand, the total surface of the oral cavity is now available for absorption. Drug loss to the saliva may be decreased by using an adhesive protective shield (Case b) or a nonpermeable backing layer (Case d); however, the main absorption site now remaining is the rather limited mucosal area covered by the dosage form itself. Further spreading of the drug across the buccal mucosa may increase the effective area for peptide absorption. This may happen either by squeezing-out effects upon individual jaw movements or may be due to a slow floating motion of the device across the mucosal surface.

The size of such systems is variable, but the maximum size suitable for buccal admin-

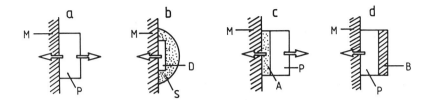

FIGURE 1. Schematic view of four different types of adhesive patches for buccal peptide delivery. Case a: bidirectional release from adhesive patch by dissolution or diffusion. Case b: unidirectional release from patch embedded in adhesive shield. Case c: bidirectional release from laminated patch. Case d: unidirectional release from laminated patch. M, mucosa; P, polymer with peptide; D, drug depot; S, adhesive shield; A, adhesive layer; B, impermeable backing layer.[13,17,27,33,34,45-47] (From Merkle, H. P. et al., in *Delivery Systems for Peptide Drugs* (NATO ASI Series A), Vol. 125, Davis, S. S., Illum, L., and Tomlinson, E., Eds., Plenum Press, New York, 1986, 161. With permission.)

istration will be around 10 to 15 cm² at the most. Much more convenient and comfortable are patches of about 1 to 3 cm².

Due to the impermeable backing layer design, there is no excessive washout of the drug by saliva, so a maximum drug activity gradient to the mucosa is established. The washout of the adhesive is also diminished, which minimizes the amount of adhesive necessary to ensure adhesion.

Depending on the size and the shape of the systems, a number of different administration sites is possible. Patches near the maximum size mentioned can be administered at the central position of the buccal mucosa only. Ellipsoid-shaped patches seem to be most suitable for this size. Small patches may be attached to variable sites on the buccal, labial, sublingual, or gingival mucosa. The labial, sublingual, and the gingival sites require rather small patches with a maximum of 1 to 3 cm². It has to be pointed out that different sites are most likely to result in differences in drug dissolution and drug release that might affect drug absorption.

To improve acceptance and compliance of the patches, a moderate size and high flexibility of the patches is required. This is a prerequisite for perfect adhesion and prevention of any local discomfort.

All systems may be additionally loaded with any additive needed. A major advantage of those systems carrying a nonpermeable protective shield or layer is that the effect of the additives can be restricted to the very site of application. A local microenvironment may thus be created between the dosage form and the mucosa, which may establish more favorable absorption conditions than the natural mucosal site, e.g., by adjustment of a specific pH, or by providing an absorption promotor, if available. Furthermore, any irritation or damage exerted to the mucosa by the drug or any of the dosage form excipients is restricted to a rather limited area and not to the complete surface of the oral mucosa as it would be the case without the protective shield or layer. Subsequent recoverage of reversibly damaged sites appears to be possible, even during long-term treatments, since the application site may be varied across the total surface available, and damaged areas will be relatively small. Anyway, all additives released to the oral cavity have to be rather critically evaluated, since the oral mucosa is the site of a vulnerable and complex bacterial microflora whose composition and viability is essential for its health and appearance.

The choice of polymers for oral mucosal patches follows the lines given by Table 1. A variety of polymers can be used, including water-soluble and insoluble hydrocolloid polymers from both the ionic and nonionic type. Drug release from soluble polymers is accompanied by the gradual erosion-type dissolution of the polymer. Polymer dissolution and drug diffusion may, therefore, determine the overall release mechanism. Drug release from nonsoluble hydrogels follows fickian or nonfickian diffusion kinetics.[49] The most common polymer applied is the anionic polyacrylate-type hydrogel.[49]

TABLE 2
Molecular Weights and Specific Viscosity of Water-Soluble Hydrocolloids

Polymer	Trade name	Molecular weight[a]	Viscosity[b] mPa·s
Hydroxyethylcellulose (HEC)	Natrosol® 250 L	80,000	14 (2%)
	Natrosol® 250 G	300,000	300 (2%)
	Natrosol® 250 K		2,000 (2%)
	Natrosol® 250 M	650,000	6,000 (2%)
	Natrosol® 250 H	900,000	30,000 (2%)
Hydroxypropylcellulose (HPC)	Klucel® EF (E)	60,000	500 (10%)
	Klucel® JF (J)		30 (2%)
	Klucel® MF (M)		5,000 (2%)
	Klucel HF (H)	1,000,000	2,000 (1%)
Poly(vinylpyrrolidone) (PVP)	Kollidon® 17	9,500	2 (10%)
	Kollidon® 25	27,000	4 (10%)
	Kollidon® 30	49,000	7 (10%)
	Kollidon® 90	1,100,000	500 (10%)
Poly(vinylalcohol) (PVA)	Mowiol® 4-88	23,300	4 (4%)
	Mowiol® 40-88	114,400	40 (4%)
	Mowiol® 4-98	23,300	4 (4%)
	Mowiol® 56-98	202,400	56 (4%)

[a] Mean molecular weight as given by the producer.
[b] Viscosity at a given concentration of polymer in water (in parenthesis); Brookfield method for HEC and HPC (25°C), Hoppler method for PVP and PVA (20°C); data as provided by the producer.

From Anders, R. and Merkle, H. P., *Int. J. Pharm.*, 49, 233, 1989. With permission.

Depending on the pharmacodynamics of the peptides, various buccal dosage forms of different release rates may be designed. In some cases, fast release of the peptide may be required; for other peptides, a sustained release may be desirable. To achieve sustained release, a number of standard strategies are at hand, e.g., matrix diffusion control, membrane-controlled transport of the peptide, or polymer erosion control. In many cases, however, instantaneous release of the peptide may be desired, which requires rapidly eroding or highly permeable carriers. The maximum application time span for adhesive mucosal dosage forms reported is in the order of several days.[35] In most cases, however, the maximum buccal residence time should not exceed several hours. This is due to the fact that buccal devices may possibly interfere with drinking, eating, and even talking. Longer periods appear to be practical for nighttime administration only. Buccal patches for treatments over several hours have to be perfectly formulated in order to motivate patients to comply with them. A smooth surface and good flexibility are prerequisites to prevent mechanical irritation or local discomfort.

IV. *IN VIVO* ADHESION AND RELEASE OF ADHESIVE HYDROCOLLOID PATCHES[9]

A. MATERIALS AND PATCH PREPARATION
1. Materials

The following water-soluble hydrocolloid mucoadhesives were used: hydroxyethyl cellulose (HEC, Natrosol® 250, Hercules, D-Hamburg), hydroxypropyl cellulose (HPC, Klucel®, Hercules, D-Hamburg), poly(vinylpyrrolidone) (PVP, Kollidon®, BASF, D-Ludwigshafen) and poly(vinylalcohol) (PVA, Mowiol®, Hoechst, D-Frankfurt). Further information regarding molecular weight and viscosity is given in Table 2.

The main backing layer used in this study was Multiphor® (sheets, from LKB, D-Gräfelfing). Multiphor® sheets were 168 to 176 μm thick and covered on one side with a thin layer of agarose grafted onto the polymer. This material is commonly used as backing layer for gel chromotography sheets. The material available on the market is rather stiff and not flexible enough to allow comfortable buccal use, so it should be regarded as a model. In some cases cellophane (Cellophane® 325 P10, from Kalle, D-Wiesbaden) was taken as backing layer. According to producer information, the thickness of the cellophane in the dry state was 22 μm.

Protirelin (TRH) was used as a model peptide drug. In addition, sodium salicylate was used as a marker compound instead of the peptide.

2. Preparation of Adhesive Patches

Preparation of adhesive patches was as follows: given volumes of appropriately made aqueous polymer solutions (for drug-free patches) or drug/polymer solutions (for drug-loaded patches) were cast onto a backing layer sheet mounted on top of a stainless steel plate by means of a frame. Previous to the preparation, the device was carefully rectified in a horizontal position. To ensure constant temperature for drying, the steel plate was constantly perfused by a thermostated stream of water. Drying at 38°C for about 2 h resulted in a laminate consisting of a backing layer and a hydrocolloid or hydrocolloid/drug layer. By means of a suitable punch-die set, the laminate was cut into patches of about 10 cm² and an oval form of 4 cm length and 3 cm width. If not otherwise specified, this preparation technique was used throughout. For the preparation of PVP and PVA patches 1,2-propylene glycol was used as plasticizer (PVP, 10% (w/w); PVA, 20 to 25% (w/w) of polymer content).

B. MUCOSAL ADHESION OF ADHESIVE PATCHES *IN VIVO*
1. Experimental Procedure

The duration of mucosal adhesion of drug-free adhesive patches was determined *in vivo*. The same subject was used throughout the study (26, male) if not otherwise specified. A self-adhesive patch was attached to the subject's right or left buccal mucosa and a blank backing layer (as nonadhesive control) on the other side. The size of the patches used was about the maximum size possible for buccal application as limited by the local anatomy. The duration of mucosal adhesion was the time span required until the adhesive patch completely lost its adhesive contact with the mucosa. This was assessed by continuing sensual comparison of the behavior of both patches on either side.

The test requires well-trained and motivated subjects. Three runs were made for each polymer composition. The test sequence was randomized with respect to polymer species and amount of polymer, and the subject was not given information about the polymer composition of the respective adhesive patch tested. During the test, the subject was not allowed to drink or eat.

2. General Observations with Adhesive Patches

The patches used in this study were mainly designed for the buccal delivery of oligopeptides.[9,11,13,34] There is no doubt, however, that this type of mucoadhesive patch may be useful for other drugs as well.

Due to the agarose-graft on one side of the backing layer used in the study (Multiphor®), there was perfect binding between backing layer and mucoadhesive polymer layer. No disintegration of any patch was ever observed in this investigation, neither in the hydrated nor nonhydrated state. On the other hand, the backing layer used in the study was not flexible enough to avoid local discomfort for the subjects. This backing layer (Multiphor®) is specifically designed to act as a support film for gel-chromatogoraphy sheets. Accordingly, with respect to its agarose-graft, Multiphor® is regarded as prototype material, ensuring

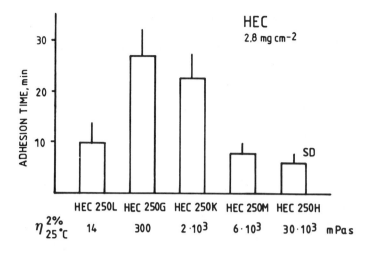

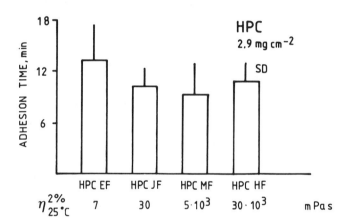

FIGURE 2.   Effect of viscosity grade of HEC and HPC on duration of mucosal adhesion *in vivo*. HEC: 2.8 mg/cm²; HPC: 2.9 mg/cm²; backing layer: cellophane. (From Anders, R. and Merkle, H. P., *Int. J. Pharm.*, 49, 235, 1989. With permission.)

permanent binding between the hydrocolloid and the water-insoluble backing layer both in a hydrated and nonhydrated state. For buccal delivery of drugs, one should use similarly coated, but more flexible and softer sheets, instead. Such material is currently being tested in this laboratory.

It is interesting that the use of Cellophane® as backing layers turned out to shorten the duration of mucoadhesion of the films. This is due to the rapid penetration of water through cellophane into the hydrocolloid in contrast to the virtually water-impermeable Multiphor® sheets allowing water uptake from the mucosal side only.

3. Duration of Mucosal Adhesion

The patches investigated were two-ply laminates with a drug-free mucoadhesive polymer. The results of a detailed adhesion study with different nonionic polymers and viscosity grades are given in Figures 2 and 3. Among the cellulose ethers previously investigated in a preliminary study,[9] it was shown that HEC and HPC possess superior mucosal adhesion as indicated by the duration of buccal adhesion in a human subject. Figure 2 shows that up to

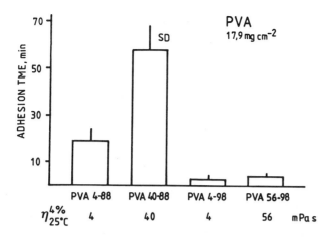

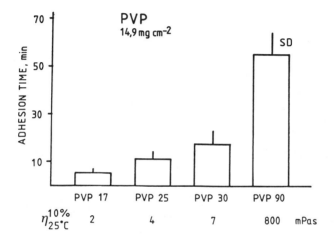

FIGURE 3. Effect of viscosity grade of PVA and PVP on duration of mucosal adhesion *in vivo*. PVA: 17.9 mg/cm²; PVP: 14.9 mg/cm²; backing layer: Multiphor®. (From Anders, R. and Merkle, H. P., *Int. J. Pharm.*, 49, 236, 1989. With permission.)

30 min of adhesion was achieved with HEC and up to about 15 min with HPC, requiring a polymer load as low as 2.8 and 2.9 mg/cm² polymer only. With HEC, the adhesion duration vs. viscosity grade relationship was found to show a maximum. HEC Natrosol® 250 G and K proved to be most adhesive. Lower and higher viscosity grades demonstrated less adhesion. It is noteworthy that an inverse relation was found with HPC, showing a minimum of adhesion at medium viscosity grades and increased adhesion at low and high viscosity grades. The mechanism of the inverse relation is not yet clear and will be further investigated.

Figure 3 shows the corresponding results with PVA and PVP. In both cases, an increase in viscosity resulted in prolonged adhesion. The adhesion of PVA (Mowiol®) patches with the high poly(vinylacetate) (PVAc) content (PVA 4-88, PVA 40-88, corresponding to 12% PVAc), lasted much longer than with the lower PVAc content (PVA 4-98, PVA 56-98, 2% PVAc content), at 17.9 and 14.9 mg/cm², respectively. Dissolution of the polymer was complete with PVA 4-88 and PVA 40-88 only; incomplete dissolution was found with both PVA patches of low PVAc content and corresponds to insignificant adhesion (PVA 4-98, PVA 56-98). With PVP (Kollidon®), only the highest molecular weight studied showed relevant buccal adhesion (PVP 90).

TABLE 3
Comparison of Adhesive Behavior of Different
Polymers *In Vivo*

Polymer/trade name	Amount of polymer mg/cm²	Duration of adhesion (min)		
		Mean	SD	N
HEC Natrosol® 250 G	2.90	32.7	5.7	3
HPC Klucel® EF	5.82	32.3	7.6	3
PVP Kollidon® 90[a]	8.81	36.3	8.1	3
PVA Mowiol® 44-88[b]	8.75	30.3	6.7	3

[a] 1,2-propylenglycol as plasticizer, 10% (w/w).
[b] 1,2-propylenglycol as plasticizer, 25% (w/w).

From Anders, R. and Merkle, H. P., *Int. J. Pharm.*, 49, 236, 1989. With permission.

HEC Natrosol® 250 G turned out to be the most effective polymer studied. This is exemplified in Table 3 comparing the amounts of polymer per square centimeter required to achieve similar durations of mucosal adhesion in the subject. As a potent mucosal adhesive, HEC 250 G was, therefore, used for a series of peptide buccal absorption studies in human subjects and in rats.[9,11,13,34]

C. *IN VIVO* DRUG AND POLYMER RELEASE FROM ADHESIVE PATCHES
1. Experimental Technique
Drug and polymer (PVP) release profiles were followed by analyzing the amount of drug and/or polymer, respectively, remaining on the patch after given contact times. As drug models, TRH and sodium salicylate (as a marker compound) were used. The procedure was as follows. The patches were attached to the buccal mucosa of human subjects, removed after given time periods and analyzed for TRH or salicylate. Excess saliva on the nonadhesive side of the patch was wiped off with a tissue. Polymer and drug remaining on the patch were dissolved in water under constant stirring for 0.5 h. TRH was analyzed by radioimmunoassay or high-performance liquid chromatography, sodium salicylate by UV spectrometry. PVP was analyzed using a colorimetric method. Further details are given elsewhere.[9]

2. *In Vivo* Drug Release
A typical example for drug release is given in Figure 4 showing the results of a study (HEC Natrosol® 250 G patch, 2.1 mg cm^{-2}) on three batches of the same composition in one subject. Each of the data points represents a complete release experiment. The profile indicates first order drug release (see inset). The variation seen in the graph represents both batch variation and within-subject variation of this dosage form remaining in a reasonable range.

a. *Effects of Polymer, Viscosity Grade of Polymer, and Polymer Load on* In Vivo *Release*
The experiments were performed with sodium salicylate (as a marker substance) loaded patches (10 mg/patch) using different polymers, viscosity grades, and polymer loads. All experiments were run in one subject.

The release profiles of the marker are demonstrated in Figures 5 and 6. It is clearly shown that *in vivo* drug release can be significantly controlled by the choice of polymers,

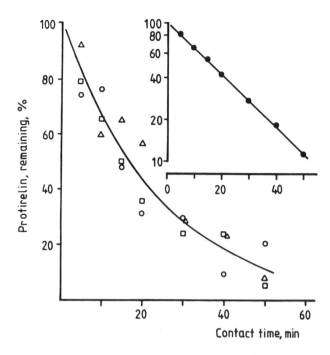

FIGURE 4. Typical profile of buccal release of protirelin from adhesive patch; Data of three batches (○, □, △); all data in one subject; 2.1 mg/cm² HEC 250 G, 1 mg protirelin per patch; inset: semilogarithmic plot. (From Anders, R. and Merkle, H. P., *Int. J. Pharm.*, 49, 237, 1989. With permission.)

viscosity grades, and polymer loads per patch. Within the range studied, drug release can be varied between 10 to 150 min required for a total of 90% of the drug released. More recent studies in this laboratory[47] indicate that drug release can be sustained for even longer periods of time (>6 h) at a more or less constant drug release rate. In most cases, however, periods of more than 3 to 4 h of release are of no practical interest for buccal patches since it may conflict with common eating intervals. Longer periods appear to be practical for nighttime administration only. Small patches attached to the gingiva of the upper incisors may be designed to adhere considerably longer and may possibly remain during meals.

b. Between-Subject Variations of **In Vivo** *Drug Release*

TRH release from adhesive patches is also demonstrated in Figure 7. The data shown are the fraction of TRH remaining in the patch after a 30-min contact with the buccal mucosa of the human subjects. Three different formulations were evaluated. Both increasing the viscosity grade and the amount of polymer is associated with an increase of the fraction of drug remaining in the patch. The between-subject variability is substantial, but within an expected range, possibly depending on the subjects' habits regarding saliva flow, talking, jaw and tongue movements, etc. The results also show that by the choice of the polymer, the release rates of adhesive patches can be individually tailored to meet the specific needs of a given therapy or drug.

Further information on between-subject variations of drug release is given in Figure 8. Here the release of sodium salicylate as a marker was studied in five subjects. Complete release profiles were recorded based on separate release experiments for each of the data points shown in the graph. As before, there is a substantial variability between the subjects, which, however, stays within a reasonable and acceptable range.

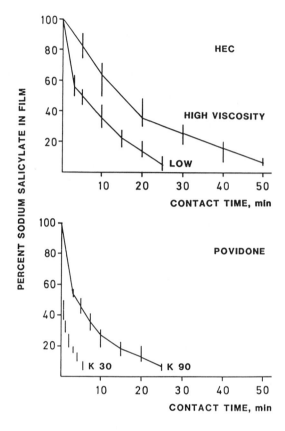

FIGURE 5.   Effect of viscosity grade of HEC and PVP on buccal release of mucoadhesive patch; all data in same subject; 2.0 to 2.1 mg polymer per patch; 10 mg sodium salicylate per patch as marker; bars indicate full range of data; HEC: high viscosity Natrosol® 250 G, low viscosity 250 L; PVP: high viscosity Kollidon® 90, low viscosity Kollidon® 30. (From Anders, R. and Merkle, H. P., *Int. J. Pharm.*, 49, 237, 1989. With permission.)

c. Correlation of Polymer Dissolution and Drug Release

A comparison of polymer dissolution and drug release from PVP 30 and PVP 90 patches using sodium salicylate as a marker is given in Figure 9. The graphs show the percentage of drug and polymer, respectively, remaining in the patch after given periods of time. The data demonstrate that both processes proceed at congruent speed, thus indicating a close correlation between drug release and polymer dissolution. It is, therefore, concluded that drug release from such patches is controlled by the dissolution kinetics of the polymeric carrier. Drug diffusion out of the swollen polymeric matrix of the patch appears to play no significant mechanistic role in the overall drug release. This is in agreement with results of Simonelli et al.[50] and Merkle[51] for drug/PVP coprecipitates where the polymer dissolution was the rate controlling step of drug release. It is assumed that the release from patches made of other water-soluble polymers than PVP 30 and 90 is governed by the same mechanism.

V. *IN VITRO* ADHESION TECHNIQUES

In the literature, a number of techniques are described to measure the adhesion force of bioadhesive polymers to natural and synthetic membranes. These techniques are thoroughly

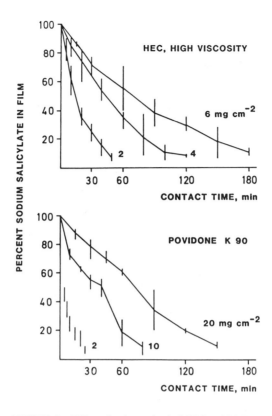

FIGURE 6. Effect of polymer load of HEC and PVP on buccal release of mucoadhesive patch; all data in same subject; 10 mg sodium salicylate per patch as marker; HEC: high viscosity Natrosol® 250 G, PVP: high viscosity Kollidon® 90; bars indicate full range of data. (From Anders, R. and Merkle, H. P., *Int. J. Pharm.*, 49, 238, 1989. With permission.)

reviewed by Peppas and Buri.[37] In a method reported by Smart and Kellaway[52] and by Smart et al.,[53] a glass plate is coated with the adhesive material to be tested. Then the force required to lift the plate out of a mucus containing beaker is measured. The design of the experiment is analogous to the Wilhelmi-plate method to measure surface tension.

A microbalance system was described by Gurny et al.[32] The system consisted of a specially designed cell, which was mounted to a typical tensile tester. The setup was mainly used to measure the adhesiveness of sublingual controlled release systems. Another approach was taken by Park and Robinson and Ch'ng and co-workers.[36,49] They studied adhesion by measuring the force required to separate a polymer specimen from freshly excised rabbit stomach tissue as model mucous membrane. These studies were aimed at polymer/mucus interaction as a means to slow GI transit.

A specific method to study the bond strength between adhesive polymers and certain functional groups of the mucus was presented by Park and Robinson[54] using a fluorescence probe technique. The result is restricted to molecular interactions, and no information can be derived for the adhesive force between polymer and mucus on a macroscopic level. The technique of Peppas and Buri[37] utilizes the movement of a bioadhesive particle across a pipe coated with artificial mucin or natural mucus. The bioadhesive behavior is assumed to relate to the motion of the particle due to a stream of air or of a second viscoelastic solution flowing over the particle.

The technique developed in this laboratory is especially designed to test mucoadhesive

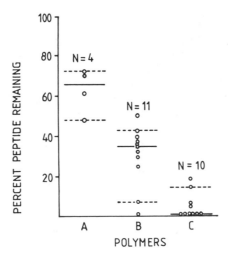

FIGURE 7. Release of protirelin from mucoadhesive patches in human subjects after 30 min; (A) 19.9 mg protirelin per patch, 6.2 mg/cm² HEC 250 G; (B) 10.4 mg protirelin per patch, 2.2 mg/cm² HEC 250 G; (C) 10.1 mg protirelin per patch, 2.1 mg/cm² HEC 250 L. (From Anders, R. and Merkle, H. P., *Int. J. Pharm.*, 49, 238, 1989. With permission.)

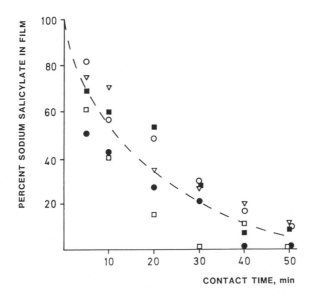

FIGURE 8. Release profile of marker (sodium salicylate) from buccal patches in five subjects; symbols indicating subjects; marker content of patch was 1 mg/cm²; 2.1 mg/cm² HEC 250 G. (From Anders, R. and Merkle, H. P., *Int. J. Pharm.*, 49, 238, 1989. With permission.)

patches.[55] A description of the adhesion test and some results of a recent adhesion study is given below. A similar technique has been approached by Peppas et al.,[56] but with no detailed information available at this time. Boddé[57] developed an alternative technique by measuring the force required to achieve shear flow of an adhesive sample across a test surface. In contrast, the stress data measured in our study were recorded normal to the surface of the sample.

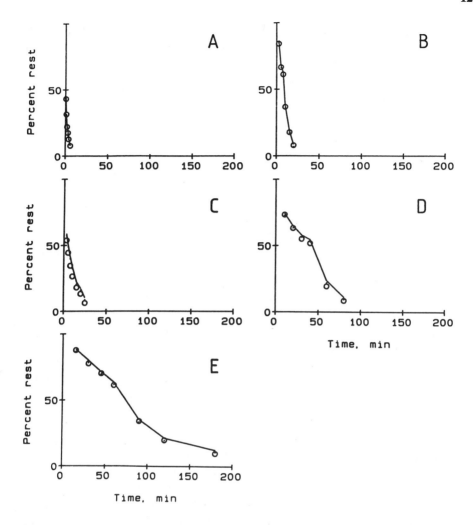

FIGURE 9. Correlation of *in vivo* polymer dissolution and marker release from PVP 30 and PVP 90 patches; all data in same subject; (A) PVP 30, 2.0 mg/cm² (B) PVP 30, 20.5 mg/cm² (C) PVP 90, 2.0 mg/cm² (D) PVP 90, 10.7 mg/cm² (E) PVP 90, 20.5 mg/cm² 10 mg marker per patch; ○, marker release; − −, polymer dissolution. (From Anders, R. and Merkle, H. P., *Int. J. Pharm.*, 49, 236, 1989. With permission.)

VI. *IN VITRO* ADHESION OF ADHESIVE HYDROCOLLOID PATCHES[47]

The technique developed in our laboratory was designed to test adhesive binding and relaxation under dynamic conditions until fracture of the adhesive bond. Adhesive patches were brought in contact with a fully hydrated test membrane and allowed to establish adhesive contact. Then the samples were displaced at constant speed, and the resulting stress/displacement profiles continuously recorded by means of an electronic balance. The stress measured was normal to the surface of the patch. By this setup, the type of adhesive flow and the maximum adhesive stress could be determined, whereas most other techniques are restricted to the maximum stress recorded at fracture of the adhesive bond only, except for Gurny et al.[32] who report on a stress/displacement profile being quite similar to those in our studies. The formulation investigated in this study was a controlled release preparation consisting of sodium carboxymethyl cellulose, gelatine, and polyethylene. In our study, various pure hydrophilic polymers were tested after different contact periods, which was to demonstrate the effect of the degree of swelling and dissolution of the polymer on its adhesive behavior.

In addition to the adhesion test under dynamic conditions, a limited number of experiments were also carried out under constant displacement of the sample, i.e., static conditions. This set-up was to obtain further information on the viscous relaxation upon adhesive stress.

A. MATERIALS AND PATCH PREPARATION

The materials tested were the same as described in Table 2. For preparation of the patches, a knife casting device was applied using appropriate aqueous polymer solutions and Multiphor® as impermeable backing layer. Patches of 1.13 cm² were prepared by means of a suitable punch-die set. Higher polymer loads required repeated casting until the desired polymer load was achieved. Drying of the laminates was on top of the casting plate at 37°C, except for PVP patches, which were dried at 25°C in order to prevent blister formation. Throughout no plasticizers were used. A detailed description is given by Wermerskirchen.[58]

B. *IN VITRO* ADHESIVE STRESS MEASUREMENT

1. Adhesion Test

Adhesion of buccal patches was tested *in vitro* by recording stress/displacement profiles of patches staying in contact with a fully hydrated test membrane. Stress was imposed by linear displacement of the sample normal to its surface until fracture of the adhesive bond occurred. Cellophane was the most frequently used test membrane. In a number of cases, freshly excised porcine colon mucosa was used as a natural mucosal membrane, taken from the distal part of the colon, approximately 20 to 70 cm above the rectum. The material was washed and stored in water at 5°C. Use was completed within 24 h.

The test configuration used included an electronic balance (maximum load <300 g) connected on-line to a suitable computer for data monitoring. Previous to the test, the dry two-ply buccal patch (1.13 cm², consisting of a Multiphor® backing layer and the hydrocolloid layer) was firmly glued onto an aluminum disk holder attached to a hook. Then contact was established between the hydrocolloid layer and the previously hydrated test membrane, which was stretched across the aperture of a suitable beaker (4 cm diameter) completely filled with pH 6.8 buffer (ionic strength of 0.1) at 37°C without any air remaining in the beaker. The beaker itself was fully submerged in water by means of another water-filled beaker at 37°C. Uptake of water by the hydrocolloid polymer leads to an adhesive interaction between the buccal patch and the test membrane. After given contact periods (>5 min), the sample holder was attached to the balance, and the beaker was vertically lowered at constant speed of 0.076 mm/s by means of a motor-driven platform, and the adhesive stress was simultaneously recorded. By this technique, the adhesive stress was measured under dynamic conditions.

For static stress relaxation measurements, the lowering of the platform was stopped at given displacements, and the adhesive stress remaining was further measured as a function of time.

2. Adhesion Profiles

Typical stress/displacement profiles of the adhesion of buccal patches to swollen cellophane membranes are given in Figure 10 (for HEC) and Figure 11 (for HPC). The profiles displayed are representative examples out of 5 to 11 repetitions. Variations between repetitive experiments were reasonable. For instance, the standard deviation (SD) between the peak stress values recorded was usually below 10% of the mean; in some cases variations of up to 20% were recorded. Therefore, the technique appears to be reasonably reproducible.

a. HEC

Different HEC 250 polymers of increasing viscosity grades, i.e., molecular sizes, were

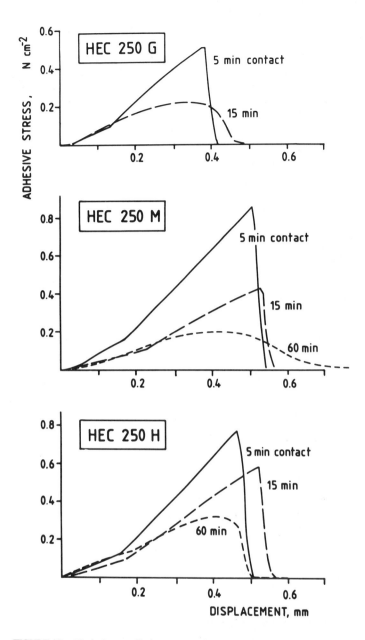

FIGURE 10. Typical stress/displacement profiles of hydroxyethyl cellulose patches (HEC Natrosol® 250 G, 250 M, 250 H) after different contact periods on cellophane; no detectable adhesion found after 60 min if not specified; polymer load: 250 G, 5.89 mg/cm²; 250 M 4.83 mg/cm²; 250 H, 5.02 mg/cm².

investigated. The profiles were recorded 5, 15, and 60 min after adhesive contact to the test membrane was established. This was in order to demonstrate the effect of simultaneous swelling and dissolution of the adhesive hydrocolloid polymer while staying in contact to the test membrane.

Examples of stress/displacement profiles in Figure 10 show that after the shortest contact time (5 min), except for an initial section, the adhesive stress curves exhibit an apparently linear course with increasing displacement of the specimen, indicating essentially elastic behavior according to Hooke's law. On the other hand, stress relaxation experiments de-

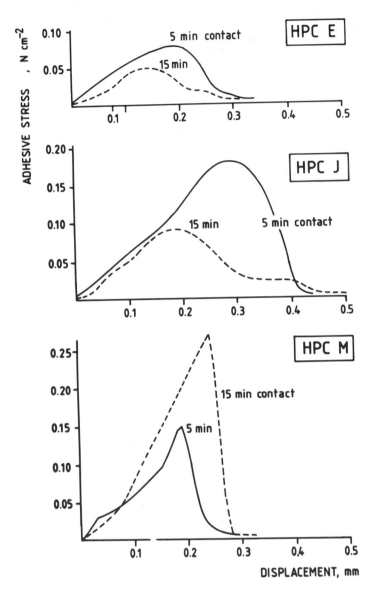

FIGURE 11.   Typical stress/displacement profiles of hydroxypropyl cellulose patches (HPC Klucel® E, J, M) after different contact periods on cellophane; no detectable adhesion found after 60 min; polymer load: E, 5.4 mg/cm²; J, 7.0 mg/cm²; M, 5.9 mg/cm².

scribed below (see Section VI.B.3.b. and Figure 14) are indicative of nonelastic viscous flow even at stress values in the essentially linear parts of the stress/displacement curves.

After the 5-min contact period, the fracture of the adhesive interaction of all HEC species is instantaneous without visible indication of viscous relaxation of the swollen adhesive. Then, after 15-min contact, in the case of HEC 250 G having the lowest molecular size among the HEC polymers applied, the linear displacement of the specimen resulted in a nonlinear increase of the adhesive stress referring to viscous relaxation of the swollen adhesive upon stress. No clear fracture point was detected, but with HEC 250 M and H, having higher molecular sizes, the increase of the adhesive stress was again almost linear but at a decreased slope. The fracture of the adhesive bond was instantaneous and not associated with viscous flow as with HEC 250 G.

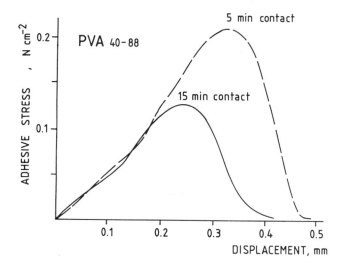

FIGURE 12.   Typical stress/displacement profiles of polyvinyl alcohol (PVA Mowiol®40-88) after different contact periods on cellophane; no detectable adhesion found after 60 min; polymer load: 10.67 mg/cm².

Finally, after 60-min contact to the test membrane, no adhesive stress was detectable with HEC 250 G. With both higher molecular size qualities, i.e., HEC 250 M and HEC 250 H, the displacement of the specimen resulted in a nonlinear increase of the adhesive stress. This is the result of a marked viscous relaxation of the adhesive polymer upon stress. No clear fracture points could be observed. Close visual inspection of the adhesion site revealed that at the end of the relaxation process viscous polymer filaments between the adhesive patches and the test membrane were formed as the process of adhesive bond separation was proceeding. Contact periods longer than 60 min were not yet tested. However, it is safe to expect that increasing water uptake will intensify viscous relaxation resulting in flatter profiles. Upon further swelling and dissolution, adhesion should become essentially zero.

b. Other Polymers: HPC, PVA, and PVP

Typical adhesion profiles of different HPC polymers of increasing molecular size are depicted in Figure 11. HPC E, i.e., the polymer with the lowest molecular size, was the least adhesive. In contrast to all HEC polymers, the stress/displacement profiles did not show essentially linear (quasi-elastic) sections; instead, the breakage of the adhesive bond was associated with strong viscous relaxation. A similar pattern was found with HPC J. Parallel to its higher molecular size, this polymer showed better adhesion, but the difference between the profiles recorded after 5 min and after 15 min contact was more pronounced with HPC J than it was with HPC E.

In contrast to any other polymer studied, HPC M showed a rather unique behavior. The most interesting point was that the maximum stress recorded after 15 min was higher than after 5 min. All other polymers showed a reverse relationship. This indicates that this polymer develops increasing adhesive capacity upon swelling, whereas in all other polymers, increasing water uptake led to decreasing adhesion. This observation should be further investigated in order to understand its mechanism.

Typical force/displacement plots of PVA 40-88 are given in Figure 12, showing a similar behavior as HPC J in Figure 11. PVP 90 is even less adhesive and not displayed in a graph.

All other polymers tested did not yield detectable adhesion. It appears that adhesion of water-soluble hydrocolloids needs a balanced relationship of polymer swelling and dissolution. Polymers of very fast dissolution rate, e.g., PVP 25 and PVP 30, did not show

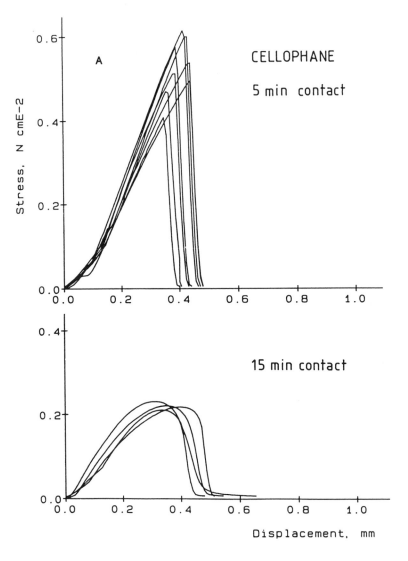

FIGURE 13.   (A) Stress/displacement profiles of HEC 250 G patches on cellophane; polymer load: 5.85 mg/cm². (B) Stress/displacement profiles of HEC 250 G patches on excised porcine colon mucosa; polymer load: 5.85 mg/cm². (C) Stress/displacement profiles of HEC 250 G patches on excised porcine colon mucosa; polymer load: 10.72 mg/cm².

detectable adhesion. The second factor, polymer swelling, appears to be equally important. PVA 56-98, a highly swellable polymer of low dissolution, did not exhibit relevant adhesion, as the result of its slow dissolution, but PVA 40-88, showing less swelling but better dissolution, was found to be an efficient adhesive.

It is obvious from these typical profiles that the test method employed represents a highly sensitive method to evaluate the dynamics of adhesive binding between a test membrane and water-soluble hydrocolloid polymers. It allows discrimination between a variety of different adhesion/relaxation patterns. Its potential includes the optimization of adhesive dosage forms as well as the insight into mechanistic aspects of adhesive bonds of hydrocolloids and other polymers. So far no comparison of this technique to those developed by other authors is available.

An example for the reproducibility of the technique is given in Figure 13A. It includes

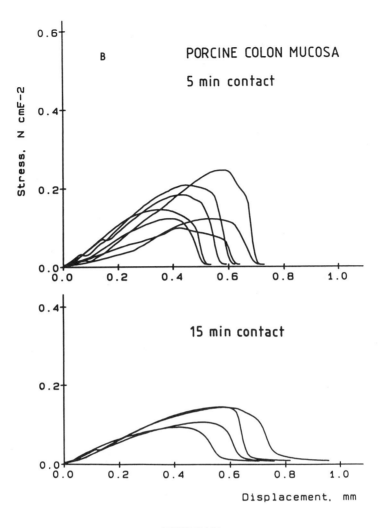

FIGURE 13B.

marked variations of slope, extension, and maximum value, but in total the variations are still in an acceptable range.

3. Mechanistic View of Adhesion Test

For a mechanistic view of the data, the theory of viscoelasticity appears to be applicable, outlines of which are given, for instance, in the principal work of Fluegge.[59] The aim would be to develop suitable composite models for viscoelastic solids and/or liquids under adhesive stress.

Two principal situations should be considered: (1) dynamic measurement of stress relaxation under a constant rate of displacement and (2) static measurement at constant displacement, both of which are the types of measurement used in this study. The simple classical Maxwell fluid and the Kelvin solid model for this situation are outlined below. More complex models[59] other than these are not yet applied.

a. Dynamic Stress Relaxation of Adhesive Polymers

Applying a simple Maxwell fluid model, consisting of one spring and one dashpot element in series, viscoelastic deformation may be described by[59]

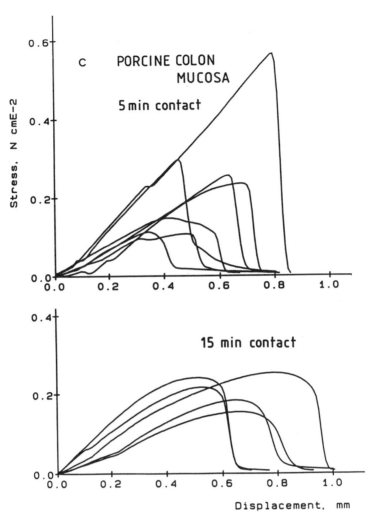

FIGURE 13C.

$$\frac{d\epsilon}{dt} = \frac{d\epsilon_{spring}}{dt} + \frac{d\epsilon_{dashpot}}{dt} \tag{1}$$

where ϵ is the strain, i.e., $\epsilon = x/1$, with $1 =$ total length and $x =$ displacement. Since according to Hooke's law for the spring element

$$\sigma = q_o\epsilon \tag{2}$$

with $\sigma =$ stress and $q_o =$ elastic modulus; and for the dashpot element with q_1 as a constant

$$\sigma = q_1 \frac{d\epsilon}{dt} \tag{3}$$

Thus one may write

$$\frac{d\epsilon}{dt} = \frac{d\sigma}{dt}\frac{1}{q_o} + \frac{\sigma}{q_1} \tag{4}$$

For a constant rate of displacement dx/dt, i.e., dϵ/dt = r we obtain

$$r = \frac{d\sigma}{dt}\frac{1}{q_o} + \frac{\sigma}{q_1} \tag{5}$$

or

$$\frac{d\sigma}{dt} = \frac{q_o}{q_1}(q_1r - \sigma) \tag{6}$$

By separation of the variables and for the initial conditions given (t = 0; σ = 0) the solution of the differential equation is simple, yielding

$$\sigma = q_1r\left[1 - \exp\left(-\frac{q_o}{q_1}t\right)\right] = q_1r\left[1 - \exp\left(-\frac{q_o}{q_1k}x\right)\right] \tag{7}$$

since according to the constant strain rate dϵ/dt, time is proportional to displacement, or t = x/k. For t $\rightarrow\infty$, i.e., increasing displacement, the stress approaches an upper limit of σ = q_1 r. For t $\rightarrow$0 and σ $\rightarrow$0 the stress change dσ/dt is constant, i.e., dσ/dt = q_o r or σ = $q_o\epsilon$, and thus approximated by Hooke's law. This means that under the dynamic conditions used for the measurements, the initial quasi-linear section of the profiles is dominated by the elastic behavior of the adhesive bond, whereas the final section is controlled by viscous flow. Moreover, the approach to the viscous flow plateau is affected by the strain rate r, i.e., by the rate of displacement selected for the adhesion test, a parameter that has not yet been studied in this work.

On the other hand, for a simple Kelvin solid model, consisting of one spring and one dashpot element in parallel, we obtain

$$\sigma = \sigma_{spring} + \sigma_{dashpot} \tag{8}$$

and from Equations 2 and 3

$$\sigma = q_o\epsilon + q_1\frac{d\epsilon}{dt} \tag{9}$$

Since the rate of displacement is constant, i.e., dϵ/dt = r, one then gets

$$\sigma = q_o\epsilon + q_1r \tag{10}$$

showing a linear relation of stress and strain (or displacement).

It is interesting to compare Equation 7 (Maxwell fluid) and Equation 10 (Kelvin solid) with the experimental profiles shown in Figures 10 to 12, for HEC, HPC, and PVA, respectively. The following discussion will be restricted to the meaningful segments excluding the lag branch at the beginning and the declining branch from the break point or maximum of the curves. This is the range of physical significance of the data with respect to the equations.

In the first place, a clear decision in favor of one of the models appears to be difficult. Quasilinear (= elastic) stress/displacement curves as predicted, for instance, by Equation 10 for Kelvin solids, are observed with all HEC polymers at short contact periods. On the

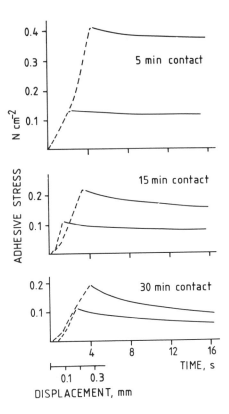

FIGURE 14.   Viscous relaxation of HEC 250 G patches on cellophane
upon constant displacement; polymer load: 16.98 mg/cm^2.

other hand, the relaxation behavior (see Section VI.B.3.b) of these polymers under constant displacement indicate that the Kelvin solid model is not applicable, since at dϵ/dt = 0, a Kelvin solid would behave strictly elastic. The pronounced relaxation phenomena shown under these conditions (see Section VI.B.3.b) make a Maxwell fluid model much more reasonable. This decision would not be contradictory since for t →0, i.e., in the initial section, the Maxwell fluid model (Equation 7) results in a quasilinear segment. Therefore, it is concluded that the linear sections observed are consistent with the Maxwell fluid model.

The profile segments of HEC for longer contact periods were typical for Maxwell fluid behavior according to Equation 7. The same type of flow was also found with the HPC polymers except for HPC M, and with PVA and PVP. Therefore, we conclude that the Maxwell fluid type is the most appropriate simple model for all polymers investigated. This observation shows that mucoadhesive binding is not only a matter of elastic binding at the boundary, but is also markedly affected by the viscous flow of the adhesive under stress.

b. Static Stress Relaxation of Adhesive Polymers

The stress/displacement profiles of HEC 250 G shown in Figure 10 were recorded under constant linear displacement of the specimen. Thus polymer relaxation was studied under dynamic conditons. Relaxation profiles under static conditions for the same polymer are presented in Figure 14. The profiles were recorded after displacement of the specimen had been stopped at a low and a high level of the adhesion stress remaining. For swelling, contact times of 5, 15, and 30 min were maintained before measurements took place.

The results (Figure 14) show that the adhesion forces decreased more or less exponentially ater displacement of the samples had been stopped. The higher the initial force, the faster the exponential decrease. Furthermore, with increasing contact times, stress relaxation became more pronounced.

For the development of a physical insight, the viscoelastic theory is once more applied. Again the simple Maxwell fluid and the Kelvin solid models are elaborated.

For constant displacement, i.e., $d\epsilon/dt = 0$, the solution of the differential equation of the Maxwell fluid model in Equation 4 is simple, resulting in

$$\sigma = \sigma_o \exp\left(-\frac{q_o}{q_1}t\right) \tag{11}$$

showing an exponential decrease of the stress remaining as a function of time. This corresponds well with the experimental profiles as demonstrated in Figure 14. Linear or nonlinear regression analysis of the data cannot lead to a determination of q_o and q_1, since the coefficients are not separable.

When the Kelvin solid model is used instead (Equation 9), $d\epsilon/dt = 0$ results in $\sigma = q_o\epsilon$, i.e., Hooke's law for a fully elastic solid. The data show clearly that the adhesive tested did not behave elastically, and the Kelvin solid model, therefore, is not suitable to describe the data. As in the previous chapter, the Maxwell fluid model is again most appropriate.

C. *IN VITRO* ADHESION TO PORCINE COLON MUCOSA

Most of the data obtained in this study refers to the use of cellophane as test membrane. Because the practical relevance of a nonbiological test membrane is limited, further studies based on excised porcine colon mucosa were also undertaken. HEC 250 G was the only polymer evaluated. The results obtained are given in Figure 13B and C for two polymer loads (high, low) and two contact times (5 min, 15 min). Corresponding results using cellophane were displayed in Figure 13A.

It is interesting to note that the variability of the mucosa experiments after the short contact period was higher as compared to the longer period. Especially at the high polymer load a dramatic variability of both the shape of the profiles and of the maximum stress value was observed. When compared to the results obtained on cellophane (Figure 13A), the mucosa experiments were found to vary much more and to remain at much lower maximum adhesion values, especially after the short contact period. After the 15-min contact, the mucosa results still showed more variation and lower adhesion than the corresponding profiles on cellophane membrane (Figure 13A). The differences of the variability and of the adhesive capacity, however, were not as marked as found after the 5-min contact.

The most reasonable explanation for the higher degree of variability comes from the different nature of the cellophane and the colon mucosa. The establishment of strong adhesive binding between the adhesive polymer and the cellulose matrix of cellophane or the glycoproteins of the mucosa, respectively, requires a dense intercalation of the polymer species upon mutual diffusion. It is not surprising that, as corresponds to the variability of a natural membrane, this process proceeds at a locally different rate and extent. As a result, adhesion on natural mucosa may vary considerably, whereas adhesion on a synthetic membrane like cellophane is more reproducible.

The generally lower adhesive capacity also needs to be interpreted. Because of the thick mucus layer covering the mucosa, this process is supposed to take more time until full adhesive contact between both polymer species can be built up. In addition, the mucus layer is partly viscous, whereas cellophane is a swollen but firm solid. Therefore, the maximum values achieved on the mucosa are to be lower than on cellophane.

A most remarkable difference in profile shape between the mucosa and cellophane was found, for instance, for the profiles recorded after 5-min contact. The breakage of the adhesive bond was instantaneous with cellophane, but showed viscous relaxation when porcine mucosa

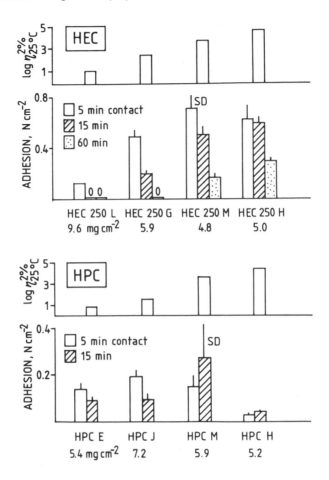

FIGURE 15.   Maximum adhesive stress of hydroxyethyl cellulose (HEC) and hydroxypropyl cellulose (HPC) polymers after different contact periods in comparison to their viscosity grades.

was used instead. This is obviously due to the viscous nature of the mucus. Thus the relaxation found is most likely the result of the natural mucus flowing under adhesive stress.

D. EVALUATION OF POLYMERS FOR MAXIMUM ADHESION CAPACITY
1. Effect of Polymer
A comparative evaluation of the adhesive capacity of the different hydrocolloid polymers on cellophane was given previously (see Sections VI.B.2.a and B.2.b). It was demonstrated that, in general terms, HEC was the most adhesive type of polymer studied, followed by HPC and PVA 40-88. A more detailed comparison of HEC and HPC, supporting this conclusion, is given in Figure 15. PVP 90 was the least adhesive polymer. All other polymers investigated did not show significant adhesive capacity.

2. Effect of Polymer Load
Examples of the effect of the polymer load on the maximum adhesive stress on cellophane are demonstrated in Figure 15. It is interesting to see that with HEC 250 G a twofold increase of the polymer content resulted in a minor increase of the maximum adhesive stress only. With HPC E and PVP 90, increasing amounts of polymer led to a more pronounced effect on the adhesive stress. As compared to the effects of the polymer itself (see Section VI.D.1) and its viscosity grade (see Section VI.D.3), the polymer load appears to have less influence on the adhesive capacity.

3. Effect of Viscosity Grade of Polymer

The effects of the viscosity grade of two series of polymers, HEC 250 and HPC, respectively, are given in Figure 15. The plots include maximum adhesion values found on cellophane after given contact periods and, for comparison, the log of the viscosity of solutions of a given concentration as a molecular size parameter. The data show a marked molecular size influence on the adhesive stress at all contact periods studied. It is interesting to note that, for instance, maximum HEC adhesion after 5-min contact was found with HEC 250 M, whereas HEC 250 H is the best adhesive after a 60-min contact time. The decrease of the adhesive stress with increasing contact times was found to be clearly less with the higher molecular weight HEC 250 H as compared to the much larger drop for the lower molecular size polymers HEC 250 G and 250 M.

With HPC the adhesion optimum achieved after the 5 min contact period was found with HPC J, but after 15 min the optimum was with HPC M. In more general terms, we observe a shift of the optimum of adhesion towards higher viscosity grades as contact times are increasing.

This result again indicates that adhesion is influenced by an interplay of both swelling and dissolution of the polymers, depending on their molecular size. At low viscosity, i.e., low molecular size, good adhesion may be achieved already after very short contact periods. This is attributed to a fast swelling process of low molecular size polymers, which leads to immediate adhesive interaction between the polymer and the test membrane. However, after longer contact periods, the process of dissolution of a low molecular size polymer during the test is responsible for a significant loss of adhesive binding. If polymers of higher viscosity grade are taken, initial adhesion may be somewhat lower because the swelling process of a high molecular weight polymer is slower. After sufficient swelling has been reached, however, an adequate degree of adhesive binding is achieved, which can be preserved for an even longer period, because polymer dissolution proceeds at a much slower dissolution rate.

E. COMPARISON OF *IN VIVO* AND *IN VITRO* ADHESION DATA

In order to compare the adhesive capacity investigated (1) in a human subject (see Section IV.B.3) and (2) by the *in vitro* technique described using a cellophane membrane, one has to be aware of the following facts. In the first case, the adhesion parameter studied was the duration of adhesion, which was determined by personal judgment of the subject. On the other hand, the parameter of the *in vitro* study was the adhesive stress measured by a physically more or less exact technique.

In a general sense, there is some correlation of both sets of data, but conflicting points are also apparent. In the *in vivo* study, the most adhesive polymer was HEC. HPC, PVA, and PVP were less adhesive or required higher amounts of polymer to achieve comparable adhesive effects. This is more or less what has been found in the *in vitro* study. On the other hand, it is interesting to look into some discrepanices. For instance, HEC 250 G was the most adhesive HEC polymer in the *in vivo* study. *In vitro*, however, HEC 250 M and H were clearly more adhesive than HEC 250 G. Moreover, in the *in vivo* study of the HPC group, a flat minimum of adhesive capacity was observed with the medium molecular size HPC M, whereas in the *in vitro* study, exactly this polymer showed an optimum adhesion among its group, with the lower and higher molecular size polymers having less adhesive capacity.

Good correlation is seen with PVA and PVP: with both methods PVA 40-88 was the most adhesive PVA polymer, and PVP 90 was the best in the PVP group. This leads to the conclusion that the data obtained from the *in vitro* test do indeed carry some relevant information for the *in vivo* adhesion behavior of buccal patches. Therefore, the test is regarded as being of practical relevance for the formulation of adhesive mucosal preparations.

Since the *in vivo* test included a personal judgment of the duration of adhesion rather than an exact measurement, some of the conflicting facts may be due to experimental variation. However, the discrepancy between *in vivo* and *in vitro* concerning the optimum HEC polymer remains an open question. It is assumed that this gap is due to the different supply of saliva and water, respectively, to the hydrocolloid polymer during both types of tests. In the *in vivo* test, the supply by the mucosa is restricted, whereas practically unlimited supply of water is available in the *in vitro* test. This may lead to different swelling and dissolution kinetics of the polymers in both environments. For full interpretation of the discrepancies found between the two test methods, further investigations need to be undertaken.

REFERENCES

1. **Su, K. S. E. and Campanale, K. M.,** Nasal drug delivery systems requirements, development and evaluations, in *Transnasal Systemic Medications,* Chien, Y. W., Ed., Elsevier, Amsterdam, 1985, 139.
2. **Su, K. S. E.,** Intranasal delivery of peptides and proteins, *Pharm. Int.,* 7, 8, 1986.
3. **Van de Donk. H. J. M., Van den Heuvel, A. G. M., Zuidema, J., and Merkus, F. W. H. M.,** The effects of nasal drops and their additives on human, nasal mucociliary clearance, *Rhinology,* 20, 127, 1982.
4. **Stratford, R. E. and Lee, V. H. L.,** Aminopeptidase activity in albino rabbit extraocular tissues relative to the small intestine, *J. Pharm. Sci.,* 74, 731, 1985.
5. **Lee, V. H. L.,** Enzymatic barriers to peptide and protein absorption and use of penetration enhancers to modify absorption, *Proc. NATO Ad. Res. Workshop: Adv. Drug Delivery Syst. Peptides Proteins* NATO ASI series, Davis, S. S., Illum, L. E., and Tomlinson, E., Eds., Plenum Press, New York, 1986, 87.
6. **Wespi, H. J. and Rehsteiner, H. P.,** Erfahrungen mit Synthocinon und ODA-Buccaltabletten, *Gynaecologia,* 162, 414, 1966.
7. **Bergsjö, P. and Jenssen, H.,** Nasal and buccal oxytocin for the introduction of labour: a clinical trial, *J. Obstet. Gynaecol. Br. Commonw.,* 76, 131, 1969.
8. **Sjöstedt, S.,** Induction of labor: a comparison of intranasal and transbuccal administration of oxytocin, *Acta Obstet. Gynaecol. Scand.,* 48 (Suppl. 7), 3, 1969.
9. **Anders, R.,** Selbsthaftende Polymerfilme zur bukkalen Applikation von Peptiden, Ph.D. thesis, Universität Bonn, Germany, 1984.
10. **Anders, R., Merkle, H. P., Schurr, W., and Ziegler, R.,** Buccal absorption of protirelin: an effective way to stimulate thyrotropin and prolactin, *J. Pharm. Sci.,* 72, 1481, 1983.
11. **Merkle, H. P., Anders, R., Sandow, J., and Schurr, W.,** Self-adhesive patches for buccal delivery of peptides, in *Proc. Int. Symp. Controlled Release Bioact. Mater.,* 12, 85, 1985.
12. **Merkle, H. P., Anders, R., and Sandow, J.,** Buccal Absorption of Peptides in Rats, in *Proc. 32nd Annu. Congr. Int. Assoc. Pharm. Technol.,* Leiden, 1986, 57.
13. **Merkle, H. P., Anders, R., Sandow, J., and Schurr, W.,** Drug delivery of peptides: the buccal route, in *Delivery Systems for Peptide Drugs* (NATO ASI Series A), Vol. 125, Davis, S. S., Illum, L., and Tomlinson, E., Eds., Plenum, New York, 1986, 159.
14. **Veillard, M. M., Longer, M. A., Tucker, I. G. and Robinson, J. R.,** Buccal controlled delivery of peptides, in *Proc. Int. Symp. Controlled Release Bioact. Mater.,* 14, 22, 1987.
15. **Earle, Sr. M. P.,** Experimental use of oral insulin, *Isr. J. Med. Sci.,* 8, 899, 1972.
16. **Laczi, F., Mezei, G., Julesz, J., and Laszlo, F. A.,** Effects of vasopressin analogues (DDAVP, DVDAVP) in the form of sublingual tablets in central diabetes insipidus, *Int. J. Clin. Pharmacol. Ther. Toxicol.* 18, 63, 1980.
17. **Ishida, M., Machida, Y., Nambu, N., and Nagai, T.,** New mucosal dosage form of insulin, *Chem. Pharm. Bull.,* 29, 810, 1981.
18. **Ho, N. H. F. and Higuchi, W. I.,** Quantitative interpretation of in vivo buccal absorption of n-alkanoic acids by the physical model approach, *J. Pharm. Sci.,* 69, 537, 1971.
19. **Schürmann, W. and Turner, P.,** The buccal absorption of atenolol and propranolol, and their physico-chemical characteristics, *Br. J. Clin. Pharmacol.,* 4, 655P, 1977.
20. **Jarrett, A.,** *The Physiology and Pathophysiology of the Skin,* Vol. 6, Academic Press, London, 1980, 1871.
21. **Ho, N. H. F., Park, J. Y., Ni, Ph. I., and Higuchi, W. I.,** Advancing quantitative and mechanistic approaches in interfacing gastrointestinal drug absorption studies in animals and humans, in *Animal Models for Oral Drug Delivery in Man: In Situ and In Vivo Approaches,* Crouthamel, W. and Sarapu, A. C., Eds., American Pharmaceutical Association, Washington D. C., 1983, 27.

22. **Tolo, K.,** A study of permeability of gingival pocket epithelium to albumin in guinea pigs and Norwegian pigs, *Arch. Oral Biol.,* 16, 881, 1971.
23. **Tolo, K. and Jonsen, J.,** In vitro penetration of tritiated dextrans through rabbit oral mucosa, *Arch. Oral Biol.,* 20, 419, 1975.
24. **Lee, V. H. L., Kashi Dodda, Patel, R. M., Hayakawa, E., and Inagaki, K.,** Mucosal peptide and protein delivery: proteolytic activities in mucosal homogenates, *Proc. Int. Symp. Controlled Release Bioact. Mater.,* 14, 23, 1987.
25. **Machida, Y. and Nagai, T.,** Application of hydroxypropyl cellulose to peroral controlled release dosage forms, *Chem. Pharm. Bull.,* 26, 1652, 1978.
26. **Machida, Y., Masuda, H., Fujiyama, N., Iwata, M., and Nagai, T.,** Preparation and phase II clinical examination of topical dosage form for the treatment of carcinoma colli containing bleomycin, carboquone, or 5-fluorouracil with hydroxypropyl cellulose, *Chem. Pharm. Bull.,* 28, 1125, 1980.
27. **Ishida, M., Nambu, N., and Nagai, T.,** Mucosal dosage form of lidocain for toothache using hydroxypropyl cellulose and Carbopol, *Chem. Pharm. Bull.,* 30, 980, 1982.
28. **Ishida, M., Nambu, N., and Nagai, T.,** Highly viscour gel ointment containing Carbopol for application to the oral mucosa, *Chem. Pharm. Bull.,* 31, 4561, 1983.
29. **Bremecker, K. D., Klein, G., Strempel, H., and Rübesamen-Vokuhl, A.,** Formulierung und klinische Erprobung einer neuartigen Schleimhauthaftsalbe, *Arzneim. Forsch./Drug. Res.,* 33, 591, 1983.
30. **Bremecker, K. D.,** Modell zur Bestimmung der Haftdauer von Schleimhauthaftsalben in vitro, *Pharm. Ind.,* 45, 417, 1983.
31. **Bremecker, K. D., Strempel, H., and Klein, G.,** Novel concept for a mucosal adhesive ointment, *J. Pharm. Sci.,* 73, 548, 1984.
32. **Gurny, R., Meyer, J. M., and Peppas, N. A.,** Bioadhesive intraoral release systems: design, testing and analysis, *Biomaterials,* 5, 336, 1984.
33. **Anders, R. and Merkle, H. P.,** Evaluation of laminated muco-adhesive patches for buccal drug delivery, *Int. J. Pharm.,* 49, 231, 1989.
34. **Merkle, H. P., Anders, R., Wermerskirchen, A., and Raehs, S.,** Buccal route of peptide and protein drug delivery, in *Peptide and Protein Drug Delivery,* Lee, V. H. L., Ed., Marcel Dekker, New York, to be published.
35. **Nagai, T.,** Adhesive topical drug delivery system, in *Advances in Drug Delivery Systems* (Controlled Release Series), Vol.1, Anderson, J. M. and Kim, S. W., Eds., Elsevier, Amsterdam, 1986, 121.
36. **Park, H. and Robinson, J. R.,** Physico-chemical properties of water insoluble polymers important to mucin/epithelial adhesion, in *Advances in Drug Delivery Systems* (Controlled Release Series), Vol.1, Anderson, J. M. and Kim, S. W., Eds., Elsevier, Amsterdam, 1986, 47.
37. **Peppas, N. A. and Buri, P. A.,** Surface, interfacial and molecular aspects of polymer bioadhesion on soft tissues, in *Advances in Drug Delivery Systems Controlled Release Series,* Vol.1, Anderson, J. M. and Kim, S. W., Eds., Elsevier, Amsterdam, 1986, 257.
38. **Manly, R. S., Ed.,** *Adhesion in Biological Systems,* Academic Press, New York, 1970.
39. **Anderson, G. P., Bennet, S. J., and DeVries, K. L.,** *Analysis and Testing of Adhesive Bonds,* Academic Press, New York, 1977.
40. **Davis, S. S., Daly, P. B., Kennerley, J. W., Frier, M., Hardy, J. G., and Wilson, C. G.,** Design and evaluation of sustained release formulations for oral and buccal administration, in *Controlled Release Nitroglycerin in Buccal and Oral Form, Advances in Pharmacotherapy,* Vol. 1, Bussmann, W. -D., Dries, R. -R., and Wagner, W., Eds., S. Karger, Basel, 1982, 17.
41. **Schor, J. M., Davis, S. S., Nigalaye, A., and Bolton, S.,** Susadrin transmucosal tablets, *Drug Dev. Ind. Pharm.,* 9, 1359, 1983.
42. **Erb, R. J.,** Bioavailability of controlled release buccal and oral nitroglycerin by digital plethysmography, in *Controlled Release Nitroglycerin in Buccal and Oral Form, Advances in Pharmacotherapy,* Vol. 1, Bussmann, W.-D., Dries, R.-R., and Wagner, W., Eds., S. Karger, Basel, 1982, 35.
43. **Chien, Y. W.,** Potential developments and new approaches in oral controlled-release drug delivery systems, *Drug. Dev. Ind. Pharm.,* 9, 1291, 1983.
44. **Ishida, M., Nambu, N., and Nagai, T.,** Ointment-type oral mucosal dosage form of Carbopol containing prednisolon for treatment of aphta, *Chem. Pharm. Bull.,* 31, 1010, 1983.
45. **Nagai, T., Machida, Y., and Suzuki, Y.,** Offenl. DE 2908847, 1980.
46. **Kissel, Th. and Bergauer, R.,** Offenl. DE 3237945 A 1, 1983.
47. **Wermerskirchen, A. and Merkle, H. P.,** unpublished data, 1986.
48. **Lee, P. I.,** Kinetics of drug release from hydrogel matrices, in *Advances in Drug Delivery Systems* (Controlled Release Series), Vol.1, Anderson, J. M. and Kim, S. W., Eds., Elsevier, Amsterdam, 1986, 277.
49. **Ch'ng, H. S., Park, H., Kelly, P., and Robinson, J. R.,** Bioadhesive polymers as platforms for oral controlled drug delivery. II. Synthesis and evaluation of some swelling, water-insoluble bioadhesive polymers, *J. Pharm. Sci.,* 74, 399, 1985.

50. **Simonelli, A. P., Mehta, S. C., and Higuchi, W. I.,** Dissolution rates of high energy polyvinylpyrrolidone(PVP)-sulfathiazole coprecipitates, *J. Pharm. Sci.,* 58, 538, 1969.
51. **Merkle, H. P.,** Untersuchungen an Einbettungen von Arzneistoffen in Polyvinylpyrrolidon, Habilitation thesis, University of Heidelberg, 1979.
52. **Smart, J. D. and Kellaway, I. W.,** In vitro techniques for measuring bioadhesion, *J. Pharm. Pharmacol.,* 34, 70P, 1982.
53. **Smart, J. D., Kellaway, I. W., and Worthington, H. E. C.,** An in vitro investigation of mucosa-adhesive materials for use in controlled drug delivery, *J. Pharm. Pharmacol.,* 36, 295, 1984.
54. **Park, K. and Robinson, J. R.,** Bioadhesive polymers as platforms for oral-controlled drug delivery: method to study bioadhesion, *Int. J. Pharm.,* 19, 107, 1984.
55. **Wermerskirchen, A. and Merkle, H. P.,** Adhesive capacity of self-adhesive buccal patches, in Proc. 34th Annu. Congr. Int. Assoc. Pharm. Technol., Hamburg, *Acta Pharm. Technol,* 34, (Suppl.), 115, 1988.
56. **Peppas, N. A., Ponchel, G., and Duchêne, D.,** The time-dependent behavior of the adhesive interactions between poly(acrylic acid) and buccal tissue, in *Proc. Int. Symp. Controlled Release Bioact. Mater.,* 14, 10, 1987.
57. **Boddé, H. E.,** unpublished data, 1987.
58. **Wermerskirchen, A.,** Haftvermögen und Freigabeverhalten von selbsthaftenden Bukkalfilmen in vitro und in vivo, Ph.D. thesis, University of Bonn, Bonn, West Germany, 1989.
59. **Fluegge, W.,** *Viscoelasticity,* Springer-Verlag, Berlin, 1975.

Chapter 7

BIOADHESIVE DOSAGE FORMS FOR BUCCAL/GINGIVAL ADMINISTRATION

Tsuneji Nagai, Yoshiharu Machida, and Ryoji Konishi

TABLE OF CONTENTS

I. INTRODUCTION

Mucosal adhesive dosage forms are a new type of external preparation that can render treatment more effective and safe, not only for topical diseases, but also for systemic ones. These unique dosage forms, which can be applied on such a wet tissue, are formulated utilizing the adhesive properties of some water-soluble polymers.

There are various mucosae at different positions in the living body. From the viewpoint of drug administration, oral mucosa is located at a convenient place for any type of dosage form. The drug is absorbed from conventional oral dosage form after it is released in saliva, while it is done directly through mucosa from a mucoadhesive dosage form. In other words, the drug absorption may take place on a triple interaction among drug, mucoadhesive base, and mucosa in the latter case. Therefore, the latter can make the drug more concentrated for absorption. Additionally, the interaction in the latter, though it is quite complicated, may be modified with the dosage form more than in the former case; this offers various possibilities of modification of drug release and absorption. When design of some oral drug delivery systems is attempted, the taste of the drug in administration must be considered. This constitutes a limitation to the application of drugs in oral systems.

Buccal tablets, sublingual tablets, and lozenges have all been used to administer drugs to the oral cavity. Lozenges are used for the topical therapy of inflammation or infection of the oral and throat mucosa. The other two dosage forms have been used for the systemic administration of such drugs as testosterone, glyceryl trinitrate, and buprenorphine. These drugs are absorbed quickly into the reticulated vein, which lies under the oral mucosa, and reach the systemic circulation directly, bypassing the liver. Therefore, oral mucosal administration can prevent the loss of a drug by first-pass metabolism. From this point of view also, the oral mucosa may offer a useful window for the administration of drugs in the future.

In addition to the two types of oral mucoadhesive administrations, i.e., systemic and topical, it may be possible to consider an intermediate between the two, which may be called "semitopical". This paper describes one example of systemic administration, namely, systemic administration of insulin, and three examples of semitopical drug delivery systems, namely, mucosal adhesive dosage forms of lidocaine for toothache using hydroxypropyl cellulose (HPC) and carbomer (CM, Carbopol®, an adhesive topical dosage form of triamcinolone acetonide for aphthous stomatitis, and an adhesive gingival plaster of prostaglandin $F_{2\alpha}$ ($PGF_{2\alpha}$) for orthodontic tooth movement.

II. SYSTEMIC ADMINISTRATION OF INSULIN

There are many kinds of bioadhesive polymers of synthetic and natural sources. However, when we consider using some additives or excipients in pharmaceutical preparations, the numbers of such materials we may use are limited because we have to guarantee the safety of them upon administration. From this point of view, we have been interested in pharmaceutical application of HPC, which is included in Japanese Pharmacopeia.

In the course of research on HPC, we found that HCP-H (high viscosity grade, Nippon Soda Co., Japan) is suitably adhesive to topical mucosal membranes. We utilized the combination of HPC and CM (Carbopol® 934, Goodrich Co.) to make an adhesive tablet for the oral mucosal administration of insulin,[1] as this combination of polymers gave suitable adhesiveness and sustained release properties.[2] However, insulin was not absorbed from the simple disk-type dosage form, which was first prepared by direct compression of the mixture of HPC/CM and insulin. We, therefore, prepared the two-phased tablet with an adhesive peripheral layer and an oleaginous core of cocoa butter, as shown in Figure 1.[1] It has been reported that insulin is absorbed from rectal mucosal membrane from a cocoa butter suppository.[2]

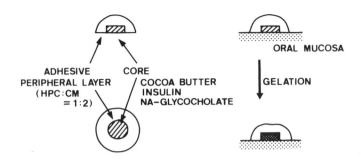

FIGURE 1. Schematic illustration of the new mucosal dosage form of insulin; left: dosage form; right: application on mucosal membrane. (From Ishida, M., Machida, Y., Nambu, N., and Nagai, T., *Chem. Pharm. Bull.*, 29, 810, 1981. With permission.)

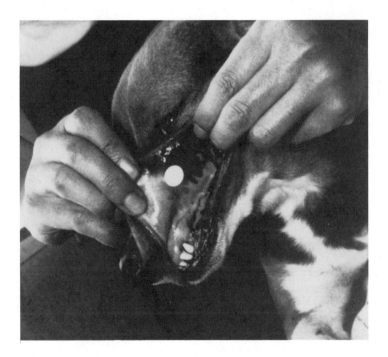

FIGURE 2. Mucosal dosage form stuck to the oral mucosa in a beagle. (From Ishida, M., Machida, Y., Nambu, N., and Nagai, T., *Chem. Pharm. Bull.*, 29, 810, 1981. With permission.)

This dosage form was administered to beagles, and the blood levels of insulin and glucose were determined. The dosage form adhered tightly to the oral mucosa of the dogs (Figure 2) in a gel-like swollen state without dispersion (Figure 3), and its shape was kept for more than 6 h.[1]

However, when the core part consisted of cocoa butter alone, insulin was not absorbed. Therefore, we investigated the use of an absorption promoter, examining the effect of various kinds of additives such as saponin, propylene glycols, and sodium glycocholate. Then we found sodium glycocholate was effective in promotion of the absorption of insulin. The mechanism of the increase with sodium glycocholate should be investigated in more detail. Glycocholate is known to act as a promoter in nasal absorption of insulin from solution.

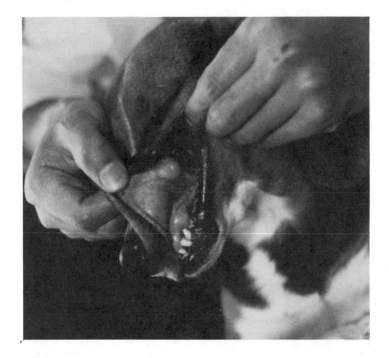

FIGURE 3.   Swollen dosage form stuck tightly at 6 h after administration. (From Ishida, M., Machida, Y., Nambu, N., and Nagai, T., *Chem. Pharm. Bull.*, 29, 810, 1981. With permission.)

Figure 4 shows the change of plasma insulin levels and plasma glucose levels after administration of the preparations.[3] It is clear that insulin was absorbed from mucosa. The bioavailability of insulin, in comparison with i.m. administration, was 0.5%. Recently, our investigation has improved it to 0.75% by using glyceride base as the core base, but this is clearly still very low. However, it should be pointed out that this was the first example of insulin absorption through the oral mucosa.

III. ADHESIVE DOSAGE FORM OF TRIAMCINOLONE ACETONIDE FOR APHTHOUS STOMATITIS

The dosage form described above has also been applied to the topical treatment of aphthous stomatitis. This disease is usually cured in 7 to 10 d if the patient is careful in eating and drinking, but it keeps him in pain until cured. An ointment preparation of triamcinolone acetonide (TAA) has already been commercially available. The dosage form we designed is a small, thin, double-layered tablet as shown in Figure 5.[3-5] The upper supporting layer, which is colored, consists mainly of lactose that has no adhesive property. TAA is included in the lower HPC/CM adhesive layer. A patient picks up the preparation by placing a wet finger tip on the upper colored surface. The adhesive side of the tablet is then held on the diseased part for several seconds, as shown in Figure 6.[5] The upper layer disintegrates soon after application and the lower layer swells gradually, covering the diseased part and releasing the drug. We found that this preparation does not cause patients any pain.

The topical concentration of the drug was determined using tritium-labeled TAA (^{3}H-TAA). The adhesive tablet and the ointment, both containing ^{3}H-TAA, were applied on the tongues of rats; the drug remained more and longer in the case of the adhesive tablet than the existing ointment on the surface of the tongue (Figure 7) and in the tissue (Figure 8).[6]

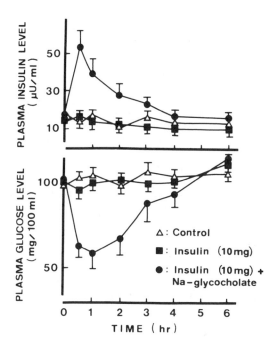

FIGURE 4. Change of plasma insulin levels and plasma glucose levels after mucosal administration of the new mucosal dosage form of insulin in beagles. Data are expressed as the mean ± SE. (n = 9). (From Ishida, M., Machida, Y., Nambu, N., and Nagai, T., *Chem. Pharm. Bull.*, 29, 810, 1981. With permission.)

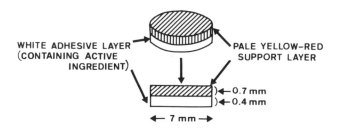

FIGURE 5. Adhesive tablet for aphtha.

Taking a microautoradiogram of tongue tissue as a function of the lapse of time after application of the adhesive tablet in comparison with the existing ointment, there was a difference in the distribution of the drug between the former and the latter, as seen in Figure 9, which shows the schematic summary of the concentration of silver particles on the microautoradiograms.[7] In the adhesive tablet, the drug stays for 30 min on the tongue surface, penetrates continuously in the connective tissue, and distributes itself in the muscular layer for a long period. On the other hand, in the existing ointment, the drug is easily removed from the tongue surface, and results in a small amount of the drug penetrating into the epidermis, the connective tissue, and the muscular layer.

Table 1 shows the result of a phase III clinical test of the adhesive preparation in comparison with the existing ointment. This adhesive dosage form was effective, with a lower dose than an ointment treatment. Additionally, a double-blind clinical test was done in comparison with the placebo; the improvement was 90.5% and 79.8% for the active

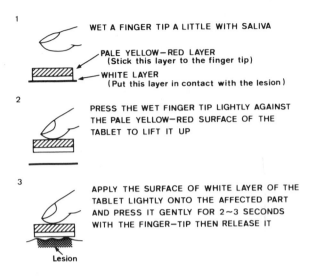

FIGURE 6.   Application of the adhesive tablet to aphtha.

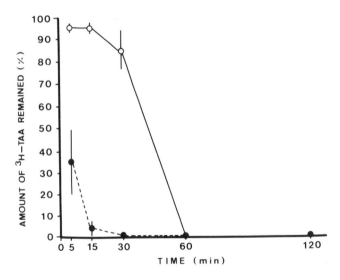

FIGURE 7.   Amount of ^{3}H-TAA that remained on the surface of the tongue in rats. Data are expressed as the mean ± SE (n = 5); -O-: adhesive tablet (25 μg ^{3}H-TAA); -●-: existing ointment (25 μg ^{3}H-TAA).

preparation and the placebo, respectively.[5] It is very interesting that the placebo is fairly effective; this may be due to the effect of the dosage form, which protects the aphtha by the swollen gel-like layer while applied. This preparation is commercially available (Aftach®).

This type of dosage form can be applied to many other drugs to be administered to the oral mucosa, such as local anesthetics for toothache or drugs easily metabolized by the liver, for example, a triple-layered mucosal dosage form containing 5 mg of lidocaine,[8] which will be described later in this chapter.

IV. SPRAY-TYPE POWDER FORM FOR STOMATITIS

Recently, a new powder dosage form for such extensive and refractory stomatitis as lichen planus and radiation stomatitis, which contains beclomethasone dipropionate and is

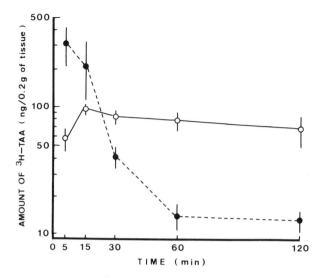

FIGURE 8. Amount of ^{3}H-TAA that remained in the tissue of the tongues in rats. Data are expressed as the mean ± SE (n = 5); -O-: adhesive tablet (25 μg ^{3}H-TAA); -●-: existing ointment (25 μg ^{3}H-TAA).

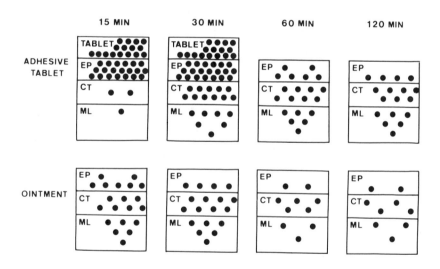

FIGURE 9. Schematic summary of concentration of silver particles on autoradiogram of the tissue of the tongue in rats with the lapse of time after application. EP: epidermis; CT: connective tissue; ML: muscular layer.

also formulated using HPC as the mucoadhesive base, has been developed as an extension of the above mentioned adhesive tablet for aphthous stomatitis.[4] This is sprayed on the affected area by a special sprayer (Puvlizer®; Figure 10) and can be used over an extensive area where the conventional ointment is not applicable.

The mucoadhesive base produces a long-lasting therapeutic effect and a covering-protecting effect on the affected area.

In clinical studies, in addition to the excellent symptom-improving effect, it achieved excellent results based on parameters including "no pain on administration", "ease of use", "no problem for continuous use", "no strange feeling", and "overall evaluation" according to a survey of the patients' impressions.

TABLE 1
Comparative Clinical Trial in Aphthous Stomatitis

	Adhesive tablet	Ointment
Average amount administered[a] (μg/day)	47.5	495.0
Side effects	None	None
Improvement (%)[b]	92.0	67.4
	$t = 3.98$	($p < 0.001$)
Usefulness (%)[c]	92.0	72.1
	$t = 3.99$	($p < 0.001$)

[a]   Average per day administered until cured.
[b]   Proportion of the number of patients whose therapeutic consequence is "effective" and "very effective".
[c]   Proportion of the number of clinicians whose global judgment is "useful" and "very useful".

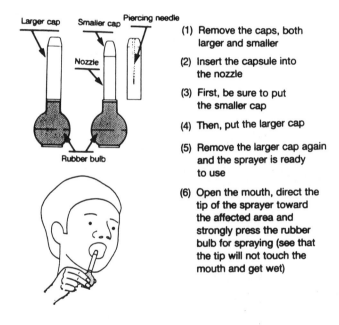

(1) Remove the caps, both larger and smaller

(2) Insert the capsule into the nozzle

(3) First, be sure to put the smaller cap

(4) Then, put the larger cap

(5) Remove the larger cap again and the sprayer is ready to use

(6) Open the mouth, direct the tip of the sprayer toward the affected area and strongly press the rubber bulb for spraying (see that the tip will not touch the mouth and get wet)

FIGURE 10.   Special sprayer for adhesive powder dosage form.

This preparation (Salcoat®) has been licensed and is on the market together with another mucoadhesive powder dosage form for nasal allergy (Rhinocort®),[3,9,10] which will be described later in a separate chapter.

V. ADHESIVE DOSAGE FORM OF LIDOCAINE FOR TOOTHACHE

At present, commercial medicines for toothache are provided in the form of lotions, viscous liquids, or ointments that are applied with a piece of cotton. However, they do not provide sustained action and there are also effects on other parts of the oral cavity.

As a continuation of the previous works on oral mucosal adhesive tablets for administration of insulin[1] and for a treatment of aphthous stomatitis,[3-5] we investigated a similar type of dosage form of lidocaine as a model drug for toothache using HPC and CM, with regard to the dissolution property and the absorption from human gingiva.[8] We anticipated

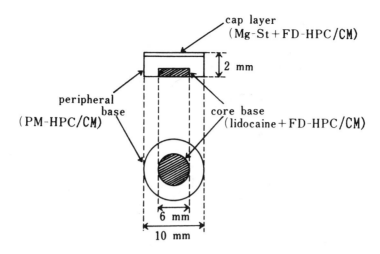

FIGURE 11. Schematic illustration of the mucosal adhesive dosage form of lidocaine. (From Ishida, M., Nambu, N., and Nagai, T., *Chem. Pharm. Bull.*, 30, 980, 1982. With permission.)

TABLE 2
Formula of the Mucosal Dosage Form of Lidocaine

Core base	Lidocaine	5 mg
	FD-HPC/CP	x mg[a]
Peripheral base	PM-HPC/CP	100 mg
Cap layer	Mg-St + FD-HPC/CP	50 mg

[a] x: 5, 10, 15, 20, 30 mg in dissolution test; 5, 10, 20 mg in absorption test.

From Ishida, M., Nambu, N., and Nagai, T., *Chem. Pharm. Bull.*, 30, 980, 1982. With permission.

that the dosage form might stick to the human gingiva, afford prolonged action, and not stimulate other parts of the oral cavity.

A schematic illustration of the mucosal dosage form of lidocaine is shown in Figure 11 and its formula in Table 2. In order to prepare a dosage form containing a small amount of lidocaine, the freeze-dried 1:2 mixture of HPC and CM (FD-HPC/CM) was used in the core. First, lidocaine and FD-HPC/CM were mixed sufficiently and compressed to make a cylindrical form of 6 mm diameter and about 1 mm thickness, which constituted the core. The core was covered with the peripheral base consisting of 100 mg of a physical mixture of HPC and CM (PM-HPC/CM) and compressed directly to make a tablet of 10 mm diameter. Finally, the tablet was covered again with 50 mg of 1:1 physical mixture of FD-HPC/CM and magnesium stearate (Mg-St) and compressed in the same way as above to make the cap layer.

This dosage form could be easily applied to the human gingiva. The lower layer of the tablet allowed the tablet to stick tightly only to the human gingiva and not to the cheek mucosa. The tablet behaved as expected in this respect; it did not stick to the oral mucosa due to the Mg-St in the cap layer.

Generally, CM is sticky and brings about a static charge, and so it is not easy to mix a small amount of drugs with CM alone. This problem was solved by using FD-HPC/CM

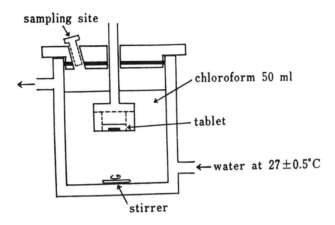

FIGURE 12.   Schematic illustration of the dissolution test apparatus for the mucosal adhesive dosage form of lidocaine. (From Ishida, M., Nambu, N., and Nagai, T., *Chem. Pharm. Bull.*, 30, 980, 1982. With permission.)

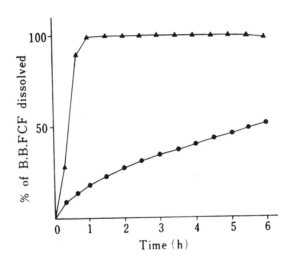

FIGURE 13.   Effect of FD-HPC on the dissolution of B.B.FCF. -▲-: FD-HPC. -●-: PM-HPC. (From Ishida, M., Nambu, N., and Nagai, T., *Chem. Pharm. Bull.*, 30, 980, 1982. With permission.)

in this study and the core of the dosage form was prepared easily. However, when the simple tablets of FD-HPC/CM and of PM-HPC/CM were applied to the human gingiva, the former was obviously less sticky than the latter. Additionally, using the dissolution test apparatus in Figure 12, the dissolution curves of brilliant blue FCF (B.B.FCF) from the dosage form in Figure 13, made it clear that the rate of gelation of FD-HPC/CM was faster than that of PM-HPC/CM. An explanation for this phenomenon may be that the viscosity of the gel layer is decreased because of the dispersion of CM in small particles by freeze-drying. The viscosities of FD-HPC/CM and PM-HPC/CM were 4 cps and 2200 cps, respectively, under the conditions used in the previous report[1] (1% solution in 1/15 M phosphate buffer, pH 7.38). Thus PM-HPC/CM was considered to be suitable as the peripheral base.

The gelation of FD-HPC/CM in the core base is necessary in the absorption of lidocaine. In the *in vitro* test, the dissolution of lidocaine was delayed as the amount of FD-HPC/CM

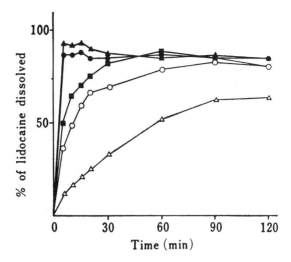

FIGURE 14.   Dissolution profile of lidocaine at various contents of FD-HPC. -●-: 5 mg; -▲-: 10 mg; -■-: 15 mg; -○-: 20
mg; -△-: 30 mg. (From Ishida, M., Nambu, N., and Nagai,
T., *Chem. Pharm. Bull.*, 30, 980, 1982. With permission.)

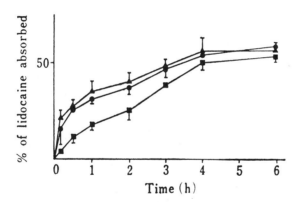

FIGURE 15.   Absorption profile of lidocaine in the mucosal adhesive dosage form from the human gingiva: -▲-: 5 mg, -●-: 10
mg, -■-: 20 mg. (Each point represents the mean ± SE of three
determinations). (From Ishida, M., Nambu, N., and Nagai, T.,
Chem. Pharm. Bull., 30, 980, 1982. With permission.)

in the core base increased, as shown in Figure 14. Therefore, it was assumed that the
dissolution rate could be controlled in the oral cavity by using various mixing ratios of FD-
HPC/CM. Lidocaine a lipophilic drug, is absorbed rapidly from the oral mucosa, in contrast
to such a hydrophilic polymer as insulin.[1] Thus, when FD-HPC/CM was used as the core
base, it was expected to obtain a rapid absorption and also a prolonged action of lidocaine.

The tablets were applied to the gingiva of each of three male volunteers for 1/6, 1/2,
1, 2, 3, 4, and 6 h, at different spaces, i.e., one tablet per run. It was confirmed by a
preliminary experiment that the order and position of application were of no significance.
The percentage of lidocaine absorbed was calculated from the amount remaining in the
dosage form after removing it completely from the gingiva.

The absorption profiles of lidocaine after application of dosage forms to the human
gingiva with various mixing ratios of FD-HPC/CM to lidocaine are shown in Figure 15.

Kiddie and Kaye[11] reported that the absorption of lidocaine by the oral mucosa was 10.5% at pH 5 and 25.6% at pH 6 in 5 min. Moreover, Beckett and Triggs[12] reported that the absorption of lidocaine increased with increase in the pH of the solution of lidocaine, though the amount absorbed was lower than that found by Kiddie and Kaye. Accordingly, the absorption of lidocaine was related closely to the pH on the oral mucosa. When PM-HPC/CM was dissolved at 1% in 1/15 M phosphate buffer (pH 7.40), the final pH changed from 7.40 to 5.80. Therefore, if this dosage form is in contact with saliva of about pH 6.2 to 7.6, the value of pH on the oral mucosa is considered to be about 5 to 6 due to the acidity of the CM gel layer. Accordingly, the present result that about 15 to 20% of lidocaine was absorbed after 10 min is almost consistent with the above reports. That is to say, it was assumed that the absorption of lidocaine from the preparations of 5 and 10 mg of FD-HPC/CM took place promptly. It was expected that the absorption of lidocaine might increase with the addition of excipients, which could increase the pH on the oral mucosa.

Regarding the relationship between the amount of lidocaine absorbed and the application period, it was found that the absorption was about 30% after 1 h and then increased by about 10% of the initial amount per hour for 4 h in the preparations of 5 and 10 mg of FD-HPC/CM. At 20 mg of FD-HPC/CM, the absorption rate was delayed, as was observed in the dissolution test.

In this dosage form, though FD-HPC/CM was used as the core base, it was assumed that lidocaine did not diffuse to the oral cavity through the gel layer of peripheral base, as lidocaine was not so much absorbed and remained in the dosage form in the period from 4 to 6 h.

From the results described above, the present dosage form may be expected to afford a prolonged anesthetic action for the treatment of toothache, beginning immediately after the application and lasting for about 4 h without anesthetizing other parts of the oral cavity.

However, lidocaine used as a model drug in this study is not exceptionally effective for toothache, and thus if a more effective drug such as dibucaine is used, the clinical utility of this dosage form might be enhanced.

VI. ADHESIVE GINGIVAL PLASTER OF PROSTAGLANDIN $F_{2\alpha}$ FOR ORTHODONTIC TOOTH MOVEMENT

Orthodontic tooth movement is accomplished by continuous application of force to the teeth. The process is rather expensive, uncomfortable, and typically requires 2 years to complete. Although orthodontic procedures are well established and produce the desired results, it would be desirable to accelerate the process.

The mechanism of tooth movement involves restructuring the alveolar bone around the tooth root. When force is continuously applied, bone is broken down and resorbed from areas of high pressure, while being formed in areas of low pressure. Workers at Ohio State University have demonstrated that prostaglandin (PG) and cyclic AMP levels increase in periodontal areas when force is applied to teeth.[13-15] Indeed, it appears that prostaglandins are necessary to accomplish tooth movement. Indomethacin, an inhibitor of prostaglandin synthesis, has been shown to inhibit orthodontic tooth movement in cats.[16]

Yamasaki and co-workers have accelerated orthodontic tooth movement by injecting PGE into the gingival tissues adjacent to the target teeth, in animals and in humans.[17-19] Although orthodontic tooth movement can be accelerated by frequent injections of PGEs, this procedure requires trained personnel and also produces pain as a direct response to high concentrations of PG.

Since we are interested in the role of $PGF_{2\alpha}$ and E_2 in the orthodontic tooth movement process, we have formulated an adhesive gingival plaster of $PGF_{2\alpha}$ that can be self-administered, and which will provide a continuous, slow release of PG into the gingival tissues

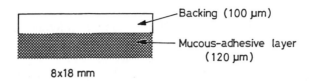

8x18 mm

FIGURE 16. Schematic illustration of the cross section of the adhesive gingival plaster of PGF$_{2\alpha}$. (From *J. Controlled Release*, 6, 357, 1987. With permisssion.)

for the purpose of accelerating tooth movement. This dosage form was examined experimentally in animals for acceleration of the tooth movement. A study using monkeys suggested that daily application of the plasters will accelerate the orthodontic process, and thereby reduce the time required for the tooth movement. Additionally, in order to investigate the tissue distribution of the active ingredient, plasters containing ^{14}C-labeled PGF$_{2\alpha}$ were applied to the cheek pouches of hamsters. Autoradiographic, histologic examination reveals that the labeled component was distributed in connective tissues and muscularis and remained for 8 h after patch application.

For delivery of bioactive substance to the gingival tissue, the design of an adhesive plaster is an important consideration. Figure 16 shows the dimension of the present system. The major components with PGF$_{2\alpha}$ in the basic formulation were synthetic resin, natural gum, hydrophobic polymers (polyvinyl alcohol, polyvinylpyrrolidone, carboxymethyl cellulose, and other polymers), polyethylene glycol, glycerine, agar, castor oil, and others.

The bioactive substance is incorporated into a water-activated adhesive layer. Water is slowly absorbed from the underlying mucosa into the adhesive, allowing the active substance to dissolve and release from the dosage form. It is also important, especially with powerful agents such as PG, to limit the release into the mouth. Therefore, a water-impermeable film serves as a backing material. The rate of adhesive hydration is thus limited, and the plaster can remain in place for many hours, without being dislodged or dissolved in the process of eating and drinking.

Although previous workers have generally concentrated on PGEs, formulating PGE as a stable dosage form is difficult. Therefore, an alternative PG was selected, that being PGF$_{2\alpha}$. Therapeutic potentials are known to be concerned with cardiovascular, respiratory, digestive, renal, endocrine, genital, nervous, connective tissue (osteoclastic and osteoblastic), and sensory cellular functions. Among them, the one concerned with connective tissue (osteoclastic and osteoblastic) is in relation to the present work. PGF$_{2\alpha}$ is physicochemically relatively stable by comparison and also shows reasonable activity with regard to osteocytes.

Table 3 shows a comparison of PGE$_1$, PGE$_2$, and PGF$_{2\alpha}$ for the effects on DNA synthesis, alkaline phosphatase production, and cyclic AMP levels in cultured osteoblasts, which were determined by the methods used by Kissane and Robins,[20] by Lowrey et al.,[21] and by Honma et al.,[22] respectively. The data obtained showed that suppressive effects were brought about by PGE$_1$ on DNA synthesis and by a higher dose of PGF$_{2\alpha}$ on alkaline phosphatase production. The mechanism of differences in these effects among PGs is not clear. The results thereby obtained suggest that PGF$_{2\alpha}$ has an effect on osteocytes, which is comparable in some ways to other PGEs.

The gingival plasters were formulated containing 50 μg/cm^2 of PGF$_{2\alpha}$. Such plasters have demonstrated good stability of PGF$_{2\alpha}$ at room temperature.

With respect to the release study, it is difficult to have an *in vitro* device that affords a reasonable model for *in vivo* release after application to buccal/gingival mucosa. However, the data obtained by *in vitro* experiments gave a useful information for formulation studies. For the *in vitro* release studies, two types of experiments were tried: (1) putting the plaster on an agar gel layer (1% agar in physiological saline), with the concentration of PGF$_{2\alpha}$ in the gel layer determined with the lapse of time; and (2) by the rotating basket dissolution

TABLE 3
Relative Increase in DNA Synthesis, Alkaline
Phosphatase Production, and Cellular Cyclic AMP
Levels in Clonal Osteoblast Cells (MC3T3-E$_1$ Cell),
Produced by Addition of PGs to the Culture Medium

PGs	E$_1$	E$_2$	F$_{2\alpha}$
DNA synthesis[a]	56.0%	728%	327%
	(2 µg/ml)	(2 µg/ml)	(20 ng/ml)
Alkaline phosphatase	160%	140%	113%[b]
production[a]	(20 ng/ml)	(20 µg/ml)	(4 ng/ml)
Cellular	Increase	Increase	No effect/
cyclic AMP			slight increase

[a]   For control: 100%.
[b]   In a higher dose than 20 ng/ml, alkaline phosphatase activity decreased
     (less than control).

From *J. Controlled Release*, 6, 358, 1987. With permission.

method in phosphate buffer solution. The *in vivo* absorption studies were done by applying four pieces of the plasters to the gingiva of each of two male volunteers, one piece of which gave one determination. The percent of PGF$_{2\alpha}$ released (i.e., to be absorbed) was calculated from the amount remaining in the plasters after removing it completely.

In order to investigate the disposition of PGF$_{2\alpha}$ in the adhesive gingival plaster, the blood concentration in monkeys was determined by radioimmunoassay, as it was not detectable otherwise. The tissue distribution of the active ingredient was investigated in plasters containing ^{14}C-labeled PGF$_{2\alpha}$, which were applied to the cheek pouches of hamsters. Autoradiographic histologic examination reveals that the labeled component distributed continuously with 5 to 8% of the total dose in connective tissues and muscularis and remained for 8 h after patch application. Interestingly, thin-layer chromatographic analysis also demonstrated that the label compound migrates into the tissue. No metabolites were detected.

No irritation of the mucosal surfaces has been found in any studies performed so far.

Toxicity testing of the plaster of PGF$_{2\alpha}$ has shown no adverse effects, even with chronic application for 2 months at dose levels substantially higher than anticipated for human application.

Preliminary studies on monkeys have demonstrated accelerated orthodontic tooth movement upon continuous application of the PGR$_{2\alpha}$ adhesive gingival plaster. Therefore, a daily application of the plasters is expected to accelerate the orthodontic process, and thereby reduce the time required for the tooth movement. The results were encouraging enough that more carefully controlled nonhuman primate studies have been initiated in the U.S.

Some clinical application of the PGF$_{2\alpha}$ adhesive gingival plaster has been evaluated in a few patients by Kawata and Yamashita.[23] These results are presented in Table 4. It appears that the PGF$_{2\alpha}$ adhesive gingival plaster does accelerate orthodontic tooth movement in at least 70% of the patients examined.

In conclusion, the plaster-type gingival therapeutic system appears to be a reasonable dosage form for gingival administration of PGs. This system may also be useful with a variety of drugs for topical/local effects in the mouth, especially for those drugs that may require a sustained tissue concentration.

ACKNOWLEDGMENT

The authors are deeply indebted to Dr. Masami Ishida, Mr. Yoshiki Suzuki, and Mr. Taichiro Iwakura for their assistance in this work.

TABLE 4
Clinical Evaluation in 11 Patients of Adhesive Gingival Plaster of $PGF_{2\alpha}$ on Orthodontic Tooth Movement

Age of patient	Distal movement of canine teeth[a]	Labial movement of anterior teeth[a]
25	+ + +	+ + +
14	+ +	+ +
10	+ + +	+ + +
14	+	+
8	+ +	+
8	+	+
14	+ + +	+ + +
11	+ +	+ +
12	+ +	+ +
10	0	0
9	+ +	+ +

[a] + + +: Tooth movement was significantly rapidly achieved (within 30 days); + +: tooth movement was rapidly achieved (within 30 days); +: tooth movement was achieved, but it was usual speed as in the case of control; 0: no effect of tooth movement was achieved.

From *J. Controlled Release*, 6, 359, 1987. With permission.

REFERENCES

1. **Ishida, M., Machida, Y., Nambu, N., and Nagai, T.,** New mucosal dosage form of insulin, *Chem. Pharm. Bull.*, 29, 810, 1981.
2. **Brahn, B. and Langer, M. T.,** Over een werkzaam insuline-suppositorium, *Tijdschr. Geneeskd.*, 83, 3784, 1939.
3. **Nagai, T., Machida, Y., Suzuki, Y., and Ikura, H.,** Method and Preparation for Administration to the Mucosa of the Oral or Nasal Cavity, Japanese Patent 1,177,734, May 13, 1983; U.S. Patent 4,226,848, October 7, 1980; U.S. Patent 4,250,163, February 10, 1981; West Germany Patent 2,908,847, August 14, 1981; French Patent 79-05,845, May 17, 1982; British Patent 2,042,888, September 28,1983; Swiss Patent 638,987, October 31, 1983.
4. **Suzuki, Y., Ikura, H., Yamashita, G., and Nagai, T.,** A Method for Treating an Injured Part on an Oral Mucosa and Covering Material for Use Thereof, Japanese Patent 1,138,989, March 11, 1983; U.S. Patent 4,292,299, September 29, 1981; E.P.C. Patent 20,777, May 23, 1984.
5. **Teijin Ltd.,** *Aftach: Adhesive Topical Preparation for Treatment of Aphthous Stomatitis,* Teijin Ltd. Pharmaceutical Division, Uchisaiwai-cho, Chiyoda-ku, Tokyo, 1982.
6. **Kubo, J., Yamamoto, M., Yamaguchi, H., Hashimoto, Y., Ikura, H., and Suzuki, Y.,** Drug sustaining effect of TN-08. I. Remaining of the preparation on the surface and concentration of active component in the tissue of tongue, *Kiso-to-Rinsho (Clin. Rep.,)* 16, 4599, 1982.
7. **Kubo, J., Yamamoto, M., Yamaguchi, H., Hashimoto, Y., Ikura, H., and Suzuki, Y.,** Drug sustaining effect of TN-08. II. Autoradiography on the penetration of active component into the tissue of tongue, *Kiso-to-Rinsho (Clin. Rep.,)* 16, 4603, 1982.
8. **Ishida, M., Nambu, N., and Nagai, T.,** Mucosal dosage form of lidocaine for toothache using hydroxypropyl cellulose and Carbopol., *Chem. Pharm. Bull.*, 30, 980, 1982.
9. **Suzuki, Y., Ikura, H., Yamashita, G., and Nagai, T.,** Powdery pharmaceutical preparation and powdery preparation to the nasal mucosa and method for administration thereof, Japanese Patent 1,286,881, October 31, 1985; U.S. Patent 4,294,829, October 13, 1981; E.P.C. Patent 23,359, July 29, 1980.
10. **Teijin Ltd.,** Rhinocort: Adhesive Topical Preparation for Nasal Allergy, Teijin Ltd. Pharmaceutical Division Uchisaiwai-cho, Chiyoda-ku, Tokyo, 1986.
11. **Kiddie, M. A. and Kaye, C. M.,** The influence of pH on the buccal absorption, and renal and plasma elimination of mexiletine and lignocaine, in *Br. J. Clin. Pharmacol.*, 3, 350, 1976.

12. **Beckett, A. H. and Triggs, E. J.,** Buccal absorption of basic drugs and its application as an *in vivo* model of passive drug transfer through lipid membranes, *J. Pharm. Pharmacol.,* 19 (Suppl.), 31s, 1967.
13. **Kiourtsis, D. J., Davidovitch, Z., Zwilling, B. S., Lanese, R. R., and Shanfeld, J. L.,** The effect of orthodontic force on peridontal PGE content, in Abstr. AADR Meeting, #1519, Washington, D.C., March 1986.
14. **Kess, B. L., Zwilling, B. S., Lanese, R. R., Shanfeld, J. L., and Davidovitch, Z.,** The effect of orthodontic force on periodontal PGE levels at tension sites, in Abstr. AADR Meeting, #1518, Washington, D.C., March 1986.
15. **Ngan, P., Crock, B., Zwilling, B. S., Shanfeld, J. L., and Davidovitch, Z.,** Effects of tension on cAMP and PGE levels in gingival fibroblasts, in Abstr. AADR Meeting, #1522, Washington, D.C., March 1986.
16. **Chumbley, A. B. and Tuncay, O. C.,** The effects of indomethacin on the rate of tooth movement in cats, *Int. Assoc. Dent. Res. Program Abst.,* 60, 596, 1981.
17. **Yamasaki, K., Miura, F., and Suda, T.,** Prostaglandin as a mediator of bone resorption induced by experimental tooth movement in rats, *J. Dent. Res.,* 59, 1635, 1980.
18. **Yamasaki, K., Shibata, Y., and Fukuhara, T.,** The effect of prostaglandins on experimental tooth movement in monkeys (Macaca fuscata), *J. Dent. Res.,* 61, 1444, 1982.
19. **Yamasaki, K., Shibata, Y., Imai, S., Tani, Y., Shibasaki Y., and Fukuhara, T.,** Clinical application of prostaglandin E, (PGE$_1$) upon orthodontic tooth movement, *Am. J. Orthod.,* 85, 508, 1984.
20. **Kissane, J. M. and Robins, E.,** The fluorometric measurement of deoxyribonucleic acid in animal tissue with special reference to the central nervous system, *J. Biol. Chem.,* 233, 184, 1958.
21. **Lowry, O. H., Roberts, N. R., Wu, M. L., Hixon, W. S., and Crawford, E. J.,** The quantitative histochemistry of brain. II. Enzyme measurements, *J. Biol. Chem.,* 207, 19, 1954.
22. **Honma, M., Satoh, T., Takezawa, J., and Ui, M.,** An ultrasensitive method for the simultaneous determination of cyclic AMP and cyclic GMP in small-volume samples from blood and tissue, *Biochem. Med.,* 18, 257, 1977.
23. **Kawata, T. and Yamashita, N.,** The effect or prostaglandin F$_{2\alpha}$ on orthdontic tooth movement, *Nippon Dent. Rev.,* 484, 10, 1983.

Chapter 8

SEMISOLID DOSAGE FORMS AS BUCCAL BIOADHESIVES

Robert Gurny and Nikolaos A. Peppas

TABLE OF CONTENTS

I. INTRODUCTION

The unique anatomy and physiology of the oral cavity with its covering mucosa makes this region liable to repeated physical insults damage of the surface epithelium. Warmth, wetness, and a high count of potentially pathogenic organisms make this part of the body very different in its response to damage and subsequent healing process.[1]

Attempts to treat oral mucus in cases of paradontoses, aphthae, and lesions by trauma have been hampered by difficulties in maintaining the medication at the site of application. An ideal bioadhesive drug delivery system should be easy to apply to the mucus and withstand salivation, tongue movement, and swallowing for a period of time, usually hours. In terms of physical and mechanical behavior, these two conditions translate into avoiding an excessive degree of swelling and withstanding shear and tensile loads.

More than 30 years ago, Rothner and co-workers[2] reported for the first time the use of sodium carboxymethylcellulose (NaCMC) in petrolatum as a vehicle for the local use of penicillin, which could provide longer contact at the site of application. In addition to NaCMC, a large number of vegetable gums and animal proteins can produce an adhesive paste when moistened or hydrated with water. The first registered products of this sort are Orahesive® powder and Orabase®. The latter consists of finely ground pectin (partially methoxylated poly[galacturonic acid]), gelatin, and NaCMC in a polyethylene/mineral oil gel base.[3,4] Early clinical experience with both these adhesives indicated that a powder product would be better. Unfortunately, application of these systems on the buccal mucus creates considerable technical problems. Another approach has been the use of NaCMC dispersed in various polymers such as polyisobutylene formulated as films and laminated with polyethylene films.[5] This type of bandage adheres to either wet or dry surfaces. Its adhesion to a dry surface occurs through a mechanism similar to those of pressure sensitive adhesives because of the presence of polyisobutylene.

There are several experimental techniques for the determination of the adhesive bond strength. Salter[6] claimed that it is difficult to assess the adhesive bond strength by a simple test and implied that it is virtually impossible to reproduce the exact conditions of the *in situ* mode of application and adhesion. Therefore, most of the techniques used till now have been devised in an effort to compare the performance rather than to measure the absolute adhesive bond strength of the hydrated hydrocolloids.

The semisolid products for the buccal cavity must have good patient compliance and so far only very few new systems have been successfully introduced.

II. MECHANISM

A. FORCES INVOLVED IN BIOADHESION

Adhesion to tissue may be effected by: (1) physical or mechanical bonds; (2) secondary chemical bonds; and/or (3) primary or covalent chemical bonds. Four possibilities of bridge formation between mucin and other molecules can be mentioned. The Van der Waals attractions between hydrophobic groups have binding energies in the region of 1 to 10 kcal/mol, for hydrogen bonds between hydrophilic groups have an energy of about 6 kcal/mol, ionic bonds (heteropolar) 100 to 200 kcal/mol and, finally, the covalent bonds (homopolar) 50 to 150 kcal/mol. Physical or mechanical bonds are obtained by deposition and inclusion of the adhesive material in the crevices of the substrate. Under these conditions, the surface roughness of the substrate may be important in the overall process. Merrill[7] has discussed the microscopic characteristics of the surface roughness in tissues. Roughness may be defined at the molecular or microscopic level. A rough surface may be defined by the ratio of maximum depth, d, to maximum width, h. This aspect ratio may be considered as insignificant roughness for adhesive purposes when it takes values of d/h <1/20. Obviously, only highly fluid products or suspensions can be incorporated in these substrates and can be considered successful adhesive systems.[8]

Secondary chemical bonds contributing to bioadhesive characteristics include hydrogen bonding and Van der Waals attraction. These forces are related to the chemical structure since, for example, hydrophilic polymers would create an interaction favorable to adhesion due to hydrogen bonding.[9] Secondary chemical bonds are important for bioadhesion in oral applications. Types of surface chemical groups that contribute to this type of adhesion include hydroxyls, carboxyls, amines, and amides.

Primary chemical bonds refer to the bonds created by chemical reaction groups. This is hardly the case with bioadhesive formulations for the intraoral applications under consideration here, and hence, they will not be discussed further.

The adherence of various oral dosage forms to the mucus layer have been investigated *in vivo* and *in vitro*.[10-12] A recent paper by Park and Robinson[13] as well as Chapter 3 in this book give an extensive overview about methods suitable for measuring bioadhesive forces. The more fundamental aspects have been recently discussed by Peppas and Buri[14] emphasizing the interfacial phenomenon related to the adhesive properties of synthetic polymers, hydrocolloids, and related systems in contact with soft, natural tissues. These aspects are also discussed in Chapter 2.

B. BIOADHESIVE MATERIALS FOR THE BUCCAL CAVITY

Appropriate materials for bioadhesive drug delivery are mainly the polymers forming hydrogels. The bioadhesive properties of a number of synthetic hydrogels were measured by a rather simple test as pointed out in Reference 15 (Table 1).

C. BIOADHESION AND DEGREE OF SWELLING

The swelling state of the polymer contributes to its bioadhesive behavior.[5,8] However, the general idea that increased swelling contributes to stronger bioadhesive bonds is not correct. For example, researches have shown in studies with hydrocolloids, more specifically with Orabase®, that, although the wet adhesive strength (measured as stress at break) that developed as the hydrocolloid components adsorbed water, increased with the increasing degree of swelling (or hydration), excessive water content led to an abrupt drop in the adhesive strength. This is clearly an indication of disentanglement at the hydrocolloid/tissue interface due to low concentration of the active components, if we accept the diffusion theories of adhesion of Bueche et al.[16] and Voyutskii,[17] according to which bioadhesion is the result of interpenetration of polymer chains through the bioadhesive interface to the substrate.

D. SWELLING TIME

The swelling time is important for assessment of adhesion. Studies have shown[5] that shortly after the beginning of swelling, adhesion does occur, but the bond formed is not very strong. The hydration of bioadhesives has been analyzed very recently by Park et al.[15] in which he points out that there is clearly an optimum water concentration needed for hydrocolloid particles to develop maximum adhesive strength (i.e., animal proteins, polycarbophil, or vegetable gums). They explained that if the adhesive becomes too susceptible to water permeation, it will eventually be displaced by water and subsequently looses its adhesiveness. Similar observation for gels have been made recently by Gurny et al.[19] Smart et al.[20] observed an increase in the adhesive strength in a mucus gel system, but a decrease in a gelatin gel system. The degradation of the adhesive bond in water or in a humid environment is another important aspect of the water in bioadhesion.

Clearly, at the molecular level, neither the necessary hydrogen bonds have been totally created nor interpenetration of the macromolecular chains of the adhesive and the substrate

TABLE 1

Potential Hydrocolloids for Bioadhesive Systems and their Evaluation *In Vivo* by Various Authors

Hydrocolloid	Adhesive properties[a] in contact with polyisobutylene[5]	P$_y$values [b]	Evaluation[c]
Acacia	P		
Agar agar	P		
Alginates			
Alginic acid	P		
Sodium alginate	E		
Carboxymethylcellulose, sodium		0.64	+ + +
Hercules Type 4	P		
Hercules Type 7,9,12	E		
Carboxymethylcellulose, calcium	P		
Dextran (Pharmachem)	P	0.67	+
Gelatin U.S.P.	F	0.73	
Guar gum (Stein Hall)			+ + +
Jaguar A-20-D 60%	S		
Jaguar A-20-D 65%	E		
Heparin		0.63	
Hyaluronic acid		0.63	
Hydroxyethylcellulose			+ +
Natrosol 250J(Hercules)	E		
Karaya gum			+ +
60%	S		
65%	E		
Methylcellulose (Dow)			
Methocel MC, 10 cps	E		
Methocel MC 15 cps	S		
Methocel MC 100 cps and higher	P		
Pectin N.F.	P		+ + +
Poly (acrylic acid)		0.62	
Poly (ethylene glycol) (Union Carbide)		0.59	
Carbowax 20 M	P		
Polyox WSR 35	P		
Poly (N-vinyl-2-pyrrolidone) (Antara)	P	0.56	
Tragacanth	E		

[a] Score *in vivo*: E = excellent ; S = satisfactory; F = fair ; P = poor.
[b] P$_y$values of polymer solutions (without cells according to Ref. 13).
[c] Score: + = poor; + + = satisfactory; + + + = good. See Ref. 13.

in the range of 150 to 200 Å has been achieved. Interpenetration can be quantified by examining the dimensionless Fourier time τ, and performing some order of magnitude calculations.[19,21-24] The Fourier number is defined as:

$$\lambda = Dt/l^2 \qquad (1)$$

For an order of magnitude analysis, one lets $\tau = 1$, which gives the following proportionality relationship:

$$l \sim \sqrt{Dt} \qquad (2)$$

If the interface between adhesive and substrate is at the early stage of swelling (hydration), a macromolecular chain from the adhesive would interpenetrate in the first layer of the substrate with a diffusion coefficient, D, of approximately 10^{-16} cm²/s, a typical value of the self diffusion of a macromolecular chain through a macromolecular system at an early stage of hydration (low solvent content).[17] Under these assumptions, after 15 min an interpenetration length, l, of 30 Å would have been obtained. In the case of a hydrated system, one could expect a diffusion coefficient of about 10^{-11} cm²/s, typical of diffusion of large molecules through a concentrated, entangled, macromolecular solution.[25,26] Then, the penetration length will be much higher, i.e., of the order of 9500 Å. Therefore, interpenetration would have occurred in 15 min (see Figure 1).

E. MOLECULAR WEIGHT OF THE BIOADHESIVES

There have been reports[27] that the adhesive strength increases as the molecular weight of adhesive polymer increases; up to 100,000 and beyond this level, there is not much effect. Although a critical length of the molecules is necessary to produce the interpenetrating layer and molecular enganglements between the bioadhesive and the substrate, one must consider also the size and the configuration of the adhesive macromolecules that interpenetrate. Thus, for example, with polyethylene oxide,[5] the adhesive strength increases even up to molecular weights of 4,000,000, since this polymer is known to contain molecules of highly linear configurations, which actually would contribute to the increase of the penetration length. On the other side, dextrans of molecular weights as high as 19,500,000 have been reported to have similar bioadhesive strength to those with molecular weight of 200,000. There, due to the coiled conformation, many of the adhesively active groups are "shielded" inside the coils and do not actively participate in the adhesion process, and also, due to the coiling, one may find intramolecular hydrogen bonds that are ineffective, rather than interfacial intramolecular hydrogen bonds that are effective. With these considerations in mind, we reproduce the Table 2 from Reference 5.

F. CONCENTRATION OF THE ACTIVE POLYMERS

There seems to exist an effective concentration for best bioadhesion.[19,28,29] Indeed, in highly concentrated systems, the adhesive strength drops significantly. In a concentrated solution, the coiled molecules become solvent-poor, the macromolecules approach the dimensions of the unperturbed state, and the available chain length for the interfacial penetration decreases significantly. It has been pointed out[30] also that excessive cross-linking of the polymer adhesive does not contribute to bioadhesion for the same reasons.

III. APPLICATIONS

An interesting study for a buccal release system has been recently published.[19] The bioadhesive polymer systems used in this study were prepared from a polyethylene gel (dispersion of polyethylene of $\overline{M}_w = 147,000$ in petrolatum at 5% wt) to which different amounts of hydrocolloids were added. The hydrocolloids used were sodium carboxymethylcellulose ($\overline{M}_n = 90,000$ Blanose Cellulose Gum 7LFD, Hercules France S.A., Rueil Malmaison, France), and hydrolyzed gelatin ($\overline{Mn} = 10,000$ to 12,000, Protein S, Croda Colloids Ltd, Cheshire, U.K.).

In a typical preparation, 66 parts (wt%) of the polyethylene gel and 34 parts of the hydrocolloids (NaCMC and gelatin in various proportions), which were previously ground and sieved to particle size smaller than 50 μm, were mixed in a mechanical mixer at 3000 rpm at 20°C. To this mixture 2% wt/wt of the active agent, febuverine hydrochloride [bis(pheny-2-butylyloxyethyl)-1,4-piperazine (MW 539.5)] (Sapos S. A. Geneva, Switzerland) was added. Upon complete mixing for 5 min at 300 rpm and room temperature, the samples were in the form of highly viscous pastes. They were stored in vials at room temperature until tested. The adhesion studies were performed with all systems prepared

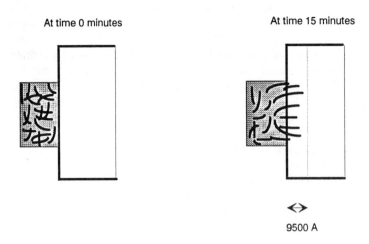

FIGURE 1.   Bioadhesive material on mucus.

Table 2
Relation between Molecular Weight of Hydrocolloids and
***In Vivo* Adhesiveness**

Hydrocolloid	Molecular weight	Adhesive property
Amylopectin	162,000-800,000	P
Guar gum	200,000	E
Karaya	9,500,000	E
Dextran	17,500-19,500,000	P
Polyethyleneglycol	200,000	P
	4,000,000	E

Note: P = poor; E = excellent

From Chen, J. L. and Cyr, C.N., in *Adhesion in Biological Systems,* Manly,
R. S., Ed., Academic Press, New York, 1970, 178. With permission,

using a tensile tester (Instron, model 1114, Instron Ltd, High Wycombe, Bucks, U.K.)
equipped with a custom-made cell for the measurement of the adhesive strength. The cell
was constructed of two Plexiglas® disks each of a diameter of 10 cm, which were connected
in their centers by permanently fixed metallic bars perpendicular to the disks. Each bar had
ends appropriately machined to fit to the clamps of the tensile tester. The two disks were
enclosed in two cylindrical chambers as shown in Figure 2.

In a typical experiment, a specific bioadhesive preparation containing the active agents
was placed between the two parallel disks held at an initial distance of 2 mm. Effort was
made to avoid inclusion of air bubbles. Then, the equipment was started, and the disk were
pulled at an extension rate of 0.1 mm/min. The stress-strain curves obtained under these
conditions are shown in Figure 3. The formulation tested in Figure 3 contains 12 wt%
NaCMC. Initially, there is an increase in the stress as a function of strain up to a yield point
where further extension does not create additional stress. This phenomenon is associated
with slippage of the macromolecular chains of the formulation, leading eventually to separation of the system between the two plates. In all mechanical tests, the available surface
area for adhesion was 0.788 cm². The initial modulus from this expermant was determined

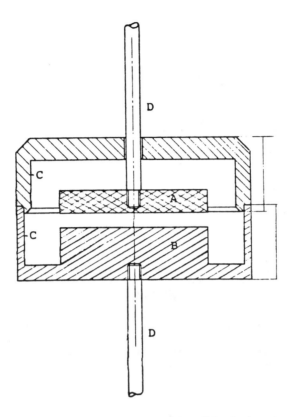

FIGURE 2. Schematic diagram of the cell for the determination of the adhesive bond strength. Major components include a movable disk (A), a lower supporting disk (B), cell enclosures (C), and metallic connecting bars (D). (From Gurny, R., Meyer, J. M., and Peppas, N. A., *Biomaterials*, 5, 336, 1984. With permission of the publishers, Butterworth & Co., Ltd. © 1984.)

as 1.24 MPa, which was reported to be higher than the values of the same formulation in artificial saliva.

Since NaCMC is the main bioadhesive component of the formulation, several additional studies of the effect of this parameter on the mechanical properties were undertaken. For example, after mixing the preparation with equal amounts of artificial saliva[31] for 120 min, the initial modulus has been plotted vs. the NaCMC concentration (Figure 4).

It can be seen that as the NaCMC concentration increases, the modulus passes through a maximum, which is characteristic of the optimum NaCMC concentration for best bioadhesion. As the amount of NaCMC increases beyond this value, either because of shielding of the active groups in the coiled molecules or because of macromolecular slippage, the molecules of NaCMC are not that effective in the bioadhesive process. These studies indicate that selection of the concentration of the active bioadhesive component is very important in these systems. It must be noted that all studies were of a comparative nature, since the only goal was to compare the effectiveness of various formulation parameters.

The same study[19] also reports the release experiments of the active agent (febuverine hydrochloride) at 37°C. Figure 5 shows a typical plot of the release of febuverine-HCl per unit area, M_t/A, as a function of time from a formulation containing 12 wt% NaCMC.

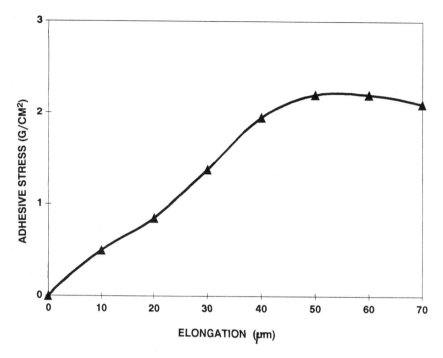

FIGURE 3.   Stress as a function of elongation for a controlled release formulation in the nonhydrated state, containing 12 wt% NaCMC, 22 wt% hydrolyzed gelatin and 66 wt% polyethylene gel. Initial disk separation was 2 mm. The results are the average of three experiments. (From Gurny, R., Meyer, J.-M., and Peppas, N. A., *Biomaterials,* 5, 336, 1984. With permission of the publishers, Butterworth & Co., Ltd. © 1984.)

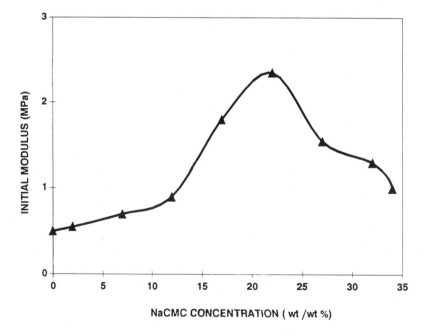

FIGURE 4.   Initial modulus of various formulations hydrated for 120 min in artificial saliva, as a function of NaCMC concentration (expressed as weight percent of the original system). The results are the average of three experiments. (From Gurny, R., Meyer, J.-M., and Peppas, N.A., *Biomaterials,* 5, 336, 1984. With permission of the publishers, Butterworth & Co., Ltd. © 1984.)

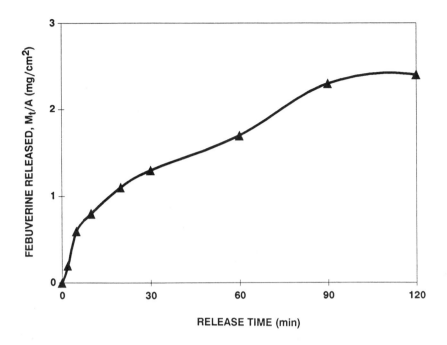

FIGURE 5. Quantity of febuverine-HCl released per unit area (mg/cm²) as a function of release time, for a preparation containing 12 wt% NaCMC on a dry base. The results are the average of three formulations. (From Gurny, R., Meyer, J.-M., and Peppas, N.A., *Biomaterials*, 5, 336, 1984. With permission of the publishers, Butterworth & Co., Ltd. © 1984.)

It is reported that the release behavior is not characteristic of the typical fickian release behavior that one obtains with conventional matrix-type controlled release systems.[32] In fact, there is a portion of the release curve between roughly 15 and 90 min, where the release behavior resembles that of zero-order release kinetics. Due to the complex macromolecular structure of the controlled release formulation, it is rather difficult to explain the mechanism of release. However, it is quite possible that the highly viscoelastic behavior of this system may create relaxational changes that lead to zero-order release, much in the same way as it has been observed with swellable systems. The effect of NaCMC concentration on the controlled release of febuverine-HCl is shown in Figure 6, where the quantity of drug released after 120 min per unit area at 37°C is given.

Since the concentration of the second swellable component (hydrolyzed gelatin) is equal to 34-x wt%, where x is the concentration of NaCMC in the preparation, the plot shows the importance of the optimal ratio of gelatin over NaCMC in the release process of the bioactive material. The plot may be separated roughly into three regions, of which the middle part (NaCMC concentrations between 12 and 25 wt%) gives the optimal release profile. The judicious design of this novel buccal release system contains an optimum concentration (20 wt%) of NaCMC, the main bioadhesive material.

In a recent study by Ishida et al.,[33] the authors reported on an ointment-type of dosage form containing Carbopol® 934 (CP) as adhesive material and prednisolone as the active ingredient (Figure 7). The local activity of this type of ointment intended for the treatment of aphthae was extensively analyzed. Three different ointments have been used, i.e., white petrolatum (WP), hydrophilic petrolatum (HP), and Lauromacrogol (Nikko Chem. Co., Ltd.) as an absorptive ointment (AO). In this study, CP was mixed completely with each base to give 0, 10, 20, or 30% CP. Then, prednisolone was added to each CP ointment at a concentration of 1%. The authors investigated the stickiness of this adhesive type of ointment in the absence and presence of water as well as the release characteristics of prednisolone from CP ointments. The interesting results are given in Figures 8 and 9.

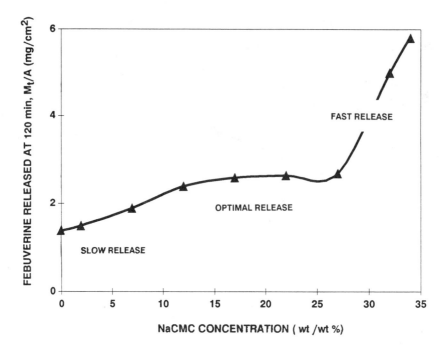

FIGURE 6.   Quantity of febuverine hydrochloride released after 120 min per unit area from prehydrated formulations as a function of the NaCMC concentration in the dry formulation. The results are the average of three runs. (From Gurny, R., Meyer, J.-M., and Peppas, N.A., *Biomaterials*, 5, 336, 1984. With permission of the publishers, Butterworth & Co., Ltd. © 1984.)

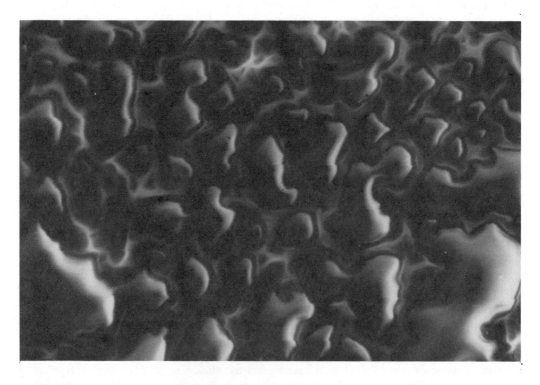

FIGURE 7.   SEM photograph of a bioadhesive gel containing adhesive particles (before contact with water).

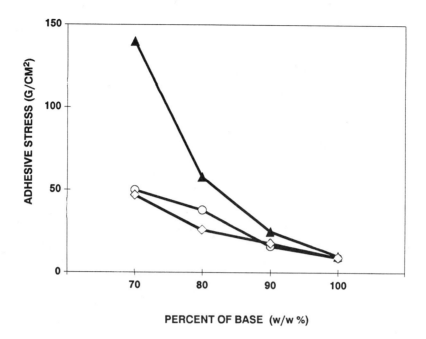

FIGURE 8.   Adhesion force of various Carbopol® containing ointments. ▲, white petrolatum; ○, hydrophilic petrolatum; and ◇ absorptive ointment. (From Ishida, M., Nambu, N., and Nagai, T., *Chem. Pharm. Bull.*, 31, 1010, 1983. With permission.)

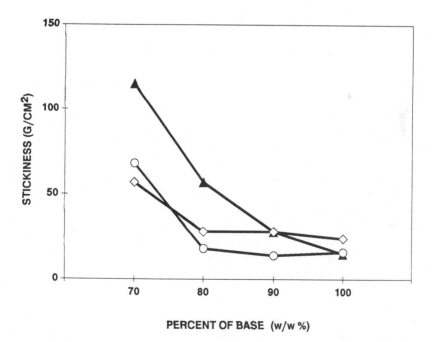

FIGURE 9.   Effect of water on the stickiness in the shearing stickiness test. ▲, white petrolatum; ○, hydrophilic petrolatum; ◇, absorptive ointment (water content: 10% in each preparation). (From Ishida, M., Nambu, N., and Nagai, T., *Chem Pharm. Bull.*, 31, 1010, 1983. With permission.)

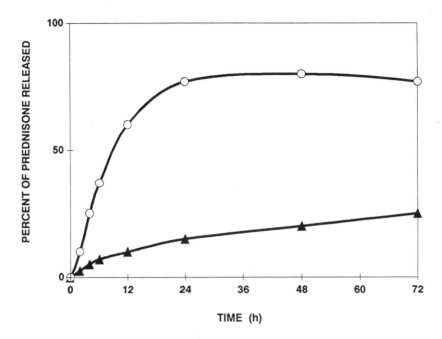

FIGURE 10.   Effect of Carbopol® on the release of prednisolone from various ointments. ○, Carbopol®30% ; ▲, Carbopol®0%. (From Ishida, M., Nambu, N., and Nagai, T., *Chem. Pharm. Bull.*, 31, 1010, 1983. With permission.)

The release behavior of the same formulations have also been analyzed for prednisolone using the HPLC method. The release profiles can be seen in Figures 10 and 11. It was considered by the authors that only in the presence of water due to the CP in the ointment, can the release of prednisolone be achieved. In the case of HP-CP ointment, the release of prednisolone was not observed since HP-CP ointment was not gelled because of its poor wettability and high consistency.

The same authors[33] investigated *in vivo* buccal absorption of prednisolone in the hamster cheek. The results for two formulations are given in Figure 12. In a recently introduced product[35-40] (Solcoseryl dental adhesive®, Solco AG, Basel, Switzerland) the effect of healing of mucosal ulcers (dental sores) was investigated in a double-blind clinical study by comparing a treatment group, a group treated with placebo, and an untreated control group. In a study on 45 persons,[40] the course of healing was evaluated on the basis of various parameters, the control group serving as "standard" reference. The area of the sore was determined as an absolute value. The other parameters were assessed on a semiquantitative basis in two or three grades. The various parameters assessed and recorded were as follows: area of sore, depth of sore, epithelization, and redness. Other, more subjective parameters such as discomfort, pain, onset of analgesic effect, duration of effect, disturbance of taste, and allergic reaction were also recorded. Figure 13 gives an overview of the first promising results of such preparations.

In another study[41] the change of the surface of the sore was followed as a function of time for a bioadhesive preparation. In Figure 14, it can be seen clearly the significant improvement of the healing process compared to the control.

Similar bioadhesive systems have been developed recently by Squibb under the name of Stomadhesive®[42] or Varihesive® for the treatment of ulceration on the surface of the skin. Efforts are made today to optimize also the supporting material for adhesive dressings. Recently, a patent application has been filed by the same company. All the systems discussed so far have been based on hydrocarbon gel ointments.[43-47] Other patents have been

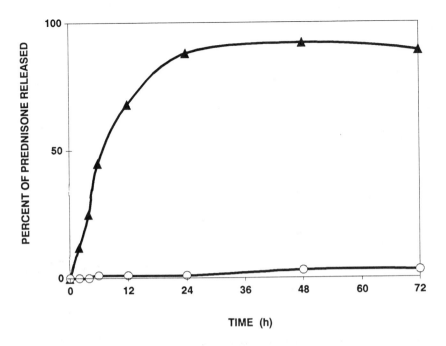

FIGURE 11. Effect of Carbopol® on the release of prednisolone in white petrolatum. ▲, Carbopol® 30% ;○, Carbopol® 0%. (From Ishida, M., Nambu, N., and Nagai, T., *Chem. Pharm. Bull.*, 31, 1010, 1983. With permission.)

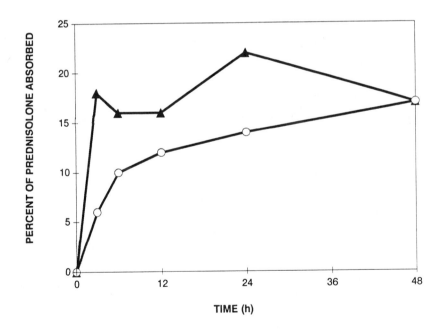

FIGURE 12. Change in absorption of prednisolone from hamster cheek pouch after administration of prednisolone in two formulations. ○, Carbopol® 30% ;▲, Carbopol® 0%. (From Ishida, M., Nambu, N., and Nagai, T., *Chem. Pharm. Bull.*, 31, 1010, 1983. With permission.)

filed[48-49] for the treatment of aphthae using semisolid or solid preparations. Most of the inventors are using methylcellulose/poly (acrylic acid) combinations.[48] In the case of dental prosthesis creams, carboxymethylcellulose,[49] ethylcellulose, saccarose monostearate, gum arabic, cellulose acetate phthalate, shellac, and other film-forming substances are used.

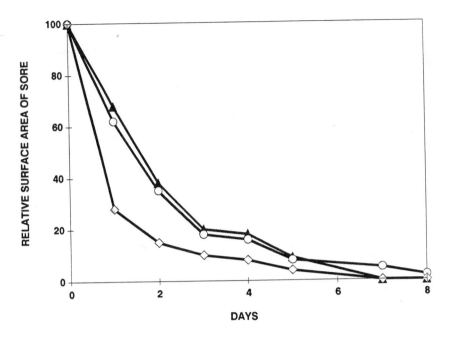

FIGURE 13.   Time lapse until complete disappearance of sore. ◇ , test preparation; ○, reference preparation; ▲, control. (From Felber, P. and Gasser, F., *Schweiz. Mschr. Zahnheilk.*, 93, 362, 1983. With permission.)

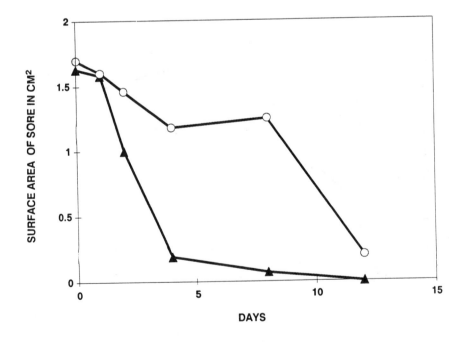

FIGURE 14.   Healing of the sore after application of bioadhesive paste compared with a control. ▲, dental adhesive; ○, control without adhesive material. (From Wunderer, S., Thams, U., and Porteder, H., *Öster. Z. Stomatologie,* 74, 62, 1982. With permission.)

REFERENCES

1. **Macalister, A. D.,** The management of oral ulceration, *Drugs,* 5, 453, 1973.
2. **Rothner, J. T., Cobe, H. M., Rosenthal, S. L., and Bailin, J.,** An adhesive penicillin ointment for topical application, *J. Dent. Res.,* 28, 544, 1949.
3. **Kanig, J. L. and Menago-Ulgado, P.,** The in vitro evaluation of orolingual adhesives, *J. Oral Ther. Pharmacol.,* 1, 413, 1965.
4. **Kutscher, A. H. Zegarelli, E. V. Benbe, F. E., Chilton, N. W., Berman, C., Mercadente, J. L., Stern, I. B., and Roland, N.,** A new vehicle (Orabase) for the application of drugs to the oral mucous membranes, *Oral Surg. Oral Med. Oral Pathol.,* 12, 1080, 1959.
5. **Chen, J. L. and Cyr, C. N.,** Composition producing adhesion through hydration, in *Adhesion in Biological Systems,* Manly, R. S., Ed., Academic Press, New York, 1970, 163.
6. **Salter, R.,** *Aspects of Adhesion,* Vol. 1, Oxford University Press, London, 1965, 81.
7. **Merrill, E. W.,** Properties of materials affecting the behavior at their surface, *Ann. N.Y. Acad. Sci.,* 283, 6, 1977.
8. **Huntsberger, J. R.,** Surface energy, wetting and adhesion, *J. Adhesion,* 6, 11, 1971.
9. **Pritchard, W. H.,** The role of hydrogen bonding in adhesion, *Proc. Conf. Aspects Adhes.,* 6, 11, 1971.
10. **Swisher, D. A., Sendelbeck, S. L., and Fara J. W.,** Adherence of various oral dosage forms to the esophagus, *Int. J. Pharm.,* 22, 219, 1984.
11. **Marvola, M., Rajaniemi, M., Marttila, E., Vahervuo, K., and Sothmann, A.,** Effect of dosage from and formulation factors on the adherence of drugs to the esophagus, *J. Pharm. Sci.,* 72, 1034, 1983.
12. **Marrola, M., Vahervuo, K., Sothmann, A., Marttila, E., and Rajaniemi, M.,** Development of a method for study of the tendency of drug product to adhere to the esophagus, *J. Pharm. Sci.,* 71, 975, 1982.
13. **Park, K. and Robinson, J. R.,** Bioadhesive polymers as platforms for oral-controlled drug delivery: method to study bioadhesion, *Int. J. Pharm.,* 19, 107, 1984.
14. **Peppas, N. A. and Buri, P. A.,** Surface, interfacial and molecular aspects of polymer bioadhesion on soft tissues, *J. Controlled Release,* 2, 257, 1985.
15. **Park, K., Cooper, S. L.,and Robinson, J. R.,** Bioadhesive hydrogels, in *Hydrogels in Medicine and Pharmacy,* Vol. 2, Peppas, N. A., Ed., CRC Press, Boca Raton, FL, 1987.
16. **Bueche, F., Cashin, W. M., and Debye, P.,** The measurement of self-diffusion in solid polymers, *J. Chem. Phys.,* 20, p. 1950, 1952.
17. **Voyutskii, S. S.,** *Autoadhesion and Adhesion of High Polymers,* Interscience, New York, 1963.
18. **Baier, R. E., Shafrin, E. G., and Zisman, W. A.,** Adhesion: mechanisms that assist or impede it, *Science,* 162, 1360, 1968.
19. **Gurny, R., Meyer, J.-M., and Peppas, N. A.,** Bioadhesive intraoral release systems: design, testing and analysis, *Biomaterials,* 5, 336, 1984.
20. **Smart, J. D., Kellaway, I. W., and Worthington, H. E. C.,** An in vitro investigation of mucosa-adhesive materials for use in controlled drug delivery, *J. Pharm. Pharmacol.,* 36, 295, 1984.
21. **De Gennes, P. G.,** Couéles de polymers compatibles: propriétés spéciales en diffusion et en adhesion, *C. R. Acad. Sci. Paris Ser. B.,* 292, 1505, 1981.
22. **Prager, S. and Tirrell, M.,** The healing processing at polymer-polymer interfaces, *J. Chem. Phys.,* 75, 5194, 1981.
23. **Ponchel, G., Touchard, F., Duchêne, D., and Peppas, A. N.,** Bioadhesive analysis of controlled-release systems. I. Fracture and interpenetration analysis in poly(acrylic acid)-containing systems, *J. Controlled Release,* 5, 129, 1987.
24. **Peppas, N. A., Ponchel, G., and Duchêne, D.,** Bioadhesive analysis of controlled-release systems. II. Time dependent bioadhesive stress in poly (acrylic acid)-containing systems, *J. Controlled Release,* 5, 143, 1987.
25. **Gilmore, P. T. and Laurence, R. L.,** Diffusion of miscible binary polymer-mixtures, *Proc. IUPAC Symp. Macromol.,* 26, 1086, 1979.
26. **Peppas, N. A., Hansen, P. J., and Buri, P. A.,** A theory of molecular diffusion in the intestinal mucus, *Int. J. Pharm.,* 20, 107, 1984.
27. **Huntsberger, J. R.,** Mechanisms of adhesion, *J. Paint Technol.,* 39, 199, 1967.
28. **Bremecker, K. D.,** Modell zur Bestimmung der Haftdauer von Schleimhautsalben in vitro, *Pharm. Ind.,* 45, 417, 1983.
29. **Bremecker, K. D.,** PMMA-ein bekanntes Polymer neu eingesetzt, *Acta Pharm. Technol.,* 26, 231, 1980.
30. **Kammer, H. W.,** Adhesion between polymers, *Acta Polymerica,* 34, 112, 1983.
31. **Fusayama, T., Katayori, T., and Nomoto, S.,** Artificial saliva, *J. Dent. Res.,* 42, 1183, 1963.
32. **Langer, R. and Peppas, N.,** Chemical and physical structure of polymers as carriers for controled release of bioactive agents, *J. Macromol. Sci. Rev. Macromol. Chem.,* C23, 61, 1983.

33. **Ishida, M., Nambu, N., and Nagai, T.,** Ointment-type oral mucosal dosage form of carbopol containing prednisolone for treatment of aphthae, *Chem. Pharm Bull.* 31, 1010, 1983.

34. **Ishida, M., Nambu, N., and Nagai, T.,** Mucosal dosage form of lidocaine for toothache using hydroxypropyl cellulose and carbopol, *Chem. Pharm. Bull.,* 30, 980, 1982.

35. **Thams, U. and Porteder, H.,** Ein neues Präparat zur Behandlung von Schleimhautläsionen. Doppelblinde klinische Vergleichsprüfung von "Solcoseryl - Adhäsivpaste", *Öster. Z. Stomatologie,* 79, 62, 1982

36. **Stoller, Ch. and Schär, E.,** Anwendung von Solcoseryl Dental Adhäsivpaste bei der Eingliederung von Sofortprothesen, *ZWR,* 81, 1075, 1972.

37. **Henning, G. and Przetak, Ch.,** Die Rolle der Stoffwechselerhöhung in der Mundschleimhaut bei Schmerz und Gewebsdefekten, *ZWR,* 85, 116, 1976.

38. **Vamos, I. and Kövesi, G.,** Experience with the use of Solcoseryl dental adhesive paste, *Különenyomat,* 73, 361, 1980.

39. **Röll, W.,** Klinische Erfahrungen zur Heilungsförderung auf dem Gebiete der Kiefer-und gesichtschirurgie, *Der Chirurg,* 34, 247, 1963.

40. **Felber, P. and Gasser, F.,** Double-blind clinical trial of Solcoceryl dental adhesive paste in the treatment of denture sores, *Schweiz. Mschr. Zahnheilk.,* 93, 362, 1983.

41. **Wunderer, S., Thams, U., and Porteder, H.,** *Öster. Z. Stomatologie,* 74, 62, 1982.

42. **Tudhope, M.,** Behaudlung von Druckgeschwüren, *J. Entero Stomal Ther.* 11, 102, 1984

43. **Foster, Sh., Wurster, D. E. and Higuchi, T.,** A pharmaceutical study of Jelene ointment base, *J. Am. Pharm. Assoc.,* 40, 123, 1951.

44. **Robinson, R.,** Plastibase — a hydrocarbon gel ointment base, *Bull. School Med. Univ. Maryland* 40, 86, 1955.

45. **Rachelson, M. and Pierce, H. E.,** Plasticized hydrocarbon ointment in the treatment of diaper dermatitis, *J. Nat. Med. Assoc.,* 47, 113, 1955.

46. **Jones, E. R. and Lewecki, B.,** A new hydrocarbon ointment base: Jelene 50 W, *J. Am. Pharm. Assoc.,* 40, 509, 1951.

47. **Mutiner, M.N., Riffkin, Ch., Hill, J. A., Glickman, M. E., and Cyr, G. N.,** Modern ointment base technology II, *J. Am. Pharm. Assoc.,* 45, 212, 1956.

48. **Wienecke, H.,** European Patent Appl., 81106903.8, 1981.

49. **Suzuki, Y., Ikura, H., Yamashita, G., and Nagai, T.,** French Patent Appl., 81 24423, 1981

Chapter 9

BIOADHESIVE DOSAGE FORMS FOR NASAL ADMINISTRATION

Tsuneji Nagai and Yoshiharu Machida

TABLE OF CONTENTS

I. INTRODUCTION

In humans, the area of the nasal mucosa is approximately 150 cm^2. Under this, there is a densely grown network of vein, which may offer a window for drug absorption. However, this window has been used mainly for the treatment of local diseases, such as nasal allergy or inflammation.

Recently, growing attention has been paid to the nose as an alternative route of administration for systemically active drugs such as peptide and proteins that are poorly absorbed orally and are extensively metabolized in the gastrointestinal tract (GIT) or by first-pass effect in the liver. For example, this was discussed at the Symposium on Transnasal Systemic Medication held at Rutgers University in New Jersey in 1984.[1] It has been reported that several kinds of drugs such as propranolol,[2] progesterone,[3] enkephalins,[4] luteinizing-hormone-releasing hormone,[5] tetracosactrin,[6] oxitocin,[7] and adrenocorticotropic hormone (ACTH)[8] are absorbed effectively through the nasal mucosa.

Physicochemically, the nasal mucosal membrane is considered to be essentially a lipophilic transport barrier without evidence of aqueous pore, as little is known of its nature. Therefore, a specific change in the nasal microenvironment,[9] which modifies this barrier function, may affect molecular transport, resulting in an enhancement of drug absorption.

With respect to approaches that are attempted in order to promote nasal absorption, there are reports in the literature about the nasal administration of drugs from solutions containing bile salts and surfactants.[10,11] Recently, Moses reported that the nasal administration of insulin mixed with sodium taurodihydofusidate, a derivative of fungal sterol fusidic acids that resembles bile acids, holds great promise for the therapy of diabetes mellitus.[12]

The absorption promoting effect of these additives has been considered generally to be due to their ability to enhance the membrane fluidity, for example, by extracting cholesterol, triglycerides, and proteins and by reducing the viscosity of the mucus thereby allowing for an easier penetration of a drug into the membrane.[11] Additionally, for bile acids, they have an ability to inhibit the degrading activity of enzymes in the membrane.[10,13]

However, the nasal mucosa is a very sensitive part of the body, and it may be damaged by the irritant effect of surfactants even if the drug absorption is promoted. From the therapeutic viewpoint, therefore, it might be preferable to use no absorption promoter in nasal dosage forms, especially for treatment of a chronic disease.

As another approach to enhancing the nasal absorption of a drug, there is an attempt to prevent the rapid clearance of the drug or the dosage form from the nasal cavity. Ciliated cells on the surface of the mucosa carry the secreted mucous fluid towards the throat at a speed of 5 mm/min.[14] A drug applied in simple liquid or powder form would, therefore, be cleaned rapidly from the site of absorption. Actually, the rate of clearance was found to be dependent on the method of application.[15-18] Therefore, if a dosage form could be developed with better adhesion, additionally with less irritation by using less or no absorption promoter, it might afford a useful means for the nasal administration of drugs.

Since the rapid mucociliary clearance mechanism in the nasal cavity can be considered as an important factor when low bioavailabilities are obtained for drugs administered intranasally, Illum *et al.* investigated a nasal delivery system in the form of bioadhesive microspheres, which should be cleared slowly from the nasal cavity thereby prolonging the contact between the delivery system and the mucosa.[19] For the formulation of the adhesive microsphere systems, they used albumin, starch, and DEAE-dextran as the bases, including Rose bengal and sodium cromoglycate as model drugs, and found as a result the possibility of controlling the release of the compounds from the systems.

Two examples of bioadhesive systems in nasal administration that we have investigated are discussed below: adhesive powder dosage form for intranasal systemic administration of insulin in comparison with that in liquid form [20] and adhesive powder spray for nasal

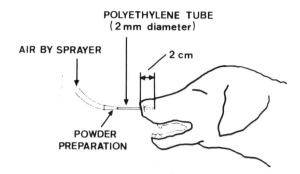

FIGURE 1. Nasal administration of powder dosage form of insulin. (From *J. Controlled Release*, 2, 131, 1985. With permission.)

allergy.[21-23] The latter may be classified into "semitopical" administration; it was mentioned earlier in Chapter 7.

It should be emphasized that bioadhesive powder dosage forms for nasal administration sometimes produce a drug absorption more effective and less irritating than liquid ones, as will be described later. However, in the case of β-interferon, the effect of the bioadhesiveness was not clear, though we were successful in its intranasal absorption from powder forms in rabbits[24] which took place with the addition of surfactants, especially sodium glycocholate.

II. ADHESIVE POWDER DOSAGE FORM FOR INTRANASAL SYSTEMIC ADMINISTRATION OF INSULIN

At present, insulin injection has been available as an effective therapy of diabetes. However, the injection causes physical discomfort and mental duress in patients. Moreover, the long-term injection of insulin may often cause an allergy and a hypotrophy of subcutaneous fat at the injection site. From this point of view, much effort has been directed towards developing new dosage forms of insulin.

Aside from injection of insulin, we can find various existing reported attempts at finding other possible routes for the administration of insulin via the intestinal tract, rectum, respiratory mucosa, oral mucosa, nasal mucosa, and skin. Additionally, there are some trials reported by ophthalmic administration. Insulin was successfully absorbed through buccal mucosa from an adhesive tablet, although the bioavailability was very low,[25] as was described in Chapter 7. At present, however, any route of administration other than injection has not materialized as a practical method for the treatment of diabetes by insulin.

Concerning the absorption of insulin from nasal mucosa in general, most of the experiments have been done in solution by spraying or recirculation in the nasal cavity. These solutions contained such absorption promoters as sodium glycocholate or surfactants. Following the previous work,[25] our intention has been to develop a powder form of dosage using bioadhesive bases that also contains as small a promoter as possible.

In the present experiments,[20] the absorption of insulin from several powder dosage forms composed of various excipients were investigated using beagles. The powder sample was compressed in a polyethylene tube of 2 mm diameter and was inserted in the nose about 2 cm from the nostril and then was sprayed by a special sprayer, as shown in Figure 1. In comparison, liquid forms were administered by dropping the sample solution from the nostril using an Eppendorf pipette.

For the first trial, we carried out the absorption experiment in comparison between powder forms (A: crystalline insulin; B: insulin freeze-dried in acidic condition; C: insulin freeze-dried in neutral conditon) and liquid forms (A': A in purified water [pH 5.7]; B': B in purified water [pH 3.4]; C': C in purified water [pH 7.4]

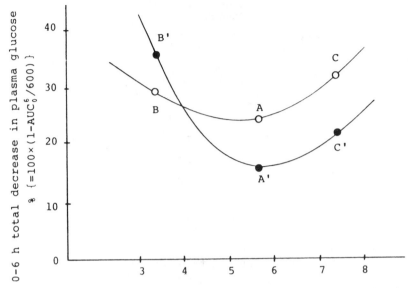

FIGURE 2. Effect of pH on the nasal absorption of insulin in dogs after administration of powder (–○–) and liquid dosage form (–●–). Data are expressed as the mean of four determinations. (From Nagai, T., et al., *J. Controlled Release*, 1, 18, 1984. With permission.)

With regard to the change in plasma glucose level after administration, it can be said that an administration of insulin in powder state may sometimes give a bioavaiability higher than that in complete solution. When the integrated decrease in plasma glucose level over a period of 6 h was calculated, which corresponds to the area above the plasma glucose concentration curve under the 100% level, all the powder preparations tested gave a large decrease in plasma glucose level to almost the same extent, without a great pH dependency (Figure 2).

Since the freeze-dried insulin powders (B and C) gave a relatively good bioavailability, we examined the dosage forms that contained the freeze-dried insulin B with different excipients, with a view to a development of a dosage form that might be more practically available. The plasma glucose level curves were different with the excipients used (Figure 3). The lactose-containing formula (D) had the smallest decrease among the four preparations. Lactose is soluble, and thus insulin may be washed out by mucus with lactose in a relatively short time. For the crystalline cellulose (CC)-containing formula (E), the absorption was the fastest and the plasma glucose level decreased down to 49% at 30 min. Insulin in this preparation can be in direct contact with nasal mucosa without interaction with CC because CC is not soluble in mucosa. For the hydroxypropyl cellulose (HPC)-containing formula (F) and carbomer (CM)-containing formula (G), especially for CM, the effect was sustained, as both HPC and CM become viscous with mucus and form gel where insulin may be included to stay on nasal mucosa for a fairly long period. It was confirmed that the above results for plasma glucose corresponded to those for the plasma immunoreactive insulin.

As a result of these investigations, it can be said that (1) freeze-dried insulin gives a relatively good bioavailability; (2) the pH dependency of absorption is not so strict in the powder forms compared with the liquid forms; and (3) the effect is sustained in using such excipients as HPC and CM, which get viscous with mucus and form gel. Therefore, we tried to prepare the sample of neutral property by freeze-drying the aqueous solution of insulin and CM, finally containing CC of the particle size between 100 and 200 mesh; formulas and process are shown in Figure 4. The formulas I, J, and K containing CM gave quite good results, as shown in Figure 5. The effect obtained after a dose of 3 IU/kg prepared as formula I or J was about twice as large as that after I.V. administration of a dose of 0.5

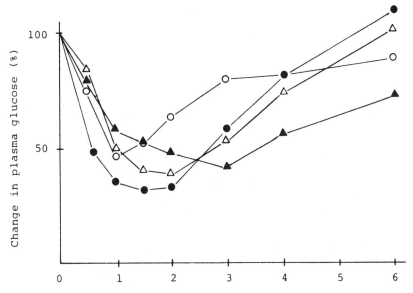

FIGURE 3.   Plasma glucose level after intranasal administration of formula D (–○–), E (–●–), F (–△–), and G (–▲–). Data are expressed as the mean of four determinations. (From Nagai, T., et al., *J. Controlled Release,* 1, 18, 1984. With permission.)

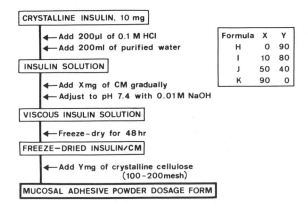

FIGURE 4.   Method of preparation of mucosal adhesive powder of insulin (formulas H, I, J, and K). (From Nagai, T., et al., *J. Controlled Release,* 1, 16, 1984. With permission.)

IU/kg. If there is a linear dose-response relation, the nasal powder would need to contain about three times the dose of insulin to produce the same effect as an I.V. administration. In other words, this final powder dosage form successfully produced hypoglycemia of one third the extent of that reached by I.V. injection, assuming that the same dose of insulin was administered.

To make sure whether the preparation was or was not inhaled to below the trachea upon administration, a sample was used in an experiment using beagles in which a cannula was inserted in the trachea by an operation, and the result was compared with that for untreated dogs. Then, there was observed no significant difference between beagles with and without tracheal cannulization as regards the change in plasma glucose level after administration of insulin in the preparation (Figure 6). Therefore, it seemed possible that the dosage form was not inhaled below the trachea while the absorption took place.

In order to make sure of the results obtained in dogs, a similar investigation was done in rabbits, because it has been known that the absorption behavior of insulin often differs

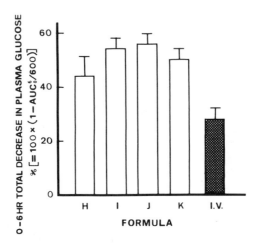

FIGURE 5.   Total decrease in plasma glucose of powder dosage forms, H-K (3 IU/kg), and i.v. administration, i.v. (0.5 IU/kg:), of insulin. Data are expressed as the mean ± SE (n = 4 to 5). (From Nagai, T., *J. Controlled Release,* 1, 19, 1984. With permission.)

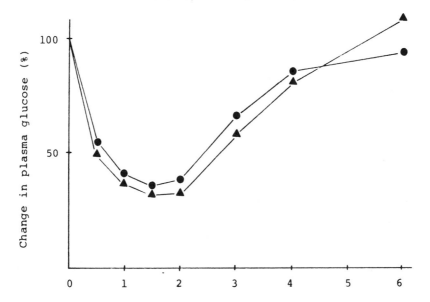

FIGURE 6.   Plasma glucose level after intranasal administration of insulin preparation with (–●–) or without (–▲–) tracheal cannulization. Data are expressed as the mean of four determinations. (From Nagai, T., *J. Controlled Release,* 1, 19, 1984. With permission.)

with animal species. Moreover, rabbits may afford a severe experimental condition for absorption of insulin because the surface area of the nasal mucosa effective for absorption is small compared with dogs. Therefore, it seemed significant to confirm whether insulin is absorbed nasally from the powder dosage form in rabbits in a way similar to the case of dogs.

The results obtained were almost similar to those obtained in dogs. Different types of enhancement and time curve for absorption of insulin in rabbits were observed with excipients. With the addition of such water insoluble excipients as crystalline cellulose and starch, the absorption became fast and was sustained in the preparation with neutralized CM (CM-Na).

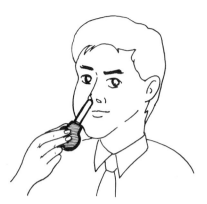

FIGURE 7.   Application of nasal powder spray by the special sprayer.
See also Chapter 7.

When we estimated the decrement of plasma glucose level at the dose of 5 IU/kg in the same way as for the nasal powder dosage form in beagles, this corresponded roughly to the result obtained previously in dogs. In other words, the powder dosage form produced hypoglycemia of about one fifth or one sixth the extent of that reached by the I.V. injection, though it was not confirmed because any comparative experiment with injection had not been done for rabbits.

Concerning the irritation to nasal mucosa by the powder preparations, the final new dosage forms created no problems when the placebo samples were administered to several volunteers. From the view point of drug safety, therefore, these preparations seemed promising for a clinical use, though more detailed studies should be carried out to clarify the influence of continuous administration on the nasal mucosa.

However, when we have examined the decrement of plasma glucose in humans using the same dosage form, the results obtained at present unfortunately are quite variable; this may be due to a difference in peptidase activities in nasal mucosa among animals.[13] Therefore, we are looking forward to having a promising absorption enhancer of insulin with a very high safety level using nasal administration.

III. ADHESIVE POWDER SPRAY FOR NASAL ALLERGY

Recently, the use of drugs for nasal allergy is increasing in Japan. A nasal spray that contains beclomethasone dipropionate (BDP) has been widely known to have an excellent therapeutic efficacy and to cause very few systemic side effects. However, a development of a new BDP preparation that permits further reduction of the BDP dose, as well as an increase in efficacy and a decrease of side effects as to severity and incidence, will be valuable in clinical treatment of nasal allergy.

For this purpose, a powder mixture preparation in capsule with HPC as the bioadhesive base, plus BDP as the active ingredient, was developed in a series of researches on bioadhesive drug delivery systems.[21-23]

As shown in Figure 7, this powder preparation is applied by a special applicator (Puvlizer®),[23] which also plays an important role in the administration of powder dosage form. The powder swells and adheres to the mucosal membrane in the same way as in the previously mentioned adhesive dosage forms. HPC stays there even at 6 h after application as confirmed by the phase I study (Figure 8).[26]

The result of the drug disposition study using tritium-labeled beclomethasone also showed that the drug remains very much longer in the body than in the case of regular nasal drops (Figure 9).[17] After a 30-day irritation test of nasal mucosa, no change was found in the tissues.[27]

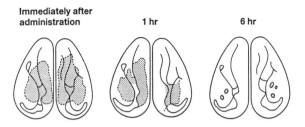

FIGURE 8.   Stay of HPC following the application in nasal cavity in phase I study.

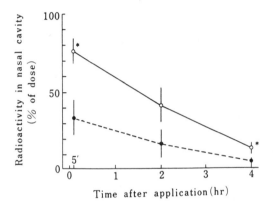

FIGURE 9.   Time course of remaining radioactivity following intranasal application of ³H-BDP preparations in nasal cavity in rabbit. —○—: nasal spray, —●—: nasal drops.

After various basic researches, the following advantages of the use of HPC were found: (1) the dose may be reduced; (2) the side effect may be lowered; and (3) a longer duration to effect is expected. Finally, the dose of BDP was decided as 100 μg/d, which is one fourth of the existing preparations.

Figure 10 shows the summary of a well-controlled clinical trial of the new one-fourth dose powder spray in comparison with three kinds of existing preparations:[23,28] (1) clemastine fumarate tablet, for which the investigation was done by double-blind clinical study in combination with the respective placebos; (2) BDP inhalation; and (3) disodium cromoglycate nasal drops.

Usefulness of the present dosage form was high compared with any of the other preparations, and the side effects were few. The incidence of side effects was especially low in the present preparation (2.6%), producing markedly little (0.5%) intranasal irritation, as compared to 9.1% for previously used inhalable steroids. Whether or not the powder might cause considerable irritation to nasal mucosa was of great concern; however, the result was low irritation compared with the other preparations. Therefore, the preparation was licensed by the Japanese government and is on the market.

ACKNOWLEDGMENT

The authors are deeply indebted to Messrs. Yoshiki Suzuki, Yuji Nishimoto, and Schoichi Narita for their assistance in this work.

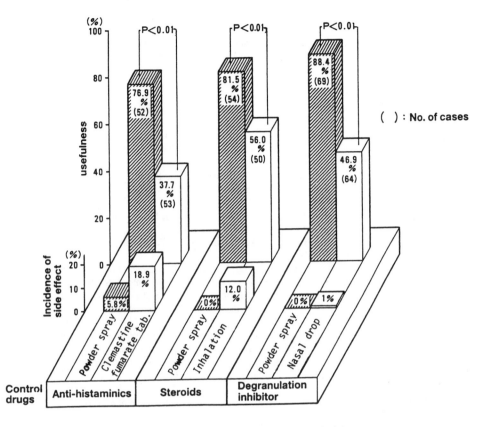

FIGURE 10. Results of comparative clinical trials.

REFERENCES

1. **Chien, Y.W.,** Ed., *Transnasal Systemic Medications — Fundamentals, Developmental Concepts and Biomedical Assessments*, Elsevier, Amsterdam, 1985.
2. **Hussain, A., Hirai, S., and Bawarshi, R.,** Nasal absorption of propranolol in rats, *J. Pharm. Sci.*, 63, 1196, 1979.
3. **Hussain, A., Hirai, S., and Bawarshi, R.,** Nasal absorption of natural contraceptive steroids in rats — progesterone absorption, *J. Pharm. Sci.*, 70, 466, 1981.
4. **Su, K. S. E., Campanale, K. M., Mendelsohn, L. G., Kerchner, G. A., and Gries, C. L.,** Nasal delivery of polypeptides. I. Nasal absorption of enkephalins, *J. Pharm. Sci.*, 74, 394, 1985.
5. **London, D. L., Butt, W. R., Lynch, S. S., Marshall, J. C., Owusu, S., Robinson, W. R., and Stephanson, J. M.,** Hormonal response to intranasal luteinizing hormone releasing hormone, *J. Clin. Endocrinol. Metab.*, 37, 829, 1973.
6. **Keenan, J. and Chamberlain, M. A.,** Nasal mucosal absorption of tetracosactrin as indicated by rise in plasma fluorogenic corticosteroids, *Br. Med. J.*, 4, 407, 1969.
7. **Mueller, K. and Osler, M.,** Induction of labour, a comparison of intravenous, intranasal and transbuccal oxitocin, *Acta Obstet. Gynecol. Scand.*, 46, 59, 1967.
8. **Bauman, G., Walser, A., Desaulles, P. A., Paesi F. J. A., and Geller, L.,** Corticotropic action of an intra-nasally applied synthetic ACTH derivative, *J. Clin. Endocrinol. Metab.*, 42, 60, 1976.
9. **Olanoff, L.,** Physical-chemical determinants of nasal drug delivery, in *Abstr. 3rd Int. Symp. Recent Adv. Drug Delivery Syst.*, Salt Lake City, Utah, February 24 to 27, 1987, 35.
10. **Hirai, S., Yashiki, T., and Mima, H.,** Mechanisms for the enhancement of nasal absorption of insulin by surfactants, *Int. J. Pharm.*, 9, 173, 1981.
11. **Lee, V. H.,** Transport and metabolic barriers to peptide and protein absorption across mucosal surfaces, in *Symp. Abstr. Jpn. - U.S. Congr. Pharm. Sci.* Honolulu, Hawaii, December 2 to 7, 1987, 89.

12. **Moses, A.C.,** Nasal absorption of insulin, in *Abstr. Int. FIP Satellite Symp. Disposition Delivery Peptide Drugs,* Leiden, The Netherlands, September 5 to 6, 1987, L17.
13. **Lee, V.H.,** Peptidase activities in various absorptive mucosae, in *Abstr. Int. FIP Satellite Symp. Disposition Delivery Peptide Drugs,* Leiden, The Netherlands, September 5 to 6, 1987, L7.
14. **Mygind, N.,** *Nasary Allergy,* Blackwell Scientific, Oxford, 1978.
15. **Aoki, F.Y. and Crawley, J. C. W.,** Distribution and removal of human serum albumin-technetium-99m instilled intranasally, *Br. J. Clin. Pharmacol.,* 3, 869, 1976.
16. **Hardy, J. G., Lee, S. W., and Wilson, C. G.,** Intranasal drug delivery by sprays and drops, *J. Pharm. Pharmacol.,* 37, 294, 1985.
17. **Yamamoto, M., Okabe, K., Kubo, J., Naruchi, T., Ikura, H., and Suzuki, Y.,** Behavior of TN-102 in nasal cavity. I. Study on adhesion and stay of active ingredient following intranasal application, *Kiso-to-Rinsho (Clin. Rep.),* 18, 4359, 1984.
18. **Yamamoto, M., Okabe, K., Kubo, J., Naruchi, T., Ikura, H., and Suzuki, Y.,** Behavior of TN-102 in nasal cavity. II. Study on distribution of active ingredient in nasal cavity by microautoradiography, *Kiso-to-Rinsho (Clin. Rep.),* 18, 4364, 1984.
19. **Illum, L., Joergensen, H., Bisgaad, H., Krogsgaad, O., and Rossig, N.,** Bioadhesive microspheres as a potential nasal drug delivery system, *Int. J. Pharm.,* 39, 189, 1987.
20. **Nagai, T., Nishimoto, Y., Nambu, N., Suzuki, Y., and Sekine, K.,** Powder dosage form of insulin for nasal administration, *J. Controlled Release,* 1, 15, 1984.
21. **Nagai, T., Machida, Y., Suzuki, Y., and Ikura, H.,** Method and preparation for administration to the mucosa of the oral or nasal cavity, Japanese Patent 1,177,734, May 13, 1983; U.S. Patent 4,226,848, October 7, 1980; U.S. Patent 4,250,163, February 10, 1981; West German Patent 2,908,847, August 14, 1981; French Patent 79-05,845, May 17, 1982; British Patent 2,042,888, September 28, 1983; Swiss Patent 638, 997, October 31, 1983.
22. **Suzuki, Y., Ikura, H., Yamashita, G., and Nagai, T.,** Powdery pharmaceutical preparation and powdery preparation to the nasal mucosa and method for administration thereof, Japanese Patent 1,286,881, October 31, 1985; U.S. Patent 4,294,829, October 13, 1981; E. P. C. Patent 23,359, July 29, 1980.
23. **Teijin Ltd.,** *Rhinocoat: Adhesive Topical Preparation for Nasal Allergy,* Teijin Ltd. Pharmaceutical Division (Uchisaiwai-cho, Chiyoda-ku, Tokyo), 1986.
24. **Maitani, Y., Igawa, T., Machida, Y., and Nagai, T.,** Intranasal administration of β-interferon in rabbits, *Drug Design Del.,* 1, 65, 1986.
25. **Ishida, M., Machida, Y., Nambu, N., and Nagai, T.,** New mucosal dosage form of insulin, *Chem. Pharm. Bull.,* 29, 810, 1981.
26. **Kuroishi, T., Asaka, H., and Okamoto, M.,** Phase I study on beclomethasone dipropionate powder preparation (TL-102) — single and repeat administrations, *Jpn. Pharmacol. Ther.,* 27, 4055, 1984.
27. **Koyama, T., Makita T., and Ichikawa, N.,** Irritating effect of TL-102 on rabbit nasal mucosa, *Kiso-to-Rinsho (Clin. Rep.),* 18, 4349, 1984.
28. **Okuda, M.,** Clinical study on beclomethasone dipropionate powder preparation (TL-102) in perennial nasal allergy, *Rhinology,* 24, 113, 1986.

Chapter 10

OCULAR BIOADHESIVE DELIVERY SYSTEMS

David L. Middleton, Sau-Hung S. Leung, and Joseph R. Robinson

TABLE OF CONTENTS

I. INTRODUCTION

The eye and precorneal surface are a unique system for the study of bioadhesive drug delivery given its accessibility. Since there is direct access to an exposed mucosal surface, evaluation of bioadhesive dosage forms can be accomplished by *in vivo* observations of a foreign body (the delivery system itself) as well as pharmacokinetic and pharmacodynamic properties.

In this chapter, there is considerable emphasis placed on preocular and ocular physiology with the intent of providing a foundation for ocular bioadhesive drug delivery systems. Subsequently, evaluation of various macromolecules that are or may be used as bioadhesive vehicles is described and, finally, the physicochemical factors that effect delivery of drug substances to the eye is considered.

II. ANATOMY AND PHYSIOLOGY OF THE PRECORNEAL AREA

This section is not intended as a comprehensive treatise on the anatomy and physiology of the eye. Rather, a brief discussion of the preocular surface pertinent to ophthalmic drug delivery is provided. For a more detailed discussion, the reader is referred to numerous texts such as *Adler's Physiology of the Eye: Clinical Application.*[1]

A. EYELIDS

The main functions of the eyelids are to protect the eye and to replenish the tear film over the exposed globe through the blinking mechanism. Located on the temporal area above each eye is the lacrimal gland, which provides the bulk of the aqueous fluid that constitutes tears. On each lid margin, located nasally toward the medial canthus, are the superior and inferior lacrimal puncta (Figure 1), which are entry points into the lacrimal drainage system and function to channel the draining tears from the preocular surface into the nasopharynx. In addition to water, tears contain a wide array of other substances including electrolytes, albumin, cell debris, etc. A thin oily monolayer, to retard tear evaporation, is provided by the meibomian glands located within the lids with secretory openings along the lid margin. Accessory lacrimal glands of Krause and Wolfring are also located within the lids (Figure 2). Like the main lacrimal gland, they secrete various protein and enzymatic components of the tear film to provide nutrition and metabolic capability to the preocular area.

During blinking, the upper lid moves vertically downward and the lower lid moves medially to direct the tear film and debris to the puncta for drainage. As the upper lid moves, it spreads and mixes the components of the tear film along the lid margin and replenishes the aqueous film over the corneal epithelium. Nonstimulated blinking occurs spontaneously at about 15 times per minute (900 times per hour) or every 2.8 to 4 s in humans and lasts 0.3 to 0.4 s.[1] This is considerably faster than the blink rate for rabbits, which is about four times per hour.[2] Since blinking spreads the tear film over the globe, any fluid dosage form instilled into the preocular area is diluted and drained markedly faster in humans than in rabbits. In addition to this involuntary reflex blinking, lid closure can be stimulated by strong light, loud noise, objects touching the cornea, or even by a perceived approaching object. When tear secretions have been stimulated, as will be seen in Section C, the lids react by adjusting their normal blinking rate to accomodate the changing tear volume.

B. CONJUNCTIVA

The conjunctiva is the mucus membrane that lines the lids and extends past the fornices onto the orbit near the junction of the cornea and sclera (Figure 3). The conjunctiva is similar to all mucus membranes, since it is a multilayered nonkeratinized columnar epithelium covering the highly vascularized substantia propria. The substantia propria near the fornices

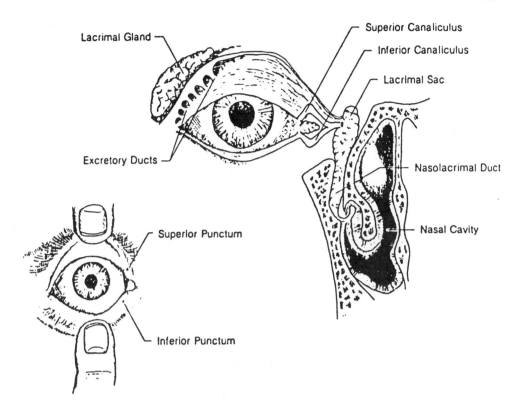

FIGURE 1. Tear drainage apparatus of the eye. (From Cunning, J. S., in *Ophthalmic Drug Delivery Systems*, Robinson, J. R., Ed., American Pharmaceutical Association, Washington, D.C., 1980. With permission. © 1980 American Pharmaceutical Association.)

is composed of loose collagen and elastic tissue containing blood and lymphatic vessels and is one of the prime locations for systemic, nonproductive ocular absorption.

The columnar epithelial cells contain numerous mucus producing goblet cells. The number of these cells increases in density in the upper and lower fornices and decreases as the palpebral conjunctiva of the inner surface of the lids becomes more keratinized near the lid margins. Marquardt[3] found an average of 25 to 40 goblet cells per square millimeter of conjunctival surface, and although variable, the cell density appears to be independent of age and sex. He also found that glaucoma patients receiving chronic administration of 2% pilocarpine solution for a number of years had a significantly higher number of goblet cells (50 to 80/mm^2). This higher number may be due to an increase in lacrimal gland secretions such that a greater number of goblet cells are needed to keep pace with the larger flow of tears. Other causes of increased goblet cell population are possible, of course, but whatever the reason, physiological changes resulting from chronic administration of drugs and/or their vehicle may change the effectiveness of the treatment and must be considered during formulation of a topical ocular product.

An important point to consider in the formulation of an opthalmic dosage form (liquid, semisolid, or device) is that while the drug entity may be extremely effective, the vehicle may be incompatible with the physiological conditions of the preocular area. As previously described, this chemical or physical incompatibility may limit chronic administration by causing physiological changes. While *in vitro* and non-human *in vivo* studies may be helpful in describing the mechanism and potential toxicity of the drug and vehicle, both short and long-term human studies are needed to fully assess physiological changes

Mucin and mucosol glycoproteins are long-chain compounds or glycoproteins charac-

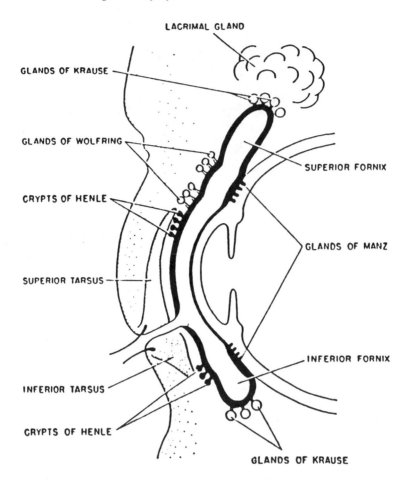

LACRIMAL GLAND

GLANDS OF KRAUSE

GLANDS OF WOLFRING

CRYPTS OF HENLE

SUPERIOR TARSUS

INFERIOR TARSUS

CRYPTS OF HENLE

SUPERIOR FORNIX

GLANDS OF MANZ

INFERIOR FORNIX

GLANDS OF KRAUSE

FIGURE 2.   Diagram of a sagittal section through the eyelids and eyeball to show the conjunctival sac and the position of its gland. (From Adler, F. H., *Physiology of the Eye: Clinical Application*, C. V. Mosby, St. Louis, 1965, 31. With permission.)

terized by numerous ionic oligosaccharide groups located at various spacings on a protein core (Figure 4). In general, mucus forms the inner layer of tear film, which is in contact with the microvilli of the corneal and conjunctival epithelium. Since these glycoproteins are more hydrophilic than the underlying epithelial cells, they appear to increase wetting and spreading of the tear film along the corneal epithelial surface.[4,5] Blinking causes sufficient shearing action to spread these glycoproteins along the corneal surface and permits continuous replenishment of the mucin layer.[6] This point is discussed further in Section E.

According to Berta and Torok,[7] tears contain acidic and neutral glycoproteins. Neutral glycoproteins are seen in the aqueous phase accompanying medium to high flow rates. At low tear flow rates, more of the acidic (sialic acid or sulfate) glycoproteins are observed. The neutral glycoproteins appear to be produced by the lacrimal gland and serum while acidic molecules are secreted from conjunctival goblet cells,[8,9] Thus at normal tear flow rates, the total glycoproteins are a mixture of all these sources, and typically constitute less than 5% of the total weight of mucus.[10]

C. LACRIMAL GLAND

The lacrimal gland is located beneath and behind the upper lid in the upper outer orbital quadrant (Figure 1) and is responsible for secretion of the major volume portion of the tear film. The rate and composition of lacrimal gland secretions are controlled primarily by

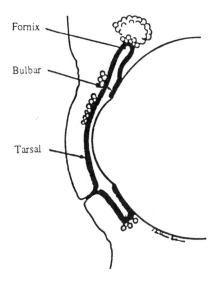

FIGURE 3. Conjunctival membrane. (From Cunning, J. S., in *Ophthalmic Drug Delivery Systems,* Robinson, J. R., Ed., American Pharmaceutical Association, Washington, D.C., 1980. With permission. © 1980 American Pharmaceutical Association.)

Oligosaccharide Side Chain with Terminal Sialic Acid ($pK_a = 2.6$)

Protein Core

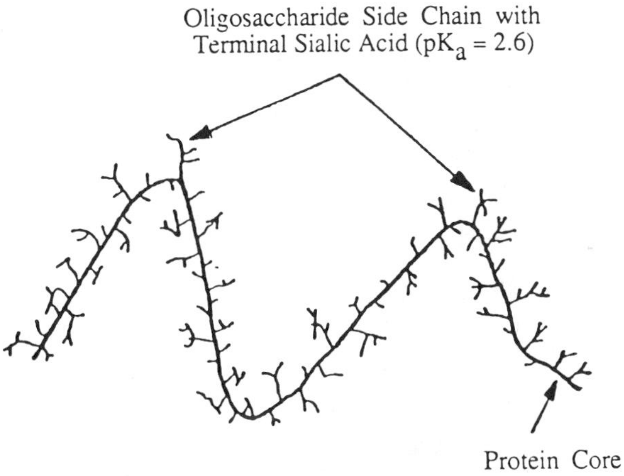

FIGURE 4. Schematic structure of mucin. (From Pigman, W., *The Glycoconjugates*, Vol. 1., Horwitz, M. I. and Pigman, W., Eds., Academic Press, New York, 1977, 132. With permission.)

cholinergic stimulation. Sympathetic innervation indirectly affects lacrimal gland secretions by changing blood flow to the gland. The changing blood flow apparently modulates the presentation rate of circulating neurotransmitters and thus alters proteinaceous secretions.

Botelho and Dartt[11] suggest that extracellular Ca^{2+} levels are directly responsible for cholinergic-activated electrolyte and water secretions. The change in water secretion (the largest component of the tear film) is also the result of electrolytes Na^+, Cl^-, and K^+ fluxes in the film. A membrane transport Na,K-ATPase pump[12] (Figure 5) common to many cell types is considered responsible for ionic movement and associated water secretion or reabsorption.

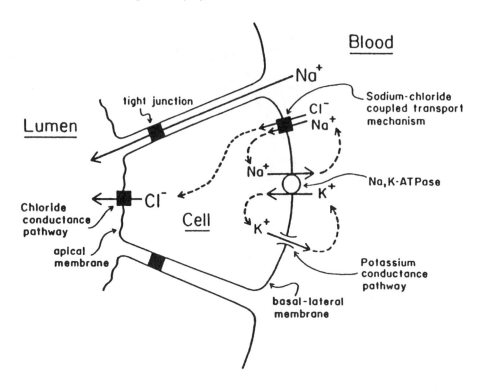

FIGURE 5.   Summary of transport mechanisms believed to be involved in formation of the NaCl-rich primary secretion in exocrine acini-intercalated ducts. (From Mircheff, A. K., *The Preocular Tear Film in Health, Disease, and Contact Lens Wear*, Holly, F. J., Ed., The Dry Eyes Institute, Lubbock, TX, 1986, 371. With permission.)

D. CORNEA

The cornea is a unique three layered membrane (Figure 6), because the special arrangement of cells, avascularity, and regularity and smoothness of the epithelium make it transparent. The epithelium is five or six layers of overlapping nonkeratinized, squamous cells approximately 60 to 65 nm thick. The aqueous corneal stroma (or substantia propria) comprises approximately 90% of the corneal thickness and is composed of layers of loosely packed parallel lamellae and holding 75 to 80% water by net weight. The single layer endothelium seves as a barrier between the hydrophilic aqueous stroma of the cornea and the aqueous humor of the anterior chamber.

For almost every drug, absorption into the cornea is limited by one of the precorneal features (i.e., tear film, conjunctiva) or the cornea itself. Water-soluble drug compounds have unfavorable partitioning characteristics into the lipophilic epithelium of the conjunctiva and cornea, but small water soluble molecules like water, methanol, ethanol, and propanol penetrate the cornea readily, presumably by a pore pathway. Absorption of lipid soluble compounds can be limited by the aqueous stromal portion of the cornea.

E. TEAR FILM

The tear film is a crucial part of the preocular area with respect to conventional and adhesive dosage systems since it is the major carrier of debris away from the eye. Although this is clearly a simplistic representation of a dynamic film, the film itself is generally described as consisting of three parts (Figure 7).[8] The outermost portion, a thin oily layer approximately 0.1 μm thick, reduces evaporation and provides a continuous covering to the tear film. Even with this protection, as much as 25% of secreted tears is lost by evaporation.[2,8] The middle portion, an aqueous layer about 7 μm thick, contains a number of salts and

Tear Film

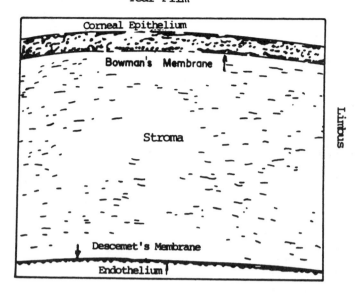

FIGURE 6. Depiction of the cornea in cross-section. (From Robinson, J. R. and Goshman, L. M., in *Pharmaceutics and Pharmacy Practice,* Banker, G. S. and Chalmers, R. K., Eds., J. B. Lippincott, Philadelphia, 1982. With permission.)

other solutes (Table 1). The aqueous protion of this layer is secreted predominantly from the lacrimal gland whereas other constituents come from the numerous accessory glands. The innermost layer, composed mostly of mucus glycoproteins, is only 0.02 to 0.05 μm thick and coats the epithelial microvilli to help hydrate and maintain a continuous film over the preocular surface. These characteristics of the tear film are common to other mucosal epithelial surfaces such as those found in the trachea, bronchi, and middle ear.[13]

Normal tear flow would facilitate drug release from a precorneal dosage form by providing a constant flow of dissolving fluid and preventing the accumulation of drug in the vicinity of the vehicle. In addition, normal tear flow continuously reduces any drug concentration established in the tear by dilution. As an example, when tear flow is suppressed by application of a topical, local anesthetic (five drops of a 0.5% tetracaine solution), the ocular bioavailability of pilocarpine in albino rabbits doubles.[14] Thus the net effect of increased tear flow is a reduction of availability of drug due to drug dilution and drainage.

1. Thickness

Tear film thickness and stability are especially important when considering topical dosage forms that may remain in contact with the precorneal area for an extended period of time. Norn[15] described the film in the lower conjunctival fornix as the final pathway for removal of foreign substances or cellular debris from the eye. Tear film mucin thus plays a role in maintenance of low surface tension by masking and removing lipid contaminants.[16] In addition, mucus glycoproteins have a high affinity for specific sites on lipid molecules and form complexes with the lipid aggregates.[17] If the mucus layer becomes too hydrophobic from the deposition of cellular debris or foreign substances, the film may become discontinuous and produce dry spots.

Foreign substances come to the surface of the mucus glycoprotein either via externaal or internal routes and cause an effective thinning of the film as they deposit on the epithelium. Thus mucus is important in removal of sloughed cells and cellular debris. Externally applied particles, whether intentional from dosage forms or accidentally from the external environ-

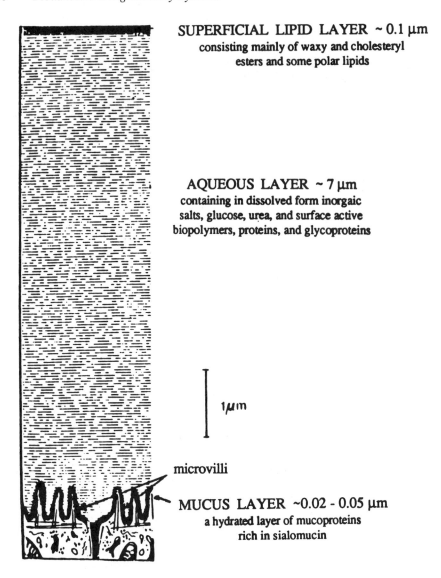

SUPERFICIAL LIPID LAYER ~ 0.1 µm
consisting mainly of waxy and cholesteryl
esters and some polar lipids

AQUEOUS LAYER ~ 7 µm
containing in dissolved form inorgaic
salts, glucose, urea, and surface active
biopolymers, proteins, and glycoproteins

1µm

microvilli

MUCUS LAYER ~0.02 - 0.05 µm
a hydrated layer of mucoproteins
rich in sialomucin

FIGURE 7.   Structure and composition of the tear film. (From Holly, F. J. and Lemp,
M. A., *Surv. Opthalmol.*, 22, 69, 1977. With permission. © 1977 Williams & Wilkins.)

ment, can migrate through the two low-viscosity upper layers to become trapped in the
mucus layer. When the tear film is sufficiently thinned, there is a physical association
between the very thin surface lipid film and the foreign substance residing on the mucus
layer, and an actual rupture or dry spot appearing in the tear film.[8] Forces generated by
blinking would cause these dry spots to ''clot'' or roll up into mucus threads with subsequent
migration of the mucin thread towards the upper and lower fornices to be removed through
the lacrimal drainage system.[2,6,16] Dosage forms with nonretentive solid particles would also
be cleared from the eye in a similar manner.

2. Osmolarity and pH

The pH of tears normally ranges between 7.3 and 7.7 and is buffered by inorganic salts[1]
(Table 1) in the aqueous layer. Reflex tearing can result from instillation of solutions outside
this range. In fact, pH-induced lacrimation can occur when the pH is ±0.5 units from 7.4[18]
Tears are poorly buffered,[19] especially at higher pHs. Mauger and Hill[20] (Figure 8) have

TABLE 1
Physical Properties and Chemical C͏͏ Human Tears

Physical properties	
Osmotic pressure	0.99
pH	7.4
Refractive index	1.
Volume	0
General chemical components	
Ash	1.05 g
Solids, total	1.8 g/100 ml
Water	98.2 g/100 ml
Electrolytes	
Bicarbonate	26 mEq/l
Chloride	120 to 135 mEq/l
Potassium	15 to 29 mEq/l
Sodium	142 mEq/l
Calcium	2.29 mg/100 ml
Nitrogenous substances	
Total protein	0.669 to 0.800 g/100 ml
Albumin	0.394 g/100 ml
Globulin	0.275 g/100 ml
Ammonia	0.005 g/100 ml
Urea	0.04 mg/100 ml
Nitrogen	
Total nitrogen	158 mg/100 ml
Nonprotein nitrogen	51 mg/100 ml
Carbohydrates	
Glucose	2.5 (0 to 5.0) mg/100 ml
Sterols	
Cholesterol and cholesterol esters	8 to 32 mg/100 ml
Miscellaneous organic acids, vitamins, enzymes	
Citric acid	0.6 mg/100 ml
Ascorbic acid	0.14 mg/100 ml
Lysozyme	800 to 2500 units/ml

From Milder, B., *Adler's Physiology of the Eye. Clinical Applications,*
8th ed., Moses, R. A. and Hart, W. M., Eds., C. V. Mosby, St. Louis,
1987. With permission.

shown that in response to titration with hydrochloric acid or sodium hydroxide, human tears have a higher buffer capacity to acids than to bases. That is, from pH~3.5 up to neutral conditions, the tears were able to buffer the titrant to ~pH 7, but with a basic challenge the effect was not as great. Carney and Hill[21] found the buffer capacity of human tears to be in the range of 10^{-5}.

Osmolarity of the ocular surface is approximately equivalent to 0.9% NaCl (300 mOsm/l) and contributes to the optical integrity of the cornea. Due to continuous evaporation of tears, actual osmolarity is 310 to 320 mOsm. It is most important to consider the tonicity of instilled preparations, since hypertonic solutions tend to cause excessive tearing. Hypotonic solutions, on the other hand, should lose water to the tear film to restore tonicity,[22] Gilbard and Dartt[23] reported that cholinergic stimulation of flow rates changes the osmolarity. At low flow rates (<0.1 μl/min), the osmolarity is high (334± 4 mOsm/l), but as flow rates increased to above 4 μl/min, osmolarity decreased to more normal levels. This suggests that an increased tear flow caused by increased tear volume, from the presence of a dosage form, may not change osmolarity significantly.

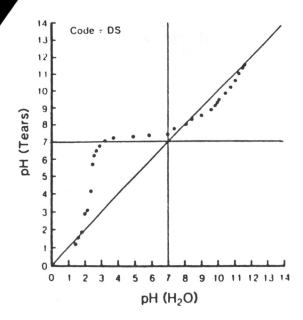

FIGURE 8. The resistance to pH change of the tears (buffering capacity) of one subject upon step-wise addition of hydrogen and hydroxlion by titration in relation to an unbuffered reference solution (degassed, demineralized distilled water). (From Mauger, T. F. and Hill, R. M., *The Preocular Tear Film in Health, Disease, and Contact Lens Wear*, Holly F. J., Ed., The Dry Eyes Institute, Lubbock, TX, 1986, 539. With permission.)

F. TEAR DRAINAGE SYSTEM

The tears, secreted and flowing predominantly from the radial sections of the upper lid, pass downward and medially over the conjunctiva and cornea to be emptied through the superior and inferior canaliculi. At this point, the tears pass into the nasal cavity via the lacrimal drainage system (Figure 1) to be eventually mixed with contents of the GI tract via the nasopharynx and oral cavity. The normal unperturbed tear volume is approximately 7 ± 2 μl and has a secretion rate of 0.5 to 2.2 μ/min,[24,25] i.e., a tear turnover rate of ~16%/min. Tear production rate can be increased several-fold by varying drug concentration or vehicle pH.[24] If the normal volume of ~ 8 μl was well distributed, Berta[26] determined that ~ 1 μl was the volume of the precorneal tear film, ~ 3 μl distributed along the lid margins and ~ 4 μl in the upper and lower fornices. In other words, the fornices can contain up to 50% of the tear volume and thus could be considered a temporary storage area for an ocular mucoadhesive drug delivery system.

The maximum fluid volume of the lower conjunctival fornix is 25 to 30 μl, if care is taken not to blink. Therefore, when drug-laden fluids are instilled, tear volume may increase to greater than the 30 μl maximum volume and rapidly exit through the drainage system and/or spill onto the cheek. The size of the punctal orifices in humans is on the order of 300 μm,[27] well above the size of most particles in ophthalmic dosage forms. Thus, preocular drug loss by an accelerated drainage rate will be significant for most ophthalmic dosage forms.

It is believed that the major loss of drugs in the precorneal area is through drainage, tear turnover, and nonproductive absorption. The losses due to drainage and tear turnover are independent of the drug when there is no induced lacrimation by the drug or its vehicle. After instillation, the diluted drug solution drains from the precorneal area at a rate that is dependent on the volume and viscosity of the ophthalmic solution.[28] Induced lacrimation can result from nonphysiologic pH and/or tonicity and from foreign body irritation.[29-31] Again, the need for dosage forms that will adhere to the preocular tissues and resist natural drainage mechanisms is obvious.

TABLE 2
Classification of Controlled Release Systems

Type	Controlling step	Drug release mechanism
Diffusion-controlled devices		
Reservoir (membrane)	Concentration difference	Diffusion
Matrix (monolithic)	Concentration difference	Diffusion
Chemically controlled devices		
Biodegradable (bioerodible)	Degradation	Reaction-dependent diffusion
Pendant chain systems	Hydrolysis	Reaction and diffusion
Solvent-activated systems		
Osmotically controlled	Osmosis	Osmotic flow
Swellable systems	Swelling	Diffusion
Swelling-controlled	Swelling front	Relaxation-dependent diffusion
Magnetically controlled devices	Diffusion	Magnetic field

From Peppas, N. A., *Recent Advances in Drug Delivery Systems*, Anderson, J. M. and Kim, S. W., Eds., Plenum Press, New York, 1984, 279. With permission.

III. CONVENTIONAL DELIVERY SYSTEMS

The major reason for failure of conventional ocular drug delivery systems is drainage of the drug substance before adequate absorption can occur. According to Maurice and Mishima,[32] ~ 2 μl is pumped from the tear film in each blink. Therefore, for a 50-μl drop, with 20 to 30 μl lost to the cheek from overflow and immediate drainage and 2 μl/blink lost continuously, only about one third of the original dose remains available for absorption after a few seconds, and even that has been diluted by tears. To overcome this great loss factor, formulators have included excess drug in their products so that a therapeutically effective dose can be achieved. The possible dangerous consequence of this, however, is that enough drained drug solution can now be absorbed from the nasolacrimal duct or GI tract after drainage through the lacrimal drainage system to present systemic side effects. Local nonproductive ocular absorption (for example into the conjunctive) also results in a decrease in available drug for corneal absorption.

IV. OCULAR MUCOADHESIVES*

In general, the classification of mucoadhesives will reflect the orientation of the classifier. Peppas,[33] and earlier with Langer,[34] classified mucoadhesive polymers as shown in Table 2. This classification was based on the release characteristics of the polymeric system and takes on the application viewpoint that will be important once a marketable system is found. In contrast, in this chapter, the chemical characterization of polymers based on the solubility of functional groups on the polymer backbone will be used. The reader should keep in mind that polymers will never dissolve completely, i.e., the interaction of their functional groups will expand their chains so that the mixture appears as a solution.

Mucoadhesive polymers are usually macromolecular hydrocolloids with numerous hydrophilic functional groups, such as carboxyl, hydroxyl, amide, and sulfate. These groups can establish electrostatic interactions, hydrophobic interactions, van der Waals intermolecular interactions, and hydrogen-bonding with underlying substrates. For many polymers, hydrogen-bonding appears to play a significant role in mucoadhesion, and thus the presence of water seems to be a prerequisite for a majority of the mucoadhesive phenomena.

---

* For purposes of this chapter, the term *mucoadhesives*, i.e., those polymers that attach to mucin, rather than the more general bioadhesive term, which implies attachment to any biological surface, will be used.

When macromolecular hydrocolloids with hydrophilic functional groups are placed in an aqueous media, they swell and expand into a gel or network. Interpentration and entanglement of this network with the mucin substrate is proposed to be partly responsible for their adhesive properties.[35,36] Therefore, mobility and flexibility of the polymer chains is a prerequisite for strong mucoadhesion.

A. SYNTHETIC MUCOADHESIVES

Synthetic mucoadhesives include water-soluble polymers that are linear, and water-insoluble polymers that are swellable networks joined by cross-linking agents.

1. Water-Soluble Mucoadhesives

The charge on water-soluble ionic polymers is important for mucoadhesion. Park et al.[37,38] measured and compared the adhesion of a series of water-soluble anionic, cationic, and neutral polymers using a cell culture-fluorescent probe technique. From their results, polyanionic polymers, which are collectively less toxic than cationic polymers, are preferred for use in humans. In addition, polycations (i.e., polylysine) can bind to negatively charged surfaces,[38] and thus can cause cell aggregation.

In some cases, corneal adsorption of some neutral polymers is reported to be comparable to the adsorption of natural mucins. Lemp and Szymanski et al.[39] measured the extent of adsorption of water-soluble polymers onto the corneal surface. This was determined by the change in contact angle compared with natural mucin (0.5% bovine submaxillary mucin[BSM]). They found that 1.4% polyvinyl alcohol, 0.5% hydroxypropyl methyl cellulose, or 0.2% hydroxyethyl cellulose vehicles have comparable corneal adsorptivity to that of BSM, and therefore, drugs contained in these vehicles should be well absorbed from topical formulations. However, the fact that in many cases only marginal improvements in bioavailability were noted suggests that the adsorbed polymer was either unable to hold the drug or was rapidly removed from the surface by the bathing tears.

Hydroxypropyl cellulose (HPC) has been used to make slowly eroding tablets and topical inserts, which swell with body fluids and slowly release their drug contents. In a recent review, Nagai[40] discusses his use of a 1:2 mixtures of HPC/Carbopol®934 compressed into tablets with drug. These tablets will swell when in contact with body fluids and adhere to a wide variety of mucosal surfaces. For example, he has had successes locally treating cervical cancer and delivering insulin nasally or buccally. The tablet or powder (in the case of nasally applied insulin) was observed at the completion of the study and consisted of a dry core of polymer and drug surrounded by a gel-like layer probably devoid of drug. Since the fluid content of the precorneal area is higher than some mucosal areas tested by Nagai, the polymer matrix reservoir for drug may remain intact long enough for extended ocular drug delivery.

Many workers have found that for water-soluble polymers, there appears to be a critical molecular weight or molecular length, which is necessary for the adhesion of polymers to a substrate. For example, the molecular weight of sodium carboxymethyl cellulose should exceed 78,600 in order to have significant bioadhesion.[35] Chen and Cyr[41] have added more information to the size characterization by showing that mucoadhesive strength increases as molecular weight of the water-soluble polymer increases above 100,000. Polymers with a highly linear configuration, like polyethylene glycols with molecular weights of 20,000, show little to no adhesive properties. However, when the molecular weight is increased to 200,000, adhesiveness is improved, and with still further increases in molecular weight (i.e., up to 4 million), an excellent mucoadhesive is obtained. For the natural polymer polysaccharide, carrageenan, they found that the degraded carrageenan is much less adhesive than the higher molecular weight potassium salt.

These workers and others have confirmed the size characterization for adhesive properties with dextrans.[38,42] Dextrans with molecular weight as high as 19,500,000 have similar mucoadhesive strength to those with molecular weights of 200,000. In this case, the helical conformation of the polymers, which could shield the adhesively active groups inside the coil may be as important as the chain length of linear polymers. Still, the effect of molecular weight can be observed, especially when the molecular weight is above 100,000. In summary, chain length, configuration, and molecular weight are important parameters for controlling the mucoadhesive strength of water-soluble polymers.

Many of these polymers have been used as drug containing vehicles. The bioadhesiveness of water-soluble polymers and their role in drug delivery can be seen when polyacrylic acid was used as a drug carrier for pilocarpine.[43] By complexing pilocarpine with polyacrylic acid, the ocular bioavailability was enhanced by a factor of two.

2. Water-Insoluble Mucoadhesives

Most water-insoluble mucoadhesive polymers have hydrophilic groups that interact with water molecules and expand the polymer network to a more flexible and mobile state. When the mucoadhesive is in contact with a hydrophilic substrate, the stretched and entangled polymer molecules can match their active adhesive sites with those on the substrate to form adhesive bonds.

The flexibility and expanded nature of the polymer network is a very important parameter for mucoadhesives.[36] There is good correlation between degree of hydration and tensile strength of polymers, and thus, greater openness of the polymer network, i.e., higher degree of hydration, results in greater mucoadhesion. In ocular drug delivery systems with mucoadhesive polymer vehicles, one has to choose polymers that can form an expanded and hydrated network to allow for sufficient interpenetration and subsequent physical entanglement. Networks may be formed by: (1) cross-linking the polymer chains with small amounts of cross-linking agents, e.g., polyacrylic acid cross-linked by 0.2% of divinyl glycol;(2) physical entanglement of the intertwined polymer chains; and (3) bridging of the polymer chains.

Cross-linked polyacrylic acid or its analogs are well known for their mucoadhesive properties, and their mechanism of bioadhesion has been extensively studied.[36,37,40,44-50] When lightly cross-linked (0.3%) polyacrylic acid was utilized in ocular drug delivery, the area under the curve was 4.2 times greater than for a conventional suspension preparation,[51] indicating prolonged residence time in the preocular area with a greater chance for ocular absorption.

Cyanoacrylates have been used to seal corneal perforations and ulcers to stop leakage of aqueous or vitreous humor and for protection against external contamination.[52,53] Cyanoacrylate monomers polymerize almost instantly upon contact with corneal tissues and adhere tenaciously. After healing of the corneal tissue, the polymer is sloughed off or can be removed by an ophthalmologist. Thus cyanoacrylates have the potential to be developed into an effective ocular mucoadhesive delivery system if monomer polymerization can be better controlled, i.e., decreasee toxicity of the polymer.

Pilocarpine has been used by many investigators to study ocular drug delivery from mucoadhesive drug delivery systems. A partially esterified acrylic acid polymer product. Piloplex®, was used to prolong the therapeutic effect of topically applied pilocarpine[54,55] It is an aqueous emulsion (dispersion) that has limited solubility in water, but which is adherent to the preocular tissue. Upon instillation of the emulsion into the eye, it appears as an opaque, visually apparent mass in the lower fornix for extended periods of time. The active ingredient, pilocarpine, via its amine group undergoes an acid-base reaction with many of the carboxylic acid groups of the polyacrylic acid-lauryl methacrylate, the polymeric carrier in Piloplex®. The release of pilocarpine from the dosage form is probably governed by entrapment of the pilocarpine in the polymer and slow dissolution of the polymer or diffusion of pilocarpine from the polymer. It is speculated that because of the unusual hydrophilic-lipophilic nature of the polymer, it undergoes a phase change of coagulation when placed in the eye (thus trapping drug), and the free carboxy groups attach to mucin for extended periods of time.[25]

Another delivery device for pilocarpine is an erodible film made of polyvinyl alcohol.[43,56] When compared to an aqueous formulation, the film showed a twofold increase in the ocular bioavailability of pilocarpine and increased the duration of miosis in the albino rabbit by a factor of five. The prolonged effect of the drug is probably due to slow dissolution of the insert, but it may also have some small mucoadhesive property.

A biocompatible, cellulose acetate hydrogen phthalate latex was used as a carrier for prolonged drug delivery by sorbing pilocarpine onto/into 0.3 mm beads of the lates,[57,58] Since the latex is highly unstable at physiological pH, it coagulates in the fornix, similar to the mechanism for Piloplex®. In this form, it cannot be readily eliminated by the tear fluid and thus remains in the fornix for an extended period of time.

Urtti et al.[59] used polyacrylamide and a copolymer of acrylamide (*N*-vinyl pyrrolidone and ethyl acrylate) as a matrix for ocular drug delivery. The increase in contact time of the vehicle with the corneal tissue resulted in a threefold increase in ocular bioavailability of pilocarpine in both albino and pigmented rabbit.

B. NATURALLY OCCURRING MUCOADHESIVES

The use of naturally occurring macromolecules as carriers in drug delivery systems has considerable potential. Fibrin[60] and collagen[61] have been used to fabricate erodible inserts for placement in the fornix for long term delivery of pilocarpine into the eye. Other natural macromolecules that have specific or nonspecific binding properties and may be used in ocular drug delivery include fibronectin, lectins, and polysaccharides. The usefulness of these macromolecules will depend on drug attachment capabilities and delivery aspects of the altered form of the natural molecule.

Fibronectin, a glycoprotein like mucin, is a component of the extracellular matrix[62] and binds certain forms of collagen,[63] glycosaminoglycans,[64] other cell surfaces, granulocytes, monocytes, and bacteria.[65] A specific area of fibronectin's backbone, i.e., a pentapeptide has been identified as having cell attachment activity.[66,67] Small synthetic peptides have also been shown to possess cellular adhesive activity.[67-69] In Japan, purified fibronectin was used to speed the healing time of corneal ulcers.[70] In this country, fibronectin and hyaluronic acid have been used in conjunction with a collagen based dressing for dermal wounds[71] to decrease healing time.

Lectins are either carbohydrate-binding proteins or glycoproteins[72] and are either divalent or polyvalent.[73] Some purified lectins were found to be specific for sialic acids,[74-77] a major component of the mucus glycoproteins.

The external surface of cells, collectively referred to as the glycocalyx,[78] are chemically polysaccharides and are partly responsible for the natural adhesive property of the cell. Clearly, these types of biopolymers would be useful mucoadhesive substances for drug delivery purposes.

V. FACTORS AFFECTING OCULAR MUCOADHESION

A. DOSAGE FORM AND VEHICLE
1. Electronic Charge

Cationic anionic, and neutral polymers have been shown to have mucoadhesive properties.[38] The mechanism of mucoadhesion for neutral polymers is not fully understood, but may involve hydrogen bonding and hydrophobic interactions. For cationic mucoadhesives, the interaction between the adhesive and substrate (e.g., mucin) is probably electrostatic in nature, because mucin is negatively charged at pH 7.4 due to the presence of sialic acids

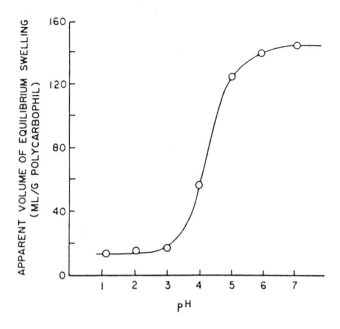

FIGURE 9. Apparent volume of equilibrium swelling of polycarbophil at various pHs. (From Park, H. and Robinson, J. R., *J. Controlled Release*, 2, 47, 1985. With permission.)

groups at the terminal ends of the oligosaccharide chains.[79,80] Electrostatic interactions at the corneal surface are also possible, and supportive evidence is the preferential corneal uptake of cationic liposomes instead of anionic and neutral liposomes.[81] For anionic mucoadhesives, e.g., cross-linked polyacrylic acid, the mucoadhesive strength is greatly increased when carboxyl groups are in an acid form,[46] thus suggesting a hydrogen-bonding mechanism for mucoadhesion.

For a macromolecular network, the number and type of charged groups, degree of hydration, and expanded nature of the network are all closely linked to adhesive strength.[49] At the physiological pH of the precorneal area (pH 7.3 to 7.7), hydration of the cross-linked polyacrylic acid is maximum[46] (Figure 9), and formation of hydrogen-bonds is less than at acidic pHs (Figure 10). These factors reflect a lower mucoadhesive strength in the preocular area[47] by virtue of pH demands for comfort. Nevertheless, even at physiological pH, attachment is firm enough to permit excellent retention of drug delivery systems in the eye. Thus, when using cross-linked polyanionic polymers in designing ocular mucoadhesive dosage forms, formation of hydrogen-bonds is only one of several stabilizing interactions needed to achieve mucoadhesion.

2. Viscosity

One of the most important properties of a mucoadhesive polymer is its aqueous viscosity. Polymer-solvent interactions and polymer-solvent-tear film interaction depend on molecular flexibility, type of solvent, degree of ionization, polymer concentration, and pH.[82] Most polymer solutions or suspensions tend to exhibit pseudoplastic behavior instead of showing Newtonian viscosity. The degree of entanglement between polymer chains affects viscosity. Thus, as demonstrated by a correlation between molecular weight and viscosity,[83] more extended polymer forms will have higher viscosities. Various polymer and copolymer suspensions exhibit different types of viscosity changes. A few examples are included to demonstrate the effect of these changes on vehicle drainage from the eye.

Methyl cellulose and polyvinyl alcohol have been used to increase the viscosity of topical

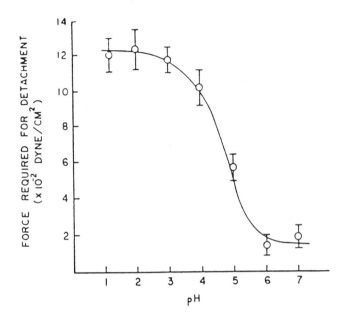

FIGURE 10.   Effect of pH on *in vitro* bioadhesion of polycabophil to rabbit stomach tissue. (From Park, H. and Robinson, J. R., *J. Controlled Release*, 2, 47, 1985. With permission.)

ocular delivery vehicles. The rate of loss of ^{99m}Tc from the preocular surface was found to be faster with saline than with higher viscosity methyl cellulose or polyvinyl alcohol solutions.[84] Thus an increase in viscosity of the vehicle may help to retain drug in the precorneal area with a subsequent increase in drug absorption and therapeutic effect.[85-89] The increase in contact time of methylcellulose ophthalmic vehicles was found to be approximately proportional to the viscosity up to about 25 cps. The contact time change was more significant in the lower viscosity ranges (5 to 25 cps), but began to level off at 55 cps.[90] A substantial improvement in vehicle retention requires several thousand cps solutions, i.e., from about 25 to ~2000 cps the gain in reduced drainage is modest and not proportional to viscosity. In humans, significant retardation of the drainage rate was noted with higher concentrations of polyvinyl alcohol (5.85%) and with 0.9% hydroxypropyl methyl cellulose.[91] Even though a tenfold reduction in the drainage rate was observed when the viscosity of the vehicle was increased from 1 to 100 cps by addition of methyl cellulose,[92] the drainage rate constant appeared to level off after the viscosity was increased to 15 cps.[93] Since higher concentrations of polyvinyl alcohol resulted in an approximate leveling off of the drainage rate constant, until very high concentrations are used, the concentration of polymer has a significant effect in decreased drainage from the eye. Thus drainage rate can be influenced by changing the viscosity and concentration of methyl cellulose and/or polyvinyl alcohol in the vehicle, but typically high viscosities are needed.

A cursory examination of the kinetics of drainage and absorption provides an explanation of the retention time requirements. Shown below is a simple model for drug disposition from an applied dose.[25]

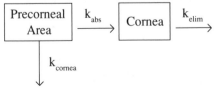

For many drugs, such as pilocarpine, k_a is one to three orders of magnitude smaller than k_{elim}, i.e., for pilocarpine $k_a = 0.001$/min and $k_{elim} = 0.024$/min. The expected behavior

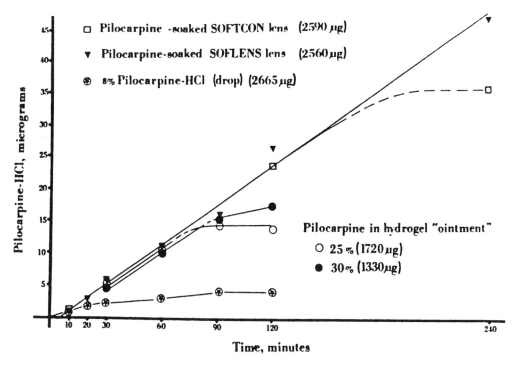

FIGURE 11. Transcorneal flux of pilocarpine-HCL *in vitro* after delivery in hydrogel "ointment" (25 and 30%), hydrogel lens buttons, and in free fluid (simulated "drops"). (From Krohn, L. and Breitfeller, J. M., *Invest Opthalmol.*, 15, 324, 1976. With permission.)

of this small absorption rate constant is a "flip-flop" model, wherein the computed rate constants are opposite of what is expected.

The reason that a flip-flop model does not result is that

$$k_{absorption(apparent)} = k_{drainage} + k_{absorption}$$

Since $k_{drainage}$ is typically 0.5 to 0.7/min, i.e., two to three orders of magnitude greater than $k_{absorption}$, the overall $k_{absorption(apparent)}$ is now much larger than k_{elim}, and hence one has traditional linear kinectic behavior.

Suppose one wished to improve the extent of drug absorption. One needs to look at the magnitude of $k_{drainage}$ relative to $k_{absorption}$ to decide on strategy. For pilocarpine in rabbits, $k_{drainage}$ is approximately 0.6/min, whereas $k_{absorption}$ is 0.001/min. The options available, therefore, are (1) increase the magnitude of $k_{absorption}$ by more than three orders of magnitude, presumably through a penetration enhancer, or (2) reduce drainage by about three orders of magnitude.

The conclusion is that to have a substantial impact on ocular drug bioavailability or duration requires an enormous reduction in precorneal drug or vehicle loss.

Pilocarpine release from vehicles composed of 25 to 30% suspensions of copolymer (hydroxymethyl methacrylate and methacrylic acid) having much higher viscosities (15,000 to 70,000, respectively) and from drug-soaked contact lenses was not significantly different up to 90 min.[94] Since the slope of the release curves were similar, a similar flux mechanism was assumed for each system (Figure 11). This is understandable in that while the apparent viscosity was quite high, the microviscosity was approximately 1 cps. Thus the equivalent of free diffusion in water occurred and no sustaining effect is expected.

Grass and Robinson[95] showed that increasing the viscosity (up to 100 cps) of vehicles containing lipid-soluble drugs did not substantially increase corneal absorption of the drug. The rate-limiting barrier for absorption of this drug type is the aqueous stroma. Therefore, there was rapid uptake by the epithelium in such a manner that increasing precorneal residence time had little effect on the ultimate bioavailability. On the other hand, for small hydrophilic drug molecules that normally penetrate the cornea with great difficulty, increasing their vehicle viscosity improved absorption by increasing precorneal residence time near the absorption-limiting epithelium. In fact, in these systems, reducing the volume to decrease the amount of spillage and any reflex-increased secretions[28] showed a greater effect than simple viscosity changes.

Finally, gets (Carbopol®940) had a great influence on the sustaining effect of the local anesthetics lidocaine and benzocaine,[96] although given the high water content of these systems, it is likely that the major sustaining effect was due to dose dumping. Therefore, increases in contact time in the precorneal area may be due to both the mucoadhesive and viscosity effects of the polymer. Finally, in choosing mucoadhesives for ocular drug delivery, it may be best to find one that has good mucoadhesive strength as well as a high viscosity at low concentration.

3. Complexing Agents, e.g., Calcium

The divalent ion, calcium, is known to precipitate mucin.[97-100] There are two mechanisms by which calcium-induced glycoprotein aggregation may occur. First, calcium can form bridges between negatively charged groups like phosphates and carboxyls of adjacent monomers or dimers, thereby reducing the normal repulsive forces and permitting an enfolding of the mucin chain, making them insoluble in the same way that other cross-linked linear polymers are insoluble. Second, calcium can cause a conformational change in the glycoprotein and expose more hydrophobic surfaces for aggregation.

The calcium-induced glycoprotein aggregation results in a reduction of the expanded nature of the mucus network. The resulting increased density of the mucus network decreases chain segment mobility of the mucin molecule and decreases interpenetration. Thus smaller physical entanglement can be shown by a reduction in mucin-mucin tangential shear stress.[36,49]

The calcium level in human tears (2.29 mg/100 ml)[101] is not high enough to elicit a significant effect on the expanded nature of mucin and entanglement with bioadhesives. It was found that at high calcium content (20% by weight), both dry and hydrated cross-linked polyacrylic acid had greater hydration volume and tensile strength than the cross-linked polymer with a lower calcium content (13% by weight). One possible reason for this is that as the calcium concentration is increased, more bridges are formed between carboxyl groups within the same or between adjacent polymer particles, resulting in a more expanded network and thus a greater hydration volume and tensile strength.[49] Thus adding a large excess of calcium to a mucoadhesive formulation may augment its mucoadhesive effect by enhancing polymer mucin bridging interactions.

4. Chelating Agents, e.g., EDTA

Chelation of free calcium in the tear film may not have a substantial effect on mucoadhesion in the precorneal area, as described above. However, 0.5% ethylenediaminetetraacetic acid (EDTA) was found to cause a transient and reversible alteration of the permeability of the corneal epithelium, thus enhancing permeability of water-soluble drugs.[102] Therefore, for some water-soluble drugs, chelating calcium (free and within the epithelial surface) with EDTA may result in an expanded mucus network and subsequent increase in shear strength. EDTA was also found to dissolve the calcium-induced precipitation of phosphoprotein,[98] thereby reversing effects of excess free calcium present in the formulation.

B. POLYMER DRUG LOADING

Loading of drug into polymer matrices for drug delivery purposes has been accomplished

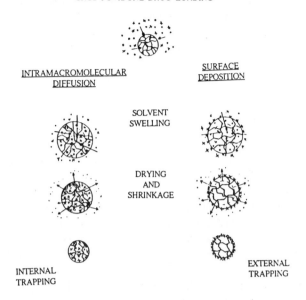

CROS POVIDONE DRUG LOADING

INTRAMACROMOLECULAR DIFFUSION

SURFACE DEPOSITION

SOLVENT SWELLING

DRYING AND SHRINKAGE

INTERNAL TRAPPING

EXTERNAL TRAPPING

FIGURE 12. Scheme of the two possible mechanisms of drug loading into crospovidone. (From Carli, F. and Garbassi, F., *J. Pharm Sci.*, 74, 963, 1985. With permission from the copyright owner, the American Pharmaceutical Association.)

by two methods: (1) synthesis of polymer with drug contained in the reaction vessel[51] and (2) hydrating or swelling the mucoadhesive polymer in a drug containing vehicle.[103] Carli and Garbassi,[104] while characterizing the loading of polymer by the swelling technique, observed that not only was there surface attachment of drug, but drug was also trapped internally when the polymer shrank as it was drying (Figure 12). Achieving high consistent loading of drug into mucoadhesives continues to be a substantial problem.

C. PHYSIOLOGICAL CONSIDERATIONS

Interdiffusion or interpenetration processes in adhesion were first discussed by Voyutskii,[105] where the chains of the adhesive and substrate penetrate into each other to a sufficient depth and create a semipermanent adhesive-bond. The representative mean diffusional path, s, for macromolecules can be estimated as:[36] $s = (2tD:)^{1/2}$ where D is the diffusion coefficient and t is time. For high molecular weight (10^4 to 10^6) polymers, the representative mean diffusional path for mucoadhesion of macromolecules at 1 s and 60 s can be estimated to be roughly 2 to 45 Å and 11 to 346 Å, respectively. Thus, although the thickness of the mucus layer in contact with the epithelial cells is quite small, it is the same magnitude as the estimated mean diffusional path, and therefore mucoadhesion (interpenetration) should occur in the preocular area.

1. Rabbits

Albino rabbits, the typical animal used to study ocular drug transport, appear to be less sensitive to viscosity changes in topical ocular vehicles than humans. Using radiolabeled polyvinyl alcohol or HPC suspensions of various viscosities in humans and rabbits, Zaki et al.[91] showed that while both polymers were retained longer on the cornea than saline controls, increasing the viscosity had less effect in rabbits than humans. Since the blink rate of rabbits (four times per hour)[2] is significantly less than that of humans (15 times per minute),[1] humans will commonly require higher viscosities than rabbits to retain drug on the cornea. In observing loss rates from precorneal ^{9m}Tc labeled vehicles, Hardberger et al.[84] found that even normal saline levels (compared to ointments) were reduced with spontaneous blinking after initial volume excesses were removed. An important issue with rabbits vs. man and mucoadhesives is the size of the drainage apparatus. Rabbits have one large puncta, capable of accomodating a large particle, whereas humans have two smaller puncta in each eye. Cross-linked mucoadhesives must be cleared from the eye, and thus the drainage opening is important.

2. Disease States

Many physiological factors of normal and diseased eyes affect the secretion rate and composition of the preocular tear film. In addition, systemic or locally administered drugs, whether salts, small organic molecules, macromolecules, or proteins may affect lacrimal gland function. Inert vehicle composition may directly stimulate or affect the epithelial layers of the cornea or conjunctiva and cause release of enzymes, glycoproteins, or immunological factors. Since the lacrimal gland and other tear-producing cells produce slightly different secretions, the various preocular areas may have different compositions. Blinking mixes secretions and removes tear film debris. An adhesive dosage form's location will contribute to the local composition and ultimately to the rate of tear secretions by both a local "irritant" effect and drug-induced and/or vehicle composition effect. Finally, in many disease conditions, there may be a change in membrane permeability (usually an increase) during disease states. Thus, in both normal and diseased eyes, the effects of the adhesive dosage form on the preocular area may decide the ultimate therapeutic outcome.

3. Dosage Form Effects

The first and most easily recognized problem with instillation of drops is that the increased volume of tears stimulates a reflex change in secretion, drainage, and blinking rates that also depends on the chemistry of the instilled drop. Since most ophthalmic products have a dose considerably larger (30 to 50 μl) than the maximum capacity of the preocular surface including the upper and lower fornices, a large portion will immediately spill onto the cheek. The remaining volume, depending on its physicochemical composition, may flush normally through the lacrimal drainage system, increase tear secretions to adjust the instilled drop to physiological pH, or change the temperature or tonicity. Dilution of the drop with tears will decrease the drug concentration and affect the amount of drug available for absorption within the first few seconds postinstillation.[22]

VI. CONCLUSION

The eye is unique, and it should be possible to design mucoadhesive delivery systems that will not interfer with the organ's natural functions. Formulators must be especially cognizant of irritant effects of the formulation as well as interference with the vision process when designing their products. Finally, care must be taken when using the rabbit model for dosage form evaluation since blinking is significantly slower than in humans even though most other physiological features are similar. This results in differences in drug or dosage form clearance from the eye between rabbits and humans.

REFERENCES

1. **Moss, R. A.,** The eyelids, *Adler's Physiology of the Eye; Clinical Applications,* 8th ed., Moses, R. A. and Hart, W. M., Jr., Ed., C. V. Mosby, St. Louis, 1987, 1.
2. **Mishma, S.,** Some physiological aspects of the precorneal tear film, *Arch. Opthalmol.,* 73, 233, 1965.
3. **Marquardt, R.,** Histological studies of goblet cell counts in human conjunctiva, in, *The Preocular Tear Film in Health, Disease, and Contact Lens Wear,* Holly, F. J., Ed., The Dry Eyes Institute, Lubbock, TX, 1986, 312
4. **Holly, J. F. and Lemp, M. A.,** Wettability and wetting of corneal epithelium, *Exp. Eye Res.,* 11, 239, 1971.
5. **Lemp, M. A., Holly, F. J., Iwata, S., and Dohlman, C. H.,** The precorneal tear film. I. Factors in spreading and maintaining a continuous tear film over the corneal surface, *Arch. Opthalmol.,* 33, 39, 1970.
6. **Adams, A. D.,** The morphology of human conjunctival mucus, *Arch. Ophthalmol.,* 97, 930, 1979.
7. **Berta, A. and Torok, M.,** Soluble glycoproteins in aqueous tears, in *The Preocular Tear Film in Health, Disease, and Contact Lens Wear,* Holly, F. J., Ed., The Dry Eyes Institute, Lubbock, TX, 1986, 506.
8. **Holly, F. J. and Lemp, M. A.,** Tear physiology and dry eyes, *Surv. Ophthalmol.,* 22, 69, 1977.
9. **Schacter, H. and Williams, D.,** Biosynthesis of mucus glycoproteins, *AEMB,* 144, 3, 1982.
10. **Allen, A. and Garner, A.,** Progress report: mucus and bicarbonate secretion in the stomach and their possible role in mucosal protection, *Gut,* 21, 249, 1980.
11. **Botelho, S. Y. and Dartt, D. A.,** Effect of calcium antagonism or chelation on rabbit lacrimal gland secretion and membrane potentials, *J. Physiol.,* 304, 397, 1980.
12. **Mircheff, A. K.,** Comprehensive subcellular fractionation of rat exorbital glands: an approach to studying lacrimal gland fluid formation, in *The Preocular Tear Film in Health, Disease, and Contact Lens Wear,* Holly, F. J., Ed., The Dry Eyes Institute, Lubbock, TX, 1986, 371.
13. **Sade, J., Eliezer, N., Silberberg, A., and Nevo, J.,** The role of mucins in transport by cilia, *Am. Rev. Respir. Dis.,* 102, 48, 1970.
14. **Patton, T. F. and Robinson, J. R.,** Influence of topical anesthesia on tear dynamics and ocular bioavailability in albino rabbits, *J. Pharm. Sci.,* 64, 267, 1975.
15. **Norn, M. S.,** Mucus on conjunctiva and cornea, *Acta Ophthalmol.,* 41, 13, 1963.
16. **Holly, F. J., Patten, J. T., and Dohlman, C. H.,** Surface activity determination of aqueous tear components in dry eye patients and normals, *Exp. Eye Res.,* 24, 479, 1977.
17. **Chao, C. C. W., Vergnes, J. P., and Brown, S. I.,** Fractionation and partial characterization of macromolecular components from human ocular mucus, *Exp. Eye Res.,* 36, 139, 1983.
18. **Schoenwald, R. D.,** The control of drug bioavailability from ophthalmic dosage forms, *Control. Drug Bioavailability,* 3, 257, 1985.
19. **Keller, N., Moore, D., Carper, D., and Longwell, A.,** Increased corneal permeability induced by the dual effect of transient tear film acidification and exposure to benzalkonium chloride, *Exp. Eye Res.,* 30, 203, 1980.
20. **Mauger, T. F. and Hill, R. M.,** Buffering response observed for human tears, in *The Preocular Tear Film in Health, Disease, and Contact Lens Wear,* Holly, F. J., Ed., The Dry Eyes Institute, Lubbock, TX, 1986, 539.
21. **Carney, L. G. and Hill, R. M.,** Human tear buffering capacity, *Arch. Ophthalmol.,* 97, 951, 1979.
22. **Maurice, D. M.,** The tonicity of an eye drop and its dilution by tears, *Exp. Eye Res.,* 11, 30, 1971.
23. **Gilbard, J. P. and Dartt, D. A.,** Changes in rabbit lacrimal gland fluid osmolarity with flow rate, *Invest. Ophthalmol. Vis. Sci.,* 23, 804, 1982.
24. **Mishima, S., Gasset, A., Klyce, S. D., Jr., and Baum, J. L.,** Determination of tear volume and tear flow, *Invest. Ophthalmol.,* 5, 264, 1966,.
25. **Lee, V. H. L., and Robinson, J. r.,** Review: topical ocular drug delivery: recent developments and future challenges, *J. Ocular Pharmacol.,* 2, 67, 1986.
26. **Berta, A.,** Collection of tear samples with and without stimulation, *Am. J. Ophthalmol.,* 96, 115, 1983.
27. **Jones, L. T.,** The cure of epiphora due to canalicular disorders, trauma and surgical failures, *Trans. Am. Acad. Ophthalmol Otolaryngol.,* 66, 506, 1962.
28. **Chrai, S., Patton, T., Mehta, A., and Robinson, J. R.,** Tear and instilled fluid dynamics in the rabbit eye, *J. Pharm. Sci.,* 62, 1112, 1973.
29. **Hui, H. W., Zelezmick, L., and Robinson, J. R.,** Ocular disposition of topically applied histamine, cimetidine and pyrilamine in the albino rabbit, *Curr. Eye Res.,* 3, 321, 1984.
30. **Holly, F. J. and Lamberts, D. W.,** Effect of nonisotonic solutions on tear film osmolality, *Invest. Ophthalmol. Vis. Sci.,* 20, 236, 1981.
31. **Conrad, J. M., Reay, W. A., Polcyn, E., and Robinson, J. R.,** Influence of tonicity and pH on lacrimation and ocular drug bioavailability, *J. Parent. Drug. Assoc.,* 32, 149, 1978.

32. **Maurice, D. M. and Mishima, S.,** Ocular pharmacokinetics, in *Handbook of Experimental Pharmacology,* Vol. 69, Sears, M. L., Ed., Springer-Verlag, Basel, 1984, 19.

33. **Peppas, N. A.,** Release of bioactive agents from swellable polymers: theory and experiments, in *Recent Advances in Drug Delivery Systems,* Anderson, J. M. and Kim, S. W., Eds. Plenum Press, New York, 1984, 279.

34. **Langer, R. S. and Peppas, N. A.,** Present and future applications of biomaterials in controlled drug delivery systems, *Biomaterials,* 2, 201, 1981.

35. **Smart, J. D., Kellaway, I. W., and Worthington, H. E. C.,** An in-vitro investigation of mucosa-adhesive materials for use in controlled drug delivery, *J. Pharm. Pharmacol.,* 36, 295, 1984.

36. **Leung, S. H. S. and Robinson, J. R.,** The contribution of anionic polymer structural features to mucoadhesion, accepted by *J. Controlled Release,* 1987.

37. **Park, K., Ch'ng, H. S., and Robinson, J. R.,** Alternative approaches to oral controlled drug delivery: bioadhesives and in-situ systems, in *Recent Advances in Drug Delivery Systems,* Anderson, J. M. and Kim, S. W., Eds., Plenum Press, 1984, 163.

38. **Park, K. and Robinson, J. R.,** Bioadhesive polymers as platforms for oral-controlled drug delivery: method to study bioadhesion, *Int. J. Pharm.,* 19, 107, 1984.

39. **Lemp, M. A. and Szymanski, E. S.,** Polymer adsorption at the ocular surface, *Arch. Ophthalmol.,* 93, 134, 1975.

40. **Nagai, T.,** Topical mucosal adhesive dosage forms, *Med. Res. Rev.,* 6, 227, 1986.

41. **Chen, J. L. and Cyr, G. N.,** Compositions producing adhesion through hydration, in *Adhesive Biological System,* Manly, R. S., Ed., Academic Press, New York, 1970, chap. 10.

42. **Gurny, R., Meyer, J. M., and Peppas, N. A.,** Bioadhesive intraoral release systems: design, testing, and analysis , *Biomaterials,* 5, 336, 1984.

43. **Saettone, M. F., Giannaccini, B., and Chetoni, P.,** Vehicle effects in ophthalmic bioavailability: an evalution of polymeric inserts containing pilocarpine, *J. Pharm. Pharmacol.,* 36, 229, 1984.

44. **Park, H., and Robinson, J. R.,** Physico-chemical properties of water insoluble polymers important to mucin/epithelial adhesion, *J. Controlled Release,* 2, 47, 1985.

45. **Ch'ng, H. S., Park, H., Kelly, P., and Robinson, J. R.,** Bioadhesive polymers as platforms for oral controlled drug delivery. II. Synthesis and evaluation of some swelling, water-insoluble bioadhesive polymers, *J. Pharm. Sci.,* 74, 399, 1985.

46. **Park, H.,** Synthesis and Evaluation of Some Bioadhesive Hydrogels, M.S. thesis, University of Wisconsin, Madison, 1984.

47. **Park, H.,** On Mechanism of Bioadhesion, Ph.D. thesis, University of Wisconsin, Madison, 1986.

48. **Leung, S.,** The Determination of Charge Density for Water-Soluble and Water-Insoluble Anionic Bioadhesives, M.S. thesis, University of Wisconsin, Madison, 1985.

49. **Leung, S.,** Polymer Structural Features Contributing to Mucoadhesion, Ph.D. thesis, University of Wisconsin, Madison, 1987.

50. **Nagai, T. and Machida, Y.,** Advances in drug delivery, mucosal adhesive dosage forms, *Pharm. Int.* August, 196, 1985.

51. **Hui, H-W. and Robinson, J. R.,** Ocular delivery of progesterone using a bioadhesive polymer , *Int. J. Pharm.* , 26, 203, 1985.

52. **Refojo, M. F.,** Current status of biomaterials in ophthalmology, *Surv. Ophthalmol.,* 26, 257, 1982.

53. **Refojo, M. F., Dohlman, C. H., and Koliopoulos, J.,** Adhesives in ophthalomology: a review, *Surv. Ophthalmol.,* 15, 217, 1971.

54. **Ticho, U., Blumenthal, M., Zonis, S., Gal, A., Blank, I., and Mazor, Z. W.,** A clincial trial with piloplex — a new long-acting pilocarpine compound: preliminary report, *Ann. Ophthalmol.* April, 555, 1979.

55. **Robinson, J. R. and Li, V. H. K.,** Ocular disposition and bioavailability of pilocarpine from piloplex and other sustained release drug delivery systems, in *Recent Advances in Glaucoma,* Ticho, U. and David, R., Eds., Excerpta Medica, Amsterdam, 1984, 231.

56. **Grass, G. M., Cobby, J., and Makoid, M. C.,** Ocular delivery of pilocarpine from erodible matrices, *J. Pharm. Sci.,* 73, 618, 1984.

57. **Gurny, R.,** Preliminary study of prolonged acting drug delivery system for the treatment of glaucoma, *Pharm. Acta Helv.,* 56, 130, 1981.

58. **Vanderdoff, J., El-Asser, E. R., and Ungerstad, J.,** U.S. Patent, 8f67031, 1977.

59. **Urtti, A., Salminen, L., Kujari, H., and Jantti, V.,** Effect of ocular pigmentation on pilocarpine pharmacology in the rabbit eye. II. Drug response, *Int. J. Pharm.,* 19, 53, 1984.

60. **Miyazaki, S., Ishii, K., and Takada, M.,** Use of fibrin film as a carrier for drug delivery: a long-acting delivery system for pilocarpine into the eye, *Chem. Pharm. Bull.,* 30, 3405, 1982.

61. **Bloomfield, S. E., Miyata, T., Dunn, M. W., Bueser, N., Stenzel, K. H., and Rubin, A. L.,** Soluble gentamicin ophthalmic inserts as a drug delivery system, *Arch. Opthalmol.,* 96, 885, 1978.

62. **Hedman, K., Vaheri, A., and Wartiovaara, J.,** External fibronectin of cultured human fibroblasts is predominantly a matrix protein, *J. Cell Biol.,* 67, 748, 1978.

63. **Dessau, W., Jilek, F., Adelman, B. C., and Hormann, H.,** Similarity of antigelatin factor and cold insoluble globulin, *Biochim. Biophys. Acta,* 533, 227, 1978.

64. **Stathakis, N. E. and Mosesson, M. W.,** Interaction among heparin, cold insoluble globulin, and fibrinogen in formation of the heparin-precipitate fraction of plasma , *J. Clin. Invest.,* 60, 855, 1977.

65. **Snyder, E. L. and Luban, N. L. C.,** Fibronectin: applications to clinical medicine, *CRC Cri. Rev. Clin. Lab. Sci.,* 23, 15, 1986.

66. **Hynes, R. O. and Yamada, K. M.,** Fibronectins: multifunctional modular glycoproteins, *J. Cell Biol.* 95, 369, 1982.

67. **Ruoslahti, E., Pierschbacher, M. D., Oldberg, A., and Hayman, E. G.,** Synthetic peptides causing cellular adhesion to surfaces, *Biotechniques,* 2, 38, 1984.

68. **Pierschbacher, M., Hayman, E. G., and Ruoslahti, E.,** Synthetic peptide with cell attachment activity of fibronectin, *Proc. Natl. Acad. Sci.* 80, 1224, 1983.

69. **Humphries, M. J., Olden, K., and Yamada, K. M.,** A synthetic peptide from fibronectin inhibits experimental metastasis of murine melanoma cells, *Science,* 233, 467, 1986.

70. **Nishida, T., Ohashi, Y., Awanta, T., and Manabe, R.,** Fibronectin, a new therapy for corneal trophic ulcer, *Arch. Ophthalmol.,* 101, 1046, 1983.

71. **Doillon, C. J. and Silver, F. H.,** Collagen-based wound dressing: effects of hyaluronic acid and fibronectin on wound healing, *Biomaterials,* 7, 3, 1986.

72. **McCoy, J. P., Jr.,** Contemporary laboratory applications of lectins, *Biotechniques,* 4, 252, 1986.

73. **Barondes, S. H.,** Soluble lectins: a new class of extracellular proteins, *Science,* 223, 1259, 1984.

74. **Marchalonis, J. J. and Edelman, G. M.,** Isolation and characterization of hemagglutinin from Limulus polyphemus, *J. Molec. Biol.,* 32, 453, 1968.

75. **Bishayee, S. and Dorai, D. T.,** Isolation and characterization of a sialic acid-binding lectin (carcinoscoporin) from Indian horseshoe crab Carcinoscoporus rotunda cauda, *Biochim. Biophys. Acta,* 623, 89, 1980.

76. **Miller, R. L., Colawn, J. F., Jr., and Fish, W. W.,** Purification and macromolecular properties of a sialic acid-specific lectin from the slug Limax flavus, *J. Biol. Chem.,* 257, 7574, 1982.

77. **Iguchi, S. M. M., Momoi, T., Egawa, K., and Matsumoto, J. J.,** An N-acetylneuraminic acid-specific lectin from the body surface mucus of African giant snail, *Comp. Biochem. Physiol.,* 81B, 897, 1985.

78. **Ito, I.,** Structure and function of the glycocalyx, *Fed. Proc.,* 28, 12, 1969.

79. **Gottschalk, A.,** in *The Chemistry and Biology of Sialic Acid and Related Substances.* Cambridge University Press, London, 1960.

80. **Jeanloz, R. W.,** in *Glycoprotein, Their Composition, Structure and Function,* Gottschalk, A., Ed., Elsevier, Amsterdam, 1972.

81. **Schaeffer, H. E. and Krohn, D. L.,** Liposomes in topical drug delivery, *Invest Ophthalmol. Vis. Sci.,* 22, 220, 1982.

82. **Florence, A. T. and Attwood, D.,** Polymeric system, in *Physicochemical Principles of Pharmacy,* 3rd ed., Chapman & Hall, New York, 1982, chap. 8.

83. **Hiemenz, P. C.,** The viscous state, in *Polymer Chemistry,* Hiemenz, P. C., ed., Marcel Dekker, New York, 1984, chap. 2.

84. **Harberger, R., Hanna, C., and Boyd, C. M.,** Effects of drug vehicles on ocular contact time, *Arch. Ophthalmol.,* 93, 42, 1975.

85. **Barsam, P. C.,** The most commonly used miotic now longer acting, *Ann. Ophthalmol.* 6, 809, 1974.

86. **Magder, H. and Boyaner, D.,** The use of a longer acting pilocarpine in the management of chronic simple glaucoma, *Can. J. Ophthalmol.,* 9, 285, 1974.

87. **Hardberger, R. E., Hanna, C., and Goodart, R.,** Effects of drug vehicles on ocular uptake of tetracycline, *Am. J. Ophthalmol.,* 80, 133, 1975.

88. **Haas, J. and Merrill, D. L.,** The effects of methyl cellulose on responses to solutions of pilocarpine, *Am. J. Ophthalmol.,* 54, 21, 1962.

89. **Mueller, W. H. and Deardorff, D. L..** Ophthalmic vehicle: the effect of methylcellulose on the penetration of homatropine hydrobromide through the cornea, *J. Am. Pharm. Assoc.,* 45, 334, 1956.

90. **Blaug, S. M. and Canada, A. T., Jr.,** Relationship of viscosity, contact time and prolongation of action of methylcellulose-containing ophthalmic solutions, *Am. J. Hosp. Pharm.,* 22, 662, 1965.

91. **Zaki, I., Fitzgerald, P., Hardy, J. G., and Wilson, C. G.,** A comparison of the effect of viscosity on the precorneal residence of solutions in rabbit and man, *J. Pharm. Pharmacol.,* 38, 463, 1986.

92. **Chrai, S. S. and Robinson, J. R.,** Ocular evaluation of methylcellulose vehicle in albino rabbits, *J. Pharm. Sci.,* 63, 1218, 1974.

93. **Kassem, M. A., Attia, M. A., Habib, F. S., and Mohamed, A. A.,** Activity of ophthalmic gels of betamethasone and phenylephrine hydrochloride in the rabbit's eye, *Int. J. Pharm.,* 32, 47, 1986.

94. **Krohn, L. and Breitfeller, J. M.,** Quantitation of pilocarpine delivery across isolated rabbit cornea by noncrosslinked high viscosity polymer gel, *Invest. Ophthalmol.,* 15, 324, 1976.

95. **Grass, G. M. and Robinson, J. R.,** Relationship of chemical structure to corneal penetration and influence of low-viscosity solution on ocular bioavailability , *J. Pharm. Sci.,* 73, 1021, 1984.

96. **Bottari, F., Giannaccini, B., Peverini, D., Saettone, M.F., and Tellini, N.,** Semisolid ophthalmic vehicles. II. Evaluation in albino rabbits of aqueous gel-type vehicles containing lidocaine and benzocaine, *Can. J. Pharm. Sci.,* 14, 39, 1979.

97. **Bettelheim, F. A.,** On the aggregation of a calcium precipitate glycoprotein from human submaxillary saliva, *Biochim. Biophys. Acta,* 236, 702, 1971.

98. **Boat, T. F., Wiesman, U. N., and Pallavicini, J. C.,** Purification and properties of the calcium-precipitable protein in submaxillary saliva of normal and cystic fibrosis subjects, *Pediatr. Res.,* 8, 531, 1974.

99. **Forstner, J. F. and Forstner, G. G.,** Calcium binding to intestinal goblet cell mucin, *Biochim. Biophys. Acta* 386, 283, 1975.

100. **Van Der Helm, D. and Willoughby, T. V.,** The crystal structure of $CaCl_2$, glycylglycylglycine, $3H_2o$, *Acta Cryst.,* B25, 2317, 1969.

101. **Uotila, M. H., Soble, R. E., and Savory, J.,** Measurement of tear calcium level, *Invest. Ophthalmol.,* 11, 258, 1972.

102. **Grass, G. M., Wood, R. W., and Robinson, J. R.,** Effects of calcium chelating agents on corneal permeability, *Invest. Ophthalmol. Vis. Sci.,* 26, 110, 1985.

103. **See, N. A., Russell, J., Connors, K. A., and Bass, P.,** Adsorption of inorganic ions to polycarbophil as a means of sustained-release dosage formulation, *Pharm. Res.,* 4, 244, 1987.

104. **Carli, F. and Garbassi, F.,** Characterization of drug loading in crospovidone by X-ray photoelectron spectroscopy, *J. Pharm. Sci.,* 74, 963, 1985.

105. **Voyutskii, S. S.,** *Autohesion and Adhesion of High Polymers,* John Wiley & Sons, New York, 1963.

Chapter 11

NANOPARTICLES AS BIOADHESIVE OCULAR DRUG DELIVERY SYSTEMS

Jörg Kreuter

TABLE OF CONTENTS

I. INTRODUCTION

The topical application of a drug to the eye in a conventional solution results in extensive drug loss. Indeed, usually only a very small amount (1 to 3%) actually penetrates the cornea and reaches intraocular tissues.[1,2] The reason for this is due to the complex fluid dynamics occurring in the precorneal area, such as tear turnover, lacrimal drainage, and drug dilution by tears.[3] As a consequence, most drug becomes systemically absorbed via the nose or via the gut after drainage from the eye, possibly leading to unwanted untoward side effects.

Decreasing the precorneal loss rate constant will not only result in an increase in contact time between the drug and absorbing tissue, thereby improving ocular bioavailability, but will also avoid frequent dosing, which is a major reason for noncompliance with prescribed dosage regimens.

Numerous attempts have been made to decrease the drug loss rate caused by drainage. Among others, viscous solution, suspensions, ointments, gels, polymeric inserts, as well as microparticulate systems such as microcapsules, liposomes, latices, and nanoparticles have been suggested for the prolongation of the residence time in the area of ocular absorption.[2,4-12] Ointments and especially drug inserts can very effectively prolong the absorption times. However, both systems can mechanically obscure the vision significantly, or, in the case of the inserts, many patients, especially the elderly, have problems with the insertion and removal of these inserts. Viscous solutions may lead to problems during manufacture and administration. Sterile filtration of viscous solutions, for instance, can be achieved only with great difficulties and often is impossible. Hard suspension particles of a size above 5 to 10 μm can lead to a scratching feeling in the eye.

From these experiences with various sorts of ophthalmic drug delivery systems, it can be concluded that the ideal carrier has to be an aqueous liquid of relatively low viscosity without any solid particular material of a size above 5 μm. Since most materials fulfilling these requirements are probably drained away with a rate constant similar to that of solutions, it is desirable that an optimal ocular drug delivery system would have additional slight bioadhesive properties.

II. MECHANISTIC ASPECTS AND REQUIREMENTS FOR OCULAR BIOADHESIVE SYSTEMS

Adhesion of polymers to tissue may be affected by physical or chemical bonds, secondary chemical bonds, or ionic, primary, or covalent chemical bonds.[13] Out of these bonds, the primary chemical bonds are too strong to be of relevance for ophthalmic drug delivery systems.

Physical or mechanical bond is obtained by deposition and inclusion of the adhesive material in crevices of the tissue.[13] In the eye, the drug delivery system thus may be entrapped mechanically under the eyelids and in the inner canthus. This mechanical entrapment is the more efficent the bigger the particle size. However, in order to prevent discomfort in the patient, the particle size should not exceed 5 to 10 μm. Mechanical entrapment of small particles intended as ophthalmic drug delivery systems can also occur in the gel network of the mucus present in the eye.[2]

Mechanical interaction of bioadhesives with the biological environment may also happen on a molecular scale. Interpenetration of movable chains of swellable polymers with those of the mucus network is able to form very effective adhesive bonds.[13] During this process, the chains move due to Brownian motion and, driven by the concentration gradient, penetrate at rates that are dependent on the diffusion coefficient of the macromolecules through the glycoproteinic network, and vice versa.[14] Once entangled, they are able to match their adhesive sites with those on the substrate to form an adhesive bond, or the entangled

TABLE 1
Surface Charge and Clearance Times of Liposomes

	Charge (mV)	Precorneal clearance T_{50} (min)	Inner canthus clearance T_{50} (min)
Small positively charged unilamellar vesicles	+84	3.8	7.7
Small neutral unilamellar vesicles	0	1.1	14.3
Small negatively charged unilamellar vesicles	−50	1.1	14.0
Solution		1.4	5.0

molecules are also free to form cohesive bonds.[15] In this process, the pH and the amount of water at the interface control adhesive performance.[16]

Extensive entanglement and effective bioadhesion, of course, are unsuitable for ophthalmic drug delivery systems because this would glue together various parts of the eye. For this reason, a compromise between effective retardation due to bioadhesion and patient comfort has to be found for ophthalmological purposes. With unhydrated, slightly hydrated, or cross-linked polymers, interpenetration of large chains is more difficult to attain. However, smaller chains and chain ends may still contribute to some interpenetration. As a consequence, the latter polymers are much more suitable for ophthalmic drug delivery.

Another mechanical adhesion mechanism that can be used in ophthalmology is adhesion of small particulate matter by capillary forces. Materials that are readily wetted by the tear film will be held within this film by these forces. The tear film is approximately 8 μm thick.[17] If the density difference between the particulate material and the tears is not too large, and if the particle size is small enough, blinking will hold the particles suspended in the tear film and will partly overcome the elimination due to the tear turnover.

The use of Coulomb's forces and of secondary chemical bonds are the third possibility for bioadhesive binding of ophthalmic drug delivery systems. The cornea has an electrical surface potential of −30 mv.[17] For this reason, positively charged particles should be bound efficiently to the corneal surface. Experiments with small charged liposomes, however, demonstrate that the charge of these drug carrier particles plays less of a role than would be expected.[18] Although the precorneal half-life of positively charged liposomes was doubled in comparison to solution and tripled in comparison to neutral or negatively charged liposomes, a half-life of 3 to 4 min. does not represent a major sustaining effect (Table 1). In addition, positively charged liposomes cleared much faster than neutral or negatively charged liposomes from the inner canthus region from which ocular absorption also may take place.

Secondary chemical bonds contributing to bioadhesive properties include van der Waals interactions and hydrogen bonding.[13] Both types of forces depend on the chemical nature of the adhesive materials. The van der Waals forces can be attributed to dipol-dipol interactions or Keesom forces, dipol-induced dipol interaction or Debye forces and dispersion or London forces. The binding energy of these forces lies between 1 to 500 kJ/mol.[19] The latter type of forces is weaker than the dipol forces.

Hydrogen bonding is also of importance for bioadhesion. Polycyanocrylates are used extensively as tissue and bone glues in surgery.[20-23] The cyanoacrylate monomers are able to form extremely efficient bonds. After polymerization in an aqueous medium, the resulting polymer does not appear to be sticky any longer. However, small particles made from this material and intended to be used as drug carriers still possess a strong tendency to associate with mucous membranes of the body. This tendency can be observed after peroral administration, where autoradiographs show an accumulation of radioactivity associated with or in proximity to the gastric and intestinal walls and little or no radioactivity in the lumen.[24] This tendency is also observed in normal and inflamed tissue of the eye (see below). The

TABLE 2
Methods for the Preparation of Ophthalmic
Nanoparticles

Polymer	Polymerization procedure	Ref.
Poly(methyl methacrylate)	γ-Irridiation	26,27,33
	Heat polymerization	26,27,34
Polybutylcyanoacrylate		
Polyhexylcyanoacrylate	Ionic polymerization	2,10,11,35
Albumin	Heat denaturation	36,37

reason why polyalkylcyanoacrylate nano- or microparticles seem to have a higher association tendency to mucous membranes than other similar polymer particles seems to be related to the cyano-group. This group has a strong electron-drawing effect and is able to form hydrogen bonds. These hydrogen bonds intensify the bioadhesive forces caused by van der Waals interactions of the polymer with the mucous membranes. Other polymers missing comparable groups such as hydrogen phthalate pseudolatices prior to pH-dependent coalescence or coagulation or uncharged polyacrylates seem to be nonbioadhesive.[8,25]

As a conclusion, in order to prevent discomfort for the patient, an ideal bioadhesive drug delivery system should only exhibit weak adhesive properties. For this reason, the classical bioadhesive polymers used for external, oral, or peroral purposes appear to be unsuitable for ophthalmology. Small polymeric particles, such as nanoparticles, with slight bioadhesive properties suspended in a liquid of low viscosity seem to hold promise for sustained ophthalmic drug delivery.

III. NANOPARTICLES FOR OCULAR THERAPY

A. DEFINITION OF NANOPARTICLES

Nanoparticles are solid colloidal particles ranging in size from 10 to 1000 nm (1μm). They consist of macromolecular materials in which the active principle (drug or biologically active material) is dissolved, entrapped, encapsulated, and/or to which the active principle is adsorbed or attached.[26]

B. PREPARATION METHODS

In general, five different methods for the preparation of nanoparticles exist:[26] emulsion polymerization,[26,27] desolvation of proteins,[26,28] heat denaturation,[26,29,30] electrocapillary emulsification,[26,31] and interfacial polymerization.[32] The last two methods may possibly lead to the formation of nanocapsules with a shell-like wall. Out of the above-mentioned methods, only the first two methods have been employed so far for the production of nanoparticles for ophthalmic purposes. A summary of methods that may be useful for the preparation of nanoparticles for ophthalmic use is listed in Table 2.

C. THE USE OF NANOPARTICLES FOR OPHTHALMOLOGIC PURPOSES

Two nanoparticulate systems have so far been developed for ophthalmic drug delivery, a charged polymethacrylate system with the trade names Piloplex® and Glauplex® and the polyalkylcyanoacrylate nanoparticles. The pseudolatex systems developed by Gurny and co-workers[8,9,38,39] start to dissolve at a pH above 5 and form a gel. Therefore, they do not exist in the eye as nanoparticles for a longer period and consequently exhibit a different mechanism of sustained release than nanoparticles that remain discrete particles after instillation into the eye. For this reason, the gelling pseudolatex systems will not be discussed here in further detail.

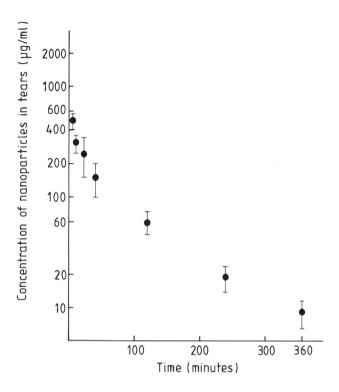

FIGURE 1. Concentration vs. time profile of nanoparticles in tear film.
(From Wood, R. W., Li, V. H. K., Kreuter, J., and Robinson, J. R., *Int.
J. Pharm.*, 23, 175, 1985. With permission.)

In the Piloplex® system, the pilocarpine is bound to charged poly(methylmethacrylate-acrylic acid) copolymer nanoparticles.[40,41] Because of this charge, the polymer particles are able to interact with mucous membranes not only via dispersion forces, but also by dipol or induced dipol interactions. In addition, the carboxyl groups present in the Piloplex® polymer will enable the formation of hydrogen bonds. Probably due to the resulting bioadhesiveness, the Piloplex® systems show a considerable retardation of the *in vitro* release of pilocarpine in comparison to a pilocarpine hydrochloride hydroxyethylcellulose (3800 cp) aqueous solution. In 6 h, 80% pilocarpine was released from the Piloplex® in comparison to 1 h for the corresponding drug solutions.[6] It should be noted, however, that pilocarpine may interact with macromolecular membranes such as dialysis bag materials.[10,42] This interaction can be changed by the presence of other macromolecules. Therefore the observed release from the dialysis bag may not represent the intrinsic release rate from the polymer.

In clinical trials, the Piloplex® systems lowered the intraocular pressure in a dose-related fashion.[7] The highest doses yielded a duration of the decreased intraocular pressure of 14 h. In addition, the fluctuations in ocular pressure, induced by multiple dosing of pilocarpine solutions, was reduced with the Piloplex® system.[40]

The second nanoparticulate ocular drug delivery system consists of the polyalkylcyanoacrylates. As discussed in Section II, nanoparticles composed of this polymer have a tendency for an accumulation with mucous membranes. Wood et al.[2] could demonstrate that ^{14}C-labeled polyhexylcyanoacrylate nanoparticles were eliminated from the tears much slower than solutions (Figure 1). The elimination kinetics was not first order, but was linear after plotting the log of the concentration over the square root of time. Nevertheless, at least an approximate half-life of 20 min could be estimated. Using another tracer technique, namely binding of ^{111}In-oxine to polybutylcyanoacrylate nanoparticles, enabled the use of gamma

TABLE 3
Concentration [μg/g] (Mean ± SD) of Poly-Hexyl-2-Cyano-[3-¹⁴C]Acrylate Nanoparticles in Healthy and Inflamed Rabbit Eyes

Time (min)	Cornea		Conjunctiva	
	Healthy	Inflamed	Healthy	Inflamed
20	3.5 ± 2.1	14.2 ± 6.9	96.7 ± 35.6	29.5 ± 24.7
60	2.4 ± 0.8	10.6 ± 6.4	5.4 ± 3.0	27.0± 16.9
240	3.5 ± 1.3	13.2 ± 4.0	6.4 ± 1.8	26.5 ± 12.1

Note: For 20 and 60 min, n = 10; for 240 min, n = 5.

Data from Diepold, R., Kreuter, J., de Burlet, G., and Robinson, J. R., unpublished data, 1987.

scintigraphy.[18] With this technique, a half-life of only 10 min was observed vs. 20 min with the ¹⁴C-labeled material. However, in comparing these somewhat contradictory results, it has to be kept in mind that while the ¹⁴C-label is incorporated covalently into the polymer chain, the ¹¹¹In-label ($^{111}In^{3+}$) is complexed by three oxime molecules, and this complex is hydrophobically attached to the nanoparticle surface. Since the tear film is quite a complex mixture, it is possible that the ¹¹¹In-label is released and cleared faster than the nanoparticles.

As shown by Wood et al.,[2] the nanoparticles also bind to the cornea and conjunctiva. Newer observations from our research group[43] indicate that the binding to these tissues may even be higher (Table 3), especially during the first 20 to 30 min. Moreover, the binding of the nanoparticles to these tissues in inflamed eyes was five times higher than the binding to these tissues in normal eyes (Table 3). The inflammation in these experiments was induced by pretreatment with clove oil 24 h prior to the application of the nanoparticles. Especially the latter experiments demonstrate that the polyalkylcyanoacrylate nanoparticles indeed seem to have bioadhesive properties: the inflamed tissue is much more hydrated and swollen than normal tissue. For this reason, bioadhesion should be much more prominent, as was in fact observed with nanoparticles.

Wood et al.[2] also carried out some preliminary experiments in order to investigate the mechanism of bioadhesion of the nanoparticles. One of the existing theories regarding the mechanism of bioadhesion is that the bioadhesive polymer adheres to the mucin-epithelial surface of cells. Therefore, the animals were predosed with the mucolytic agent N-acetyl-L-cysteine[44] prior to the instillation of the nanoparticles. There was no significant difference between treatments for the cornea and aqueous humor, suggesting that the nanoparticles were able to adhere directly to the tissue.[2] The mucin layer also did not seem to represent any barrier to the permeation of degradation products of the polymer through the cornea.

The concentration of nanoparticles at the conjunctiva was significantly higher after treatment with the mucolytic agent. However, it is possible that this higher conjunctiva concentration was caused by an artifact: upon treatment with the mucolytic agent, mucin collected in the cul-de-sac and formed a gel-like substance and also adhered somewhat to the conjunctiva. Radioactivity resulting from nanoparticles entrapped in this gel adhering to the conjunctiva may account for the higher conjunctiva levels.

Very interesting results were obtained using the polyalkylcyanoacrylate nanoparticles as drug delivery systems for pilocarpine. Previous *in vitro* release experiments in diffusion chambers with artificial membranes have shown that the results obtained with these membranes do not bear any correlation with *in vivo* observations.[12] Using bovine cornea as a membrane, consistently an increased permeability was found with pilocarpine nitrate bound to polybutylcyanoacrylate nanoparticles in comparison to pilocarpine nitrate solution.[45] The

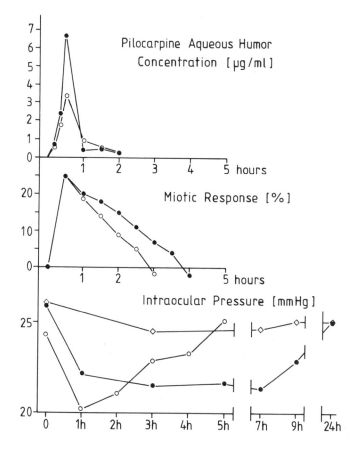

FIGURE 2.   Pilocarpine aqueous humor concentration and miotic response in normal rabbits and intraocular pressure in betamethasone-treated rabbits after instillation of pilocarpine nitrate 1% (aqueous humor and miosis) or 2% (intraocular pressure) in the form of aqueous eyedrops ○ or bound to poly-butylcyanoacrylate nanoparticles ●. Controls ◇, (Data generated by Diepold, R., Kreuter, J., Gurny, R., Schnaudigel, O. E., Saettone, F. M., and Robinson, J. R.)

difference between the two formulations was not significant and did not indicate any sustained effect of pilocarpine nanoparticles.

The aqueous humor concentration of pilocarpine observed in rabbit eyes after instillation of pilocarpine hydrochloride as a solution or bound to the same type of nanoparticles also did not indicate any sustained action of the pilocarpine nanoparticles (Figure 2). Rather, a very rapid and very pronounced invasion and a rapid elimination was obtained.[45] The peak concentrations after 30 min were more than twice as high than after instillation of a solution, whereas after 60 min the aqueous humor concentrations with the nanoparticles were even lower than those of the solution. However, the miotic response in normal rabbits was prolonged with nanoparticles from 3 to 4 h.[45] Even more important was the extreme prolongation of the reduction of the intraocular pressure in betamethasone-treated rabbits (Figure 2). Betamethasone-treated rabbits were used, because pilocarpine has very little effect on the intraocular pressure of normal rabbits. Three subconjunctival injections of 40 mg betamethasone increased the intraocular pressure over 3 weeks from 21.5 mmHg to 26 mmHg.

These very recent observations about the pronounced sustained effect with nanoparticles[45] have so far not been explained. Whether these tremendous time profile differences between the aqueous humor concentration, the miotic effect, and the reduction of the intraocular pressure are caused by special pharmacological effects or by a different ocular distribution pattern of the drug due to the nanoparticles is still an open question. Also whether these effects are caused by special thermodynamical properties or by the bioadhesive properties of these nanoparticles cannot be answered at the moment.

D. TOXICITY

As mentioned in Section II, the polycyanoacrylates have been extensively used as artificial tissue and bone glues for over 15 years.[20-23] The toxicity of the polycyanoalkylesters decreases with increasing side-chain length.[20,46,47] The histotoxicity of butyl-2-cyanoacrylate was less than that of other tissue glues such as gelatin-resorcin-formaldehyde (GRF).[48]

Couvreur et al.[24] carried out a variety of toxicity tests with cyanoacrylate nanoparticles. Mutagenicity tests were performed with both intact and degraded polymethylcyanoacrylate and polybutylcyanoacrylate nanoparticles using the Ames test.[49,50] Neither the nanoparticles nor their degradation products exerted a mutagenic effect.

In tissue cultures, a low toxicity was detected with high concentrations of the cyanoacrylates. Again this toxicity was lower with the derivatives with longer side-chain esters.[24,47,49]

Couvreur et al. also tested the acute toxicity in mice and the subacute toxicity in rats.[24] In his earlier experiments, an LD_{50} of around 200 mg/kg was determined in mice.[49] This toxicity, however, seems to be caused by the rather toxic surfactant mixture used in these earlier experiments. Later, less toxic surfactants were employed, and the results obtained later by Couvreur et al. as well as our own experiences indicate that the toxicity is above 500 mg/kg. (Various experiments were carried out with methotrexate nanoparticles using a nanoparticle dose of 500 mg/kg and no single mouse died.[51])

In the subacute toxicity tests, Couvreur et al. did not observe a significant effect on either the histological pattern of the tissues studied, the blood parameters, or on the body weight after injection of polyisobutyl- or polyhexylcyano-acrylate nanoparticles.[24]

After ocular application of polybutyl- or polyhexylcyanoacrylate nanoparticles to rabbits, no reddening of the eyes or other adverse effects were observed even after multiple dosing. The ocular application of empty polybutylcyanoacrylate nanoparticles in saline to human volunteers did not cause any adverse sensations.[42]

IV. CONCLUSION

Polyacrylic nanoparticles, especially polyalkylcyanoacrylate nanoparticles, are slightly bioadhesive to cornea and conjunctiva. These nanoparticles prolong the action of pilocarpine and demonstrate a significant tendency for an accumulation at inflamed ocular tissue. Because of these properties, polyalkylcyanoacrylate nanoparticles hold promise as bioadhesive ocular drug delivery systems for antiglaucoma and antiinflammatory drugs.

REFERENCES

1. **Patton, T. F. and Robinson, J. R.,** Quantitative precorneal disposition of topically applied pilocarpine nitrate in rabbit eyes, *J. Pharm. Sci.,* 65, 1295, 1976.
2. **Wood, R. W., Li, V. H. K., Kreuter, J., and Robinson, J. R.,** Ocular disposition of poly-hexyl-2-cyano[3-^{14}C]acrylate nanoparticles in the albino rabbit, *Int. J. Pharm.,* 23, 175, 1985.
3. **Lee, V. H. L. and Robinson, J. R.,** Mechanistic and quantitative evaluation of precorneal pilocarpine disposition in albino rabbits, *J. Pharm. Sci.,* 68, 673, 1979.
4. **Schaeffer, H. E. and Krohn, D. L.,** Liposomes in topical drug delivery, *Invest. Ophthalmol. Visual Sci.,* 22, 220, 1982.
5. **Singh, K. and Mezei, M.,** Liposomal ophthalmic drug delivery system. I. Triamcinolone acetonide, *Int. J. Pharm.,* 16, 339, 1983.

6. **Ticho, U., Blumenthal, M., Zonis, S., Gal, A., Blank, I., and Mazor, Z. W.,** Piloplex, a new long-acting pilocarpine polymer salt. A long-term study, *Br. J. Ophthalmol.,* 63, 45, 1979.

7. **Klein, H. Z., Lugo, M., Shields, M. B., Leon, J., and Duzman, E.,** A dose-response study of piloplex for duration of action, *Am. J. Ophthalmol.,* 99, 23, 1985.

8. **Gurny, R.,** Preliminary study of prolonged acting drug delivery systems for the treatment of glaucoma, *Pharm. Acta Helv.,* 56, 130, 1981.

9. **Gurny, R., Boye, T., and Ibrahim, H.,** Ocular therapy with nanoparticulate systems for controlled drug delivery, *J. Controlled Release,* 2, 353, 1985.

10. **Harmia, T., Speiser, P., and Kreuter, J.,** Optimization of pilocarpine loading onto nanoparticles by sorption procedures, *Int. J. Pharm.,* 33, 45, 1986.

11. **Harmia, T., Speiser, P., and Kreuter, J.,** A solid colloidal drug delivery system for the eye: encapsulation of pilocarpin in nanoparticles, *J. Microencaps.,* 3, 3, 1986.

12. **Harmia, T., Kreuter, J., Speiser, P., Boye, T., Gurny, R., and Kubis, A.,** Enhancement of the myotic response of rabbits with pilocarpine-loaded polybutylcyanoacrylate nanoparticles, *Int. J. Pharm.,* 33, 187, 1986.

13. **Peppas, N. A. and Buri, P. A.,** Surface, interfacial and molecular aspects of polymer bioadhesion on soft tissues, *J. Controlled Release,* 2, 257, 1986.

14. **Prager, S. and Tirrell, M.,** The healing process at polymer-polymer interfaces, *J. Chem. Phys.,* 7, 5194, 1981.

15. **Chen, J. L. and Cyr, G. N.,** Compositions producing adhesion through hydration, in *Adhesion in Biological Systems,* Manly, R. S., Ed., Academic Press, New York, 1970, chap. 10.

16. **Park, H. and Robinson, J. R.,** Physico-chemical properties of water insoluble polymers important to mucin/epithelial adhesion, *J. Controlled Release,* 2, 47, 1986.

17. **Maurice, D. M. and Mishima, S.,** Ocular pharmacokinetics, in *Pharmacology of the Eye,* Sears, M. L., Ed., Springer-Verlag, Berlin, 1984, 19.

18. **Fitzgerald, P., Hadgraft, J., Kreuter, J., and Wilson, C. G.,** A γ-scintigraphic evaluation of micro-particulate ophthalmic delivery systems: liposomes and nanoparticles, *Int. J. Pharm.,* 40, 81, 1987.

19. **Moore, W. J. and Hummel, D. O.,** *Physikalische Chemie,* de Gruyter, Berlin, 1976, 1100.

20. **Leonhard, F., Kulkarni, K., Nelson, J., and Brandes, G.,** Tissue adhesives and hemostasis-inducing compounds: the alkyl cyanoacrylates, *J. Biomed. Mater. Res.,* 1, 3, 1967.

21. **Matsumoto, T., Pani, K. C., Hardaway, R. M., and Leonhard, F.,** N-alkyl alpha cyanoacrylate monomers in surgery, *Arch. Surg.,* 94, 153, 1967.

22. **Häring, S.,** Klebstoff als Nahtersatz in der Chirurgie, *Fortschr. Med.,* 86, 179, 1968.

23. **Heiss, W. H.,** Gewebekleber, *Melsunger Med. Mitt.,* 47, 117, 1973.

24. **Couvreur, P., Grislain, L., Lenaerts, V., Brasseur, F., Guiot, P., and Biernacki, A.,** Biodegradable polymeric nanoparticles as drug carrier for antitumor drugs, in *Polymeric Nanoparticles and Microspheres,* Guiot, P. and Couvreur, P., Eds., CRC Press, Boca Raton, FL, 1986, 27.

25. **Gurny, R.,** personal communication, 1987.

26. **Kreuter, J.,** Evaluation of nanoparticles as drug-delivery systems. I. Preparation methods, *Pharm. Acta Helv.,* 58, 196, 1983.

27. **Kreuter, J.,** Poly(alkyl acrylate) nanoparticles, in *Methods in Enzymology,* Vol. 112, Widder, K. J. and Green, R., Eds., Academic Press, Orlando, 1985, 129.

28. **Marty, J. J., Oppenheim, R. C., and Speiser, P.,** Nanoparticles — a new colloidal drug delivery system, *Pharm. Acta Helv.,* 53, 17, 1978.

29. **Kramer, P. A.,** Albumin microspheres as vehicles for achieving specifity in drug delivery, *J. Pharm. Sci.,* 63, 1646, 1974.

30. **Widder, K., Flouret, G., and Senyei, A.,** Magnetic microspheres: synthesis of a novel parenteral drug carrier, *J. Pharm. Sci.,* 68, 79, 1979.

31. **Arakawa, M. and Kondo, T.,** Preparation and properties of poly(N^α, N^ϵ-L-Lysinediyl(terephthaloyl) microcapsule containing hemolysate in the nanometer range, *Can. J. Physiol. Pharmacol.,* 58, 183, 1980.

32. **Al Khouri Fallouh, N., Roblot-Treupel, L., Fessi, H., Devissaguet, J. Ph., and Puisieux, F.,** Development of a new process for the manufacture of polyisobutylcyanoacrylate nanocapsules, *Int. J. Pharm.,* 28, 125, 1986.

33. **Kreuter, J. and Zehnder, H. J.,** The use of ^{60}Co-γ-irradiation for the production of vaccines, *Radiat. Eff.,* 35, 161, 1978.

34. **Berg, U. E., Kreuter, J., Speiser, P. P., and Soliva, M.,** Herstellung und In vitro-Prüfung von polymeren Adjuvantien für Impfstoffe, *Pharm. Ind.,* 48, 75, 1986.

35. **Douglas, S. J., Illum, L., Davis, S. S., and Kreuter, J.,** Particle size and size distribution of poly(butyl-2-cyanoacrylate) nanoparticles, *J. Colloid. Interface Sci.,* 101, 149, 1984.

36. **Widder, K. J. and Green, R.,** Eds., *Methods in Enzymology,* Vol. 112, Academic Press, Orlando, 1985, chaps. 1-5.

37. **Gallo, J. M., Hung, C. T., and Perrier, D. G.,** Analysis of albumin microsphere preparation, *Int. J. Pharm.,* 22, 63, 1984.

38. **Gurny, R.,** Ocular therapy with nanoparticles, in *Polymeric Nanoparticles and Microspheres,* Guiot, P. and Couvreur, P., Eds., CRC Press, Boca Raton, FL, 1986, 127.

39. **Boye, T.,** *Nouveau Système Ophthalmologique,* Ph. D. thesis No. 7000, Université de Geneve, 1985.

40. **Andermann, G., de Burlet, G., and Cannet, C.,** Etude comparative de l'activité antiglaucomateuse de Glauplex 2 et du nitrate de pilocarpine sur le glaucome expèrimental á l'alpha-chymotrypsine, *J. Fr. Ophthalmol.,* 5, 499, 1982.

41. **Blank, I. and Fertig, J.,** U. S. Patent 4,248,855, 1981.

42. **Diepold, R. and Kreuter, J.,** unpublished data, 1987.

43. **Diepold, R., Kreuter, J., de Burlet, G., and Robinson, J. R.,** unpublished data, 1987.

44. **Swinyard, E. A. and Pathak, M. A.,** Surface-acting drugs, In *The Pharmacological Basis of Therapeutics,* 6th. ed., Gilman, A. G., Goodman, L. S., and Gilman, A., Eds., Macmillan Press, New York, 1980, 960.

45. **Diepold, R., Kreuter, J., de Burlet, G., Gurny, R., Robinson, J. R., Saetonne, M. F., and Schnaudigel, O. E.,** unpublished data, 1987.

46. **Pani, K. C., Gladieux, G., Brandes, G., Kulkarni, R. K., and Leonhard, F.,** The degradation of n-butyl alpha cyanoacrylate tissue adhesives. II, *Surgery,* 63, 481, 1987.

47. **Gipps, E. M., Groscurth, P., Kreuter, J., and Speiser, P. P.,** The effects of polycyanoacrylate nanoparticles on human normal and malignant mesenchymal cells in vitro, *Int. J. Pharm.,* 40, 23, 1987.

48. **Pigisch, E. F. and Gottlob, R.,** Vergleichende Untersuchungen zur Histotoxizität eines Butyl-2-Zyanoakrylates und eines GRF-Klebers, *Z. Exp. Chirurg.,* 3, 243, 1970.

49. **Kante, B., Couvreur, P., Debois-Krach, G., De Meester, C., Guiot, P., Roland, M., Mercier, M., and Speiser, P.,** Toxicity of polyalkylcyanoacrylate nanoparticles. I. Free nanoparticles, *J. Pharm. Sci.,* 7, 786, 1982.

50. **Ames, B. N., McCann, J., and Yamasaki, E.,** Methods for detecting carcinogens and mutagens with the Salmonella/mammalian-microsome test, *Mutat. Res.,* 31, 347, 1975.

51. **Kreuter, J. and Groscurth, P.,** unpublished data, 1983.

Chapter 12

BIOADHESIVE DOSAGE FORMS FOR VAGINAL AND INTRAUTERINE APPLICATION

Tsuneji Nagai and Yoshiharu Machida

TABLE OF CONTENTS

I. INTRODUCTION

As vagina and uterus are female sexual organs, the kinds of drugs delivered there have been limited to those related to the function or specificity of the organs, such as contraceptives, antifungals, and antibacterials.

The most sophisticated example of the dosage forms for the delivery of contraceptive is Progestasert® that was developed by the Alza Corporation. This T-shaped drug delivery system is inserted into the uterine cavity and releases progesterone for 1 year. As shown in this example, the drug delivery to the whole uterine cavity seemed easier than that to vagina, because the uterine cavity is separated from the vagina by the cervical canal. In vaginal drug delivery, usually, there are administered suppositories, gels, and vaginal effervescent tablets. However, if the drug itself is an irritant there, the dosage forms mentioned above would not be employed, and some other more site-specific dosage form would be requested. From this point of view, a bioadhesive dosage form may afford a useful means for such a drug delivery.

In this chapter, the bioadhesive dosage forms containing anticancer drugs, developed for a local chemotherapy of uterine cancer, are discussed.

II. BIOADHESIVE TABLET FOR VAGINAL APPLICATION

In Japan, uterine cervix cancer is 95% of uterine cancers. Generally, this disease is treated by an extirpation of the whole uterus, regardless of the stage of the disease. However, the cancer cells in the earliest stage of uterine cervix cancer stay in the epithelium, and it seemed possible to bring about a cure by topical application of anticancer drugs.

Therefore, we attempted to design a new topical dosage form for uterine cancer that has bioadhesive and sustained release properties.[1]

Intending to choose a suitable vehicle for the dosage form, directly compressed tablets (flat face, 13 mm in diameter) of polymers or their mixtures were put on 1% agar gel plate used as a model of mucosa, and examined for the bioadhesiveness and the drug release. The results indicated that a combination of hydroxypropyl cellulose-H (HPC) and carbomer (Carbopol®934, CM) is preferable as vehicle. Therefore, further experiments were carried out using the tablet mixture of HPC and CM.

Figure 1 shows the amounts of bleomycin (BLM) released to an agar plate from the tablets containing 30 mg of BLM and different amounts of HPC. The release of BLM increased remarkably with an increase of HPC concentration. The other experiment about the water-absorbing property of a tablet showed the increased amount of CM brought about water absorption, which seemed to relate closely to the initial bioadhesive force of the tablet.

Prior to clinical application of the bioadhesive tablet, a tablet (HPC:CM = 1:1) containing no BLM was set on *portio vaginalis* of voluntary patients for 24 h. The tablet did not give any irritant effect on the mucosa and adhered to the set place as in a swollen state; thus the safety and bioadhesive property of the tablet was confirmed.

The tablet containing 30 mg of BLM in the mixture of HPC and CM in the ratio of 1:1 or 1:2 was administered to voluntary patients with uterine cervix cancer diagnosed as stage 0 to Ib. Figure 2 shows the schematic comparisons in the focus of uterine cervix cancer before and after the administration of a bioadhesive tablet containing BLM. The circle symbolized the *portio vaginalis,* and the form of the external os of the uterus is indicated in the circle. The oblique lined part in the left circle indicates the lesion presumed from colposcopic observation, and the point in the right circle indicates the position and number of a remnant of cancerous focus observed in the histological section of the uterus removed after the local chemotherapy by a bioadhesive tablet.

In three of nine patients, any cancerous focus was not found after the local chemotherapy using a small amount of BLM as the bioadhesive tablet.

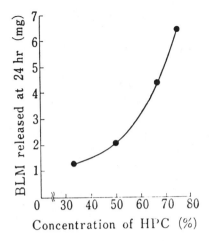

FIGURE 1. Relation between release of bleomycin from the tablet and concentration of HPC. Each symbol represents the mean of three determinations by the agar gel plate method. (From Machida, Y., et al., *Chem. Pharm. Bull.*, 27(1), 97, 1979. With permission.)

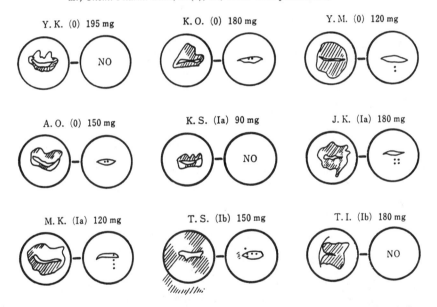

FIGURE 2. Schematic comparisons in focus of the uterine cervix cancer before (left) and after (right) the administration of a bioadhesive tablet containing bleomycin. (From Machida, Y., et al., *Chem. Pharm. Bull.*, 27(1), 99, 1979. With permission.)

The percentage of perfect disappearance of cancerous focus was 33%. The higher percent of disappearance, which means the possibility of cure of uterine cervix cancer in the earliest stage without the extirpation of uterus, might be expected by the continuous administration of BLM bioadhesive tablet for a longer period.

III. STICK-TYPE BIOADHESIVE DOSAGE FORMS FOR INTRAUTERINE APPLICATION

The bioadhesive tablet that can be applied to the *portio vaginalis,* a part of uterine cervix exposed in the vagina, seemed inconvenient for treatment of cancerous foci on the mucosa of cervical canal. Actually, many of the remnant foci were found in this part in the previous

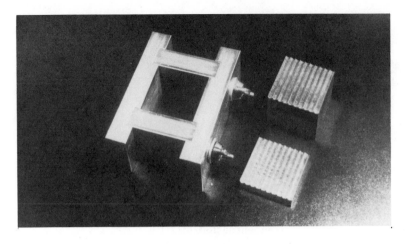

FIGURE 3.   Die and punches used for the preparation of sticks.

TABLE 1
Compositions of Sticks Used in Drug Release Test and Clinical Examination

Stick (diam)	Drug content (mg)	Total weight (mg)	Vehicle (HPC:CM)
BLM (2 mm)	25	150	3:1
(4 mm)	50	300	3:1
CQ (2 mm)	6	150	5:1
(4 mm)	12	300	5:1
5FU (2 mm)	75	225	3:1
(4 mm)	150	450	3:1

From Machida, Y., et al., *Chem. Pharm. Bull.*, 28(4), 1127, 1980. With permission.

study. Therefore, stick-type preparations (sticks) containing BLM, carboquone (CQ), or fluorouracil (5FU) were prepared.[2]

Sticks of 40 mm length and a diameter of 2 mm (150 mg) or 4 mm (300 mg) were made by compressing the mixed powder in a specially designed set of die and punches, shown in Figure 3. The sticks with the compositions shown in Table 1 were examined for their drug release properties and applied clinically. Drug release properties of sticks were measured by the Keramifilter® method[2] using an apparatus shown in Figure 4. Keramifilter® (Koshin Rikagaku Co., Japan) is a porous cylindrical filter made mainly of Al_2O_3, 100 mm in length with 4 mm of wall thickness.

This method avoided the problem of swelling of stick during the test and gave a good reproducibility of data in a short period compared with the agar gel plate method. Figure 5 shows the releasing profiles from 2 and 4 mm sticks of BLM. In the cases of BLM and 5FU, the drug release was larger from the 2 mm stick than from the 4 mm stick. The small diameter stick was considered to take up water rapidly, resulting in a rapid release of such water-soluble drugs as BLM and 5FU. In the case of CQ, there was no remarkable difference between the sticks, except at 24 h.

In the clinical application, the sticks were inserted into the cervical canal of voluntary patients, prior to surgical operations. As clinical circumstances required, two sticks or doubled sticks were used. Figure 6 shows a stick of CQ that was removed from a patient after 4 d. The stick was swollen with secreted fluid, but the shape of the preparation was

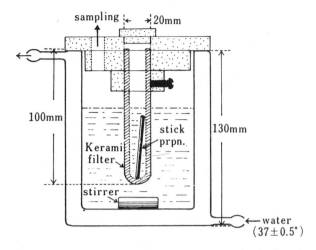

FIGURE 4. Apparatus used in the drug release test by the Kerami-filter® method. (From Machida, Y., et al., *Chem. Pharm. Bull.*, 28(4), 1126, 1980. With permission.)

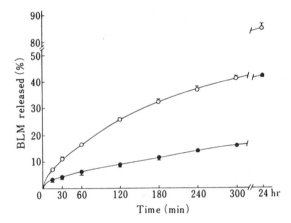

FIGURE 5. *In vitro* release profiles of bleomycin from 2 mm and 4 mm sticks. (○) 2 mm; (●) 4 mm. Each symbol represents the mean ± SD of five determinations. (From Machida, Y., et al., *Chem. Pharm. Bull.*, 28(4), 1128, 1980. With permission.)

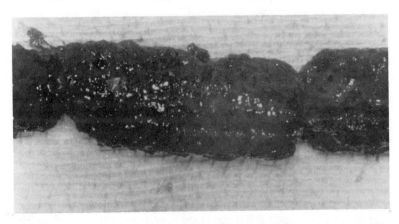

FIGURE 6. Swollen stick of carboquone removed from a patient after 4 d. (From Machida, Y., et al., *Chem. Pharm. Bull.*, 28(4), 1127, 1980. With permission.)

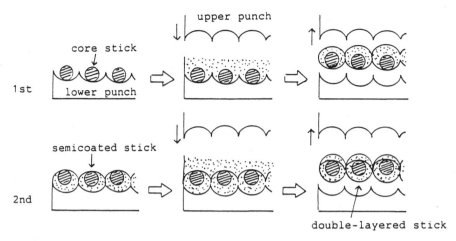

FIGURE 7.   Illustrated process of preparation of double-layered stick. (From Iwata, M., et al., *Drug Design Delivery*, 1, 254, 1987. With permission.)

well maintained. The dark color of the swollen stick indicated that some amount of CQ remained.

Generally, the stick gave a higher percentage of perfect disappearance of cancerous foci for patients with stage 0 than for stage Ia.[2,3] The stick-type bioadhesive dosage forms could reduce the cancerous foci at a low dose of anticancer drugs with lower frequency of adverse reaction compared with the stick-type suppository using Witepsol® as the base.[3]

The sticks of BLM and CQ were used clinically for the local chemotherapy of uterine body cancer by inserting the sticks into the uterine cavity.[4] The morphological changes in tumor tissue and calls indicated that it may be possible to cure early cancer of the uterine body sited only in the superficial layer. Also, no severe adverse reactions occurred and no effects on major organs, i.e., bone marrow, liver, kidney, heart, and lung, were observed.

IV. DESIGN OF DOUBLE-LAYERED STICK-TYPE BIOADHESIVE DOSAGE FORMS FOR UTERINE CANCER

In the clinical studies, the cancer cells did not disappear completely when the stick was administered only once a week. This result means that the sticks used were unable to release the drug effectively over a week. However, coming to the hospital more than once a week is rather inconvenient for the patients.

Therefore, we designed a double-layered stick-type bioadhesive dosage form, which would be able to supply the drug continuously for one week.[5]

Figure 7 shows the process for the preparation of a double-layered stick. Initially, the core stick of 40 mm in length and 2 mm in diameter was prepared by compressing 3 g of powder mixture under 400 kg/cm^2 for 2 min using a set of die and punches shown in Figure 3. A mixture of HPC and CM (3:1) was used as a vehicle for the core stick. A core stick was put on each of the grooves of the secondary lower punch with a diameter of 4 mm. Then 55% of the powder mixture for the outer layer was spread smoothly on the core sticks. The upper punch was set and the sticks were compressed for 2 min under 200 kg/cm^2. The semicoated sticks were reversed on the grooves of the lower punch, the remainder (45%) of powder mixture was spread and compressed again.

As shown in Figure 8, the release of brilliant blue FCF (BB), used as a model of an anticancer drug, from the core of a double-layered stick was delayed by increasing the weight of the outer layer. The release of BB decreased linearly by an increased weight of the outer layer from 300 to 500 mg, but no significant difference was observed between 500 and 600

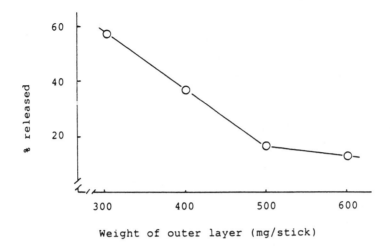

FIGURE 8.   Relationship between weight of outer layer and release of brilliant blue
FCF at 23 h. (From Iwata, M., et al., *Drug Design Delivery*, 1, 257, 1987. With
permission.)

mg. Moreover, the section of the preparation with an outer layer of 600 mg was not circular,
so the weight of the outer layer was fixed at 500 mg.

The release of BB decreased linearly with an increase of HPC in the outer layer from
approximately 1:3 to 3:1, and the increase from 3:1 to 5:1 did not affect the drug release.
However, 5:1 was chosen as the mixing ratio of HPC and CM for the outer layer because
of the greater ease in molding.

Next came the effect of coating to the core stick on the release property of the double-
layered stick. The release of BB decreased linearly with an incresed number of coatings
using 2-methyl-5-vinyl-pyridine methylacrylate-methacrylic acid copolymer. Therefore, a
double-layered stick containing 20 mg of BLM in the outer layer and 30 mg in the core
stick was prepared, and the release of BLM from the double-layered stick, which was coated
three times, and the noncoated core stick was examined.

As shown in Figure 9, the release of BLM was apparently sustained by the employment
of a double-layer, rather than a monolayered stick of the same dimensions, containing the
same quantity of BLM.[2] Moreover, coating of the core stick brought about more delayed
release compared with the double-layered stick having no core coating.

Therefore, "once-a-week" treatment of uterine cervix cancer might be possible using
a double-layered stick of BLM with or without a coating to the core stick.

V. OIL/WATER TYPE CREAM FOR INTRAUTERINE
APPLICATION

We have already described the stick-type bioadhesive dosage form for local chemotherapy of uterine body cancer. The anticancer drugs from the sticks caused the morphological
changes in tumor tissue and cells at the superficial layer. In the clinical trials, the clinician
pointed out the remarkable necrosis of the tissue observed on the lesion where the sticks
adhered.

Therefore, semisolid preparations using HPC were designed for improving the therapeutic
effect in local treatment of uterine body cancer.[6,7] An oil/water-type cream of BLM was
prepared by homogenizing the aqueous solution of HPC, BLM, and sesame oil.[6] In order
to find the optimum formula of cream, degree of penetration, spreadability, and drug release
were measured for creams. As a result, 5% was chosen as the appropriate concentration of
HPC and the ratio of HPC solution and sesame oil was decided as 5:1.

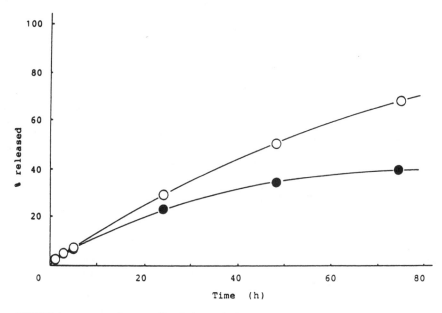

FIGURE 9. *In vitro* release profile of bleomycin from double-layered stick containing 50 mg of bleomycin. (○) noncoated; (●) coated. (From Iwata, M., et al., *Drug Design Delivery,* 1, 260, 1987. With permission.)

The cream containing 5 mg/g of BLM released approximately 40% of the drug into a 1% agar gel plate, after 24 h. This semisolid preparation had weak bioadhesive property compared with the previously described systems, but it had an advantage in causing the preparation to inject into the uterine cavity of voluntary patients with uterine body cancer without flowing out to the vagina.

Similar cream was prepared using water-insoluble CQ as an active drug.[7] Since the solubility of CQ in sesame oil was only 47.2 µg/ml, CQ was dispersed in oil by the solvent disposition method using chloroform, which gave a smaller size of CQ particle than that obtained by the mechanical crush.

Figure 10 shows the release profiles of creams containing 2 mg/g of CQ, measured by the cellulose membrane method using a specially designed diffusion cell.[6] The release of CQ increased with an increased ratio of HPC solution.

Anyway, a sufficiently sustained release of CQ was observed in the CQ cream. Clinical trials about this dosage form are not yet fully completed. However, continuous release of an anticancer drug and the intimate contact to mucosa in the semisolid dosage form seemed to bring about the effective local chemotherapy.

Furthermore, it was expected that CQ partially dissolved and dispersed in the oil phase of the cream should have a preventive effect on metastasis after carrying it into the lymphatic vessels.

ACKNOWLEDGMENT

The authors are deeply indebted to Drs. Hiroshi Masuda and Masanori Iwata for their assistance in this work.

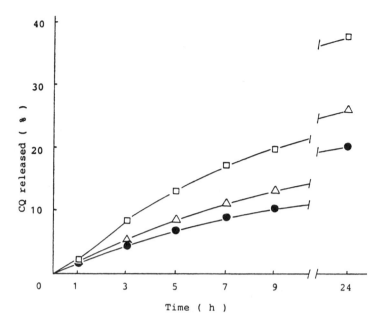

FIGURE 10. Carboquone release profiles of creams with different ratios of HPC solution and sesame oil, obtained by the cellulose membrane method. Ratio of 5% HPC solution and sesame oil; (□) 7:1; (△) 5:1; (●) 3:1. (From Iwata, M., et al., *Yakuzaigaku*, 47(1), 5, 1987. With permission.)

REFERENCES

1. **Machida, Y., Masuda, H., Fujiyama, N., Ito, S., Iwata, M., and Nagai, T.,** Preparation and phase II clinical examination of topical dosage form for treatment of *carcinoma colli* containing bleomycin with hydroxypropyl cellulose, *Chem. Pharm. Bull.*, 27, 93, 1979.
2. **Machida, Y., Masuda, H., Fujiyama, N., Iwata, M., and Nagai, T.,** Preparation and phase II clinical examination of topical dosage forms for the treatment of *carcinoma colli* containing bleomycin, carboquone, or 5-fluorouracil with hydroxypropyl cellulose, *Chem. Pharm. Bull.*, 28, 1125, 1980.
3. **Masuda, H., Sumiyoshi, Y., Shiojima, Y., Suda, T., Kikyo, T., Iwata, M., Fujiyama, N., Machida, Y., and Nagai, T.,** Local therapy of carcinoma of the uterine cervix, *Cancer*, 48, 1899, 1981.
4. **Masuda, H., Sumiyoshi, Y., Shiojima, Y., Kikyo, T., Fujiyama, N., Iwata, M., Machida, Y., and Nagai, T.,** Local therapy of carcinoma of the uterine body, *Asia-Oceania J. Obstet. Gynaecol.*, 8, 117, 1982.
5. **Iwata, M., Machida, Y., and Nagai, T.,** Double-layered stick-type formulation of bleomycin for treatment of uterine cervical cancer, *Drug Design Delivery*, 1, 253, 1987.
6. **Iwata, M., Machida, Y., Masuda, H., and Nagai, T.,** Development of cream-type preparation and device for local chemotherapy of uterine cancer, *Yakuzaigaku*, 46, 203, 1986.
7. **Iwata, M., Machida, Y., Masuda, H., and Nagai, T.,** Oil/water type cream of carboquone for local chemotherapy of uterine body cancer, *Yakuzaigaku*, 47, 1, 1987.

INDEX

C